# UCLA Symposia on Molecular and Cellular Biology, New Series

*Series Editor,* C. Fred Fox

Please contact the publisher for information about previous titles in this series.

# UCLA Symposia Board

**C. Fred Fox,** Ph.D., Director
Professor of Microbiology, University of California, Los Angeles

# Molecular Biology of the Eye

## Genes, Vision, and Ocular Disease

# Molecular Biology of the Eye

## Genes, Vision, and Ocular Disease

Proceedings of a National Eye Institute—UCLA Symposium
Held at Santa Fe, New Mexico, February 6–12, 1988

### Editors

**Joram Piatigorsky**

**Toshimichi Shinohara**

**Peggy S. Zelenka**

Laboratory of Molecular and Developmental Biology
National Eye Institute
National Institutes of Health
Bethesda, Maryland

**Alan R. Liss, Inc. • New York**

**Address all Inquiries to the Publisher**
**Alan R. Liss, Inc., 41 East 11th Street, New York, NY 10003**

---

**Copyright © 1988 Alan R. Liss, Inc.**

---

**Printed in the United States of America**

**Library of Congress Cataloging-in-Publication Data**

Molecular biology of the eye : genes, vision, and ocular disease :
    proceedings of a National Eye Institute—UCLA symposium held at Santa
    Fe, New Mexico, February 6–12, 1988 / editors, Joram Piatigorsky,
    Toshimichi Shinohara, Peggy S. Zelenka.
        p.  cm.—(UCLA symposia on molecular and cellular biology ;
    new ser., v 88)
    Includes bibliographies and index.
    ISBN 0-8451-2687-3
    1. Eye—Diseases and defects—Congresses.  2. Vision.  3. Eye.
4. Molecular genetics.  I. Piatigorsky, Joram.  II. Shinohara,
Toshimichi.  III. Zelenka, Peggy S.  IV. National Eye Institute.
V. University of California, Los Angeles.  VI. Series.
    [DNLM:  1. Eye—physiology—congresses.  2. Eye Diseases—familial
& genetic—congresses.  3. Gene Expression Regulation—congresses.
4. Vision—physiology—congresses.  W3 U17N new ser. v. 88 / WW 103
M7176 1988]
RE48.M64 1988
617.7′1—dc19
DNLM/DLC                                                          88-13557
for Library of Congress                                               CIP

# Contents

# Contributors

**H.J.M. Aarts,** Department of Molecular Biology, University of Nijmegen, 6525 ED Nijmegen, The Netherlands **[229]**

**Grazyna Adamus,** Department of Ophthalmology, University of Florida, Gainesville, FL 32610 **[35]**

**A. Albini,** Laboratory of Retinal Cell and Molecular Biology, National Eye Institute, National Institutes of Health, Bethesda, MD 20892 **[93]**

**B. Amaladoss,** Laboratory of Immunology, National Eye Institute, National Institutes of Health, Bethesda, MD 20892 **[73]**

**I. Araki,** Department of Biophysics, Faculty of Science, Kyoto University, Kyoto 606, Japan **[189]**

**Anatol Arendt,** Department of Ophthalmology, University of Florida, Gainesville, FL 32610 **[35]**

**Lyman G. Armes,** W. Alton Jones Cell Science Center, Inc., Lake Placid, NY 12946 **[107]**

**David Barrett,** Department of Ophthalmology and Medical Genetics, UCLA School of Medicine, Los Angeles, CA 90024 **[317]**

**J. Bronwyn Bateman,** Jules Stein Eye Institute and Departments of Ophthalmology and Medical Genetics, UCLA School of Medicine, Los Angeles, CA 90024 **[317,329]**

**B. Bax,** Birkbeck College, Department of Crystallography, Laboratory of Molecular Biology, London WC1 7HX, England **[419]**

**Kevin M. Bean,** Eye Research Institute of Retina Foundation and the Department of Ophthalmology, Harvard Medical School, Boston, MA 02114 **[355]**

**Andrew Becker,** Hospital for Sick Children Research Institute and the Departments of Ophthalmology and Medical Genetics, The University of Toronto, Toronto, Canada M5G 1X8 **[437]**

**David C. Beebe,** Department of Anatomy, Uniformed Services University of the Health Sciences, Bethesda, MD 20814 **[457]**

**J.W. Belmont,** Institute for Molecular Genetics and Howard Hughes Medical Institute, Baylor College of Medicine, Houston, TX 77030 **[1]**

**S.S. Bhattacharya,** M.R.C. Clinical and Population Cytogenetics Unit, Western General Hospital, Edinburgh EH4 2XU, Scotland, and the Department of Human Genetics, University of Newcastle-upon-Tyne, Newcastle-upon-Tyne NE2 4AA, England **[293]**

**M.A. Bibby,** Birkbeck College, Department of Crystallography, Laboratory of Molecular Biology, London WC1 7HX, England **[419]**

The numbers in brackets are the opening page numbers of the contributors' articles.

**A.C. Bird,** Department of Clinical Ophthalmology, University of London, Moorsfield Eye Hospital, London EC1V 2PD, England **[293]**

**H. Bloemendal,** Department of Biochemistry, University of Nijmegen, 6500 HB Nijmegen, The Netherlands **[149]**

**Brian T. Bloomquist,** Department of Biological Sciences, Purdue University, West Lafayette, IN 47906 **[117]**

**T.L. Blundell,** Birkbeck College, Department of Crystallography, Laboratory of Molecular Biology, London WC1 7HX, England **[419]**

**C. Bohan,** Department of Pathology, Emory University School of Medicine, Atlanta, GA 30322 **[365]**

**Robert Bookstein,** Experimental Pathology Program and Center for Molecular Genetics, Department of Pathology, University of California at San Diego, La Jolla, CA 92093 **[427]**

**Teresa Borrás,** Laboratory of Molecular and Developmental Biology, National Eye Institute, National Institutes of Health, Bethesda, MD 20892 **[179,197]**

**D.E. Borst,** Laboratory of Retinal Cell and Molecular Biology, National Eye Institute, National Institutes of Health, Bethedsa, MD 20892 **[93]**

**Cathy Bowes,** Jules Stein Eye Institute and Department of Ophthalmology, UCLA School of Medicine, Los Angeles, CA 90024 **[339]**

**C. David Bridges,** Department of Biological Sciences, Purdue University, West Lafayette, IN 47907 **[159]**

**Ann Bunt-Milam,** Department of Ophthalmology, University of Washington, Seattle, WA 98195 **[53]**

**Steven A. Carr,** SmithKline and French Laboratories, Swedeland, PA 19479 **[107]**

**C.T. Caskey,** Institute for Molecular Genetics and Howard Hughes Medical Institute, Baylor College of Medicine, Houston, TX 77030 **[1]**

**G.J. Chader,** Laboratory of Retinal Cell and Molecular Biology, National Eye Institute, National Institutes of Health, Bethesda, MD 20892 **[93,399]**

**S.M-W. Chang,** Institute for Molecular Genetics and Howard Hughes Medical Institute, Baylor College of Medicine, Houston, TX 77030 **[1]**

**Hai-Bao Chen,** Departments of Biology and Chemistry, Massachusetts Institute of Technology, Cambridge, MA 02139; present address: Shanghai Institute of Organic Chemistry, Academia Sinica, Shanghai, China **[23]**

**Ana B. Chepelinsky,** Laboratory of Molecular and Developmental Biology, National Eye Institute, National Institutes of Health, Bethesda, MD 20892 **[179,215]**

**R.M. Clayton,** Department of Genetics, University of Edinburgh, Edinburgh EH9 3JN, Scotland **[239]**

**John P. Coghlan,** The Howard Florey Institute for Experimental Physiology and Medicine, University of Melbourne, Parkville, Victoria, 3052, Australia **[409]**

**Victoria Cortessis,** Jules Stein Eye Institute and Department of Ophthalmology, UCLA School of Medicine, Los Angeles, CA 90024; present address: Department of Psychiatry/Biomathematics, UCLA School of Medicine, Los Angeles, CA 90024 **[329]**

**W. Maxwell Cowan,** Department of Neurosurgery, Washington University School of Medicine, St. Louis, MO 63110 **[269]**

**John W. Crabb,** W. Alton Jones Cell Science Center, Inc., Lake Placid, NY 12946 **[107]**

**I.W. Craig,** Genetics Laboratory, Department of Biochemistry, University of Oxford, Oxford OX1 3QU, England **[293]**

**R. Andrew Cuthbertson,** The Howard Florey Institute for Experimental Physiology and Medicine, University of Melbourne, Parkville, Victoria, 3052, Australia **[409]**

**W.W. de Jong,** Department of Biochemistry, University of Nijmegen, 6500 HB Nijmegen, The Netherlands **[149]**

**M. Dempster,** M.R.C. Clinical and Population Cytogenetics Unit, Western General Hospital, Edinburgh EH4 2XU, Scotland **[293]**

**Beverley Dere,** Department of Biochemistry and the Howard Hughes Medical Institute, University of Washington, Seattle, WA 98195 **[53]**

**Larry A. Donoso,** Department of Research, Wills Eye Hospital, Philadelphia, PA 19107 **[73,385]**

**H.P.C. Driessen,** Department of Crystallography, Laboratory of Molecular Biology, London WC1 7HX, England **[419]**

**Robert A. Dubin,** Laboratory of Molecular and Developmental Biology, National Eye Institute, National Institutes of Health, Bethesda, MD 20892 **[179]**

**Edmund C. Dunkel,** Eye Research Institute of Retina Foundation, Molecular Virology Laboratory, and Department of Ophthalmology, Harvard Medical School, Boston, MA 02114 **[355,379]**

**Ashley Dunn,** Ludwig Institute for Cancer Research, Melbourne Tumour Biology Branch, P.O. Royal Melbourne Hospital, 3050, Victoria, Australia **[409]**

**James M. Dunn,** Hospital for Sick Children Research Institute and the Departments of Ophthalmology and Medical Genetics, The University of Toronto, Toronto, Canada M5G 1X8 **[437]**

**H.J. Evans,** M.R.C. Clinical and Population Cytogenetics Unit, Western General Hospital, Edinburgh EH4 2XU, Scotland **[293]**

**Debora B. Farber,** Jules Stein Eye Institute and Department of Ophthalmology, UCLA School of Medicine, Los Angeles, CA 90024 **[339,349]**

**F.A. Fletcher,** Institute for Molecular Genetics and Howard Hughes Medical Institute, Baylor College of Medicine, Houston, TX 77030 **[1]**

**Shao-Ling Fong,** Department of Biological Sciences, Purdue University, West Lafayette, IN 47907 **[159]**

**Mark E. Fortini,** Howard Hughes Medical Institute and Department of Biochemistry, University of California, Berkeley, CA 94720 **[277]**

**Roland R. Franke,** Departments of Biology and Chemistry, Massachusetts Institute of Technology, Cambridge, MA 02139 **[23,45]**

**N. Fraser,** Genetics Laboratory, Department of Biochemistry, University of Oxford, Oxford OX1 3QU, England **[293]**

**Marlene Fu,** Departments of Ophthalmology, Physiology, and Biophysics, University of Washington, Seattle, WA 98195 **[305]**

**Brenda L. Gallie,** Hospital for Sick Children Research Institute and the Departments of Ophthalmology and Medical Genetics, The University of Toronto, Toronto, Canada M5G 1X8 **[437]**

**Patricia A. Geary,** Eye Research Institute of Retina Foundation and the Department of Ophthalmology, Harvard Medical School, Boston, MA 02114 **[355]**

**I. Gery,** National Eye Institute, National Institutes of Health, Bethesda, MD 20892 **[399]**

**Marie I. Girard,** Eye Research Institute of Retina Foundation and the Department of Ophthalmology, Harvard Medical School, Boston, MA 02114 **[355]**

**Audrey Goddard,** Hospital for Sick Children Research Institute and the Departments of Ophthalmology and Medical Genetics, The University of Toronto, Toronto, Canada M5G 1X8 **[437]**

**Steven Goldflam,** W. Alton Jones Cell Science Center, Inc., Lake Placid, NY 12946 **[107]**

**Y. Jerold Gordon,** Department of Ophthalmology, University of Pittsburgh, Pittsburgh, PA 15260 **[379]**

**K. Goto,** Department of Biophysics, Faculty of Science, Kyoto University, Kyoto 606, Japan **[189]**

**Robert M. Graham,** Cellular and Molecular Research Laboratories, Cardiac Unit, Massachusetts General Hospital and Harvard Medical School, Boston, MA 02114 **[45]**

**Paul A. Hargrave,** Department of Ophthalmology and Department of Biochemistry and Molecular Biology, University of Florida, Gainesville, FL 32610 **[xxv, 35]**

**Steven E. Harris,** W. Alton Jones Cell Science Center, Inc., Lake Placid, NY 12946 **[107]**

**S. Hayashi,** Department of Biophysics, Faculty of Science, Kyoto University, Kyoto 606, Japan; present address: Department of Molecular, Cellular, and Developmental Biology, University of Colorado, Boulder, CO 80309 **[189]**

**M.W. Head,** Department of Genetics, University of Edinburgh, Edinburgh EH9 3JN, Scotland **[239]**

**W. Hendriks,** Department of Biochemistry, University of Nijmegen, 6500 HB Nijmegen, The Netherlands **[149]**

**B. Hershfield,** Laboratory of Retinal Cell and Molecular Biology, National Eye Institute, National Institutes of Health, Bethesda, MD 20892 **[93]**

**Yoshihiro Hotta,** Laboratory of Mechanisms of Ocular Diseases, and Clinical Branch, National Eye Institute, National Institutes of Health, Bethesda, MD 20892 **[317]**

**L.H. Hu,** National Eye Institute, National Institutes of Health, Bethesda, MD 20892 **[399]**

**James B. Hurley,** Department of Biochemistry and the Howard Hughes Medical Institute, University of Washington, Seattle, WA 98195 **[53]**

**George Inana,** Jules Stein Eye Institute and Department of Ophthalmology, UCLA School of Medicine, Los Angeles, CA 90024 and Laboratory of Mechanisms of Ocular Diseases, and Clinical Branch, National Eye Institute, National Institutes of Health, Bethesda, MD 20892 **[317,329]**

**L. Inouye,** Laboratory of Retinal Cell and Molecular Biology, National Eye Institute, National Institutes of Health, Bethesda, MD 20892 **[93]**

**B. Jay,** Department of Clinical Ophthalmology, University of London, Moorsfield Eye Hospital, London EC1V 2PD, England **[293]**

**M. Jay,** Department of Clinical Ophthalmology, University of London, Moorfields Eye Hospital, London EC1V 2PD, England **[293]**

**Charles M. Johnson,** W. Alton Jones Cell Science Center, Inc., Lake Placid, NY 12946 **[107]**

**Muriel Kaiser,** Laboratory of Mechanisms of Ocular Diseases, and Clinical Branch, National Eye Institute, National Institutes of Health, Bethesda, MD 20892 **[317]**

**H.J. Kaplan,** Department of Ophthalmology, Washington University School of Medicine, St. Louis, MO 63110 **[365]**

**Sadashiva S. Karnik,** Departments of Biology and Chemistry, Massachusetts Institute of Technology, Cambridge, MA 02139 **[23]**

**Paul S. Kaytes,** Molecular Biology Research, The Upjohn Company, Kalamazoo, MI 49001 **[169]**

**Nancy Kennaway,** Department of Ophthalmology and Medical Genetics, Oregon Health Sciences University, Portland, OR 97201 **[317]**

**H. Gobind Khorana,** Departments of Biology and Chemistry, Massachusetts Institute of Technology, Cambridge, MA 02139 **[23,45]**

**Masahi Kitamura,** Department of Biophysics, Faculty of Science, Kyoto University, Kyoto 606, Japan **[205]**

**John F. Klement,** Laboratory of Molecular and Developmental Biology, National Eye Institute, National Institutes of Health, Bethesda, MD 20892 **[179]**

**Gordon K. Klintworth,** Duke Eye Center, Duke University Medical Center, Durham, NC 27710 **[409]**

**Barry E. Knox,** Departments of Biology and Chemistry, Massachusetts Institute of Technology, Cambridge, MA 02139 **[23]**

**H. Kondoh,** Department of Biophysics, Faculty of Science, Kyoto University, Kyoto 606, Japan **[189]**

**T. Kuwabara,** National Eye Institute, National Institutes of Health, Bethesda, MD 20892 **[399]**

**Richard A. Lang,** Ludwig Institute for Cancer Research, Melbourne Tumour Biology Branch, P.O. Royal Melbourne Hospital, 3050, Victoria, Australia **[409]**

**Eva Y.-H.P. Lee,** Experimental Pathology Program and Center for Molecular Genetics, Department of Pathology, University of California at San Diego, La Jolla, CA 92093 **[427]**

**W.H. Lee,** Experimental Pathology Program and Center for Molecular Genetics, Department of Pathology, University of California at San Diego, La Jolla, CA 92093 **[427]**

**Connie Lerea,** Department of Biochemistry and the Howard Hughes Medical Institute, University of Washington, Seattle, WA 98195 **[53]**

**J.A.M. Leunissen,** Department of Biochemistry, University of Nijmegen, 6500 HB Nijmegen, The Netherlands **[149]**

**Tom Lietman,** Laboratory of Molecular and Developmental Biology, National Eye Institute, National Institutes of Health, Bethesda, MD 20892 **[139]**

**P.F. Lindley,** Birkbeck College, Department of Crystallography, Laboratory of Molecular Biology, London WC1 7HX, England **[419]**

**N.H. Lubsen,** Department of Molecular Biology, University of Nijmegen, 6525 ED Nijmegen, The Netherlands **[229]**

**Ian Lyons,** The Howard Florey Institute for Experimental Physiology and Medicine, University of Melbourne, Parkville, Victoria, 3052, Australia **[409]**

**G.R. MacGregor,** Institute for Molecular Genetics and Howard Hughes Medical Institute, Baylor College of Medicine, Houston, TX 77030 **[1]**

**H. Margalit,** National Eye Institute, National Institutes of Health, Bethesda, MD 20892 **[399]**

**Jean-Marc Matter,** Department of Neurosurgery, Washington University School of Medicine, St. Louis, MO 63110 **[269]**

**Lidia Matter-Sadzinski,** Department of Neurosurgery, Washington University School of Medicine, St. Louis, MO 63110 **[269]**

**J. Hugh McDowell,** Department of Ophthalmology, University of Florida, Gainesville, FL 32610 **[35]**

**T. Meitinger,** Genetics Laboratory, Department of Biochemistry, University of Oxford, Oxford OX1 3QU, England **[293]**

**Carmen F. Merryman,** Department of Biochemistry, Thomas Jefferson University, Philadelphia, PA 19107 **[385]**

**Donald Metcalf,** The Walter and Eliza Hall Institute for Medical Research, P.O. Royal Melbourne Hospital, 3050, Victoria, Australia **[409]**

**B. Minke,** Departments of Biological Chemistry and Physiology, The Hebrew University of Jerusalem, 91904 Jerusalem, Israel **[125]**

**Drzislav Mismer,** Howard Hughes Medical Institute and Department of Biochemistry, University of California, Berkeley, CA 94720; present address: Synergen, Inc., Boulder, CO 80301 **[277]**

**T. Mohandas,** Jules Stein Eye Institute and Department of Ophthalmology, UCLA School of Medicine, Los Angeles, CA 90024; present address: Division of Medical Genetics, Harbor/UCLA Medical Center, Torrance, CA 90509 **[329]**

**Craig Montell,** Howard Hughes Medical Institute and Department of Biochemistry, University of California, Berkeley, CA 94720; present address: Department of Biological Chemistry, The Johns Hopkins University School of Medicine, Baltimore, MD 21205 **[117, 277]**

**K.A. Moore,** Institute for Molecular Genetics and Howard Hughes Medical Institute, Baylor College of Medicine, Houston, TX 77030 **[1]**

**A.A. Moscona,** Laboratory for Developmental Biology, Department of Molecular Genetics and Cell Biology, The University of Chicago, Chicago, IL 60637 **[259]**

**D.S. Moss,** Birkbeck College, Department of Crystallography, Laboratory of Molecular Biology, London WC1 7HX, England **[419]**

**Joel Moss,** Laboratory of Cellular Metabolism, National Heart, Lung, and Blood Institute, National Institutes of Health, Bethesda, MD 20892 **[63]**

**S. Mylvaganam,** Birkbeck College, Department of Crystallography, Laboratory of Molecular Biology, London WC1 7HX, England **[419]**

**S. Najmudin,** Birkbeck College, Department of Crystallography, Laboratory of Molecular Biology, London WC1 7HX, England **[419]**

**Akira Nakajima,** Department of Ophthalmology, Juntendo University School of Medicine, Tokyo, Japan **[317]**

**Pravendra Nath,** Laboratory of Molecular and Developmental Biology, National Eye Institute, National Institutes of Health, Bethesda, MD 20892 **[249]**

**Julielani T. Ngo,** Jules Stein Eye Institute and Department of Ophthalmology, UCLA School of Medicine, Los Angeles, CA 90024 **[329]**

**J.M. Nickerson,** Laboratory of Retinal Cell and Molecular Biology, National Eye Institute, National Institutes of Health, Bethesda, MD 20892 **[93]**

**Kenji Okazaki,** Department of Biophysics, Faculty of Science, Kyoto University, Kyoto 606, Japan; present address: Tsukuba Research Center for Life Science, The Institute of Physical and Chemical Research, Tsukuba 305, Japan **[205]**

**Daniel D. Oprian,** Departments of Biology and Chemistry, Massachusetts Institute of Technology, Cambridge, MA 02139; present address: Graduate Department of Biochemistry, Brandeis University, Waltham, MA 02254 **[23]**

**William L. Pak,** Department of Biological Sciences, Purdue University, West Lafayette, IN 47906 **[117]**

**Krzysztof Palczewski,** Department of Ophthalmology, University of Florida, Gainesville, FL 32610 **[35]**

**Luke Pallansch,** Laboratory of Molecular and Developmental Biology, National Eye Institute, National Institutes of Health, Bethesda, MD 20892 **[249]**

**Deborah Pavan-Langston,** Eye Research Institute of Retina Foundation and the Department of Ophthalmology, Harvard Medical School, Boston, MA 02114 **[355,379]**

**R. Peek,** Department of Molecular Biology, University of Nijmegen, 6525 ED Nijmegen, The Netherlands **[229]**

**Jennifer D. Penschow,** The Howard Florey Institute for Experimental Physiology and Medicine, University of Melbourne, Parkville, Victoria, 3052, Australia **[409]**

**Jay Pepose,** Department of Ophthalmology, Georgetown University Medical Center, Washington, DC 20037 **[379]**

**A. Peter,** Department of Genetics, University of Edinburgh, Edinburgh EH9 3JN, Scotland **[239]**

**Charlotte A. Peterson,** Laboratory of Molecular and Developmental Biology, National Eye Institute, National Institutes of Health, Bethesda, MD 20892 **[179,197]**

**Robert A. Phillips,** Hospital for Sick Children Research Institute and the Departments of Ophthalmology and Medical Genetics, The University of Toronto, Toronto, Canada M5G 1X8 **[437]**

**Joram Piatigorsky,** Laboratory of Molecular and Developmental Biology, National Eye Institute, National Institutes of Health, Bethesda, MD 20892 **[xxiii,139,179,197,215]**

**Jean Plouet,** U 86 INSERM, Centre Biomedical des Cordeliers, 75006 Paris, France; present address: Cancer Research Institute, University of California Medical Center, San Francisco, CA 94143 **[83]**

**Carol Raport,** Department of Biochemistry and the Howard Hughes Medical Institute, University of Washington, Seattle, WA 98195 **[53]**

**T.M. Redmond,** Laboratory of Retinal Cell and Molecular Biology, National Eye Institute, National Institutes of Health, Bethesda, MD 20892 **[93,399]**

**R.A. Robinson,** Department of Microbiology, University of Texas Southwestern Medical Center, Dallas, TX 75235 **[365]**

**H. John Roth,** Laboratory of Molecular and Developmental Biology, National Eye Institute, National Institutes of Health, Bethesda, MD 20892 **[179]**

**Gerald M. Rubin,** Howard Hughes Medical Institute and Department of Biochemistry, University of California, Berkeley, CA 94720 **[117,277]**

**John C. Saari,** University of Washington, Seattle, WA 98195 **[107]**

**Thomas P. Sakmar,** Departments of Biology and Chemistry, Massachusetts Institute of Technology, Cambridge, MA 02139 **[23,45]**

**H. Sanui,** National Eye Institute, National Institutes of Health, Bethesda, MD 20892 **[399]**

**P. Vijay Sarthy,** Departments of Ophthalmology, Physiology, and Biophysics, University of Washington, Seattle, WA 98195 **[305]**

**J.G.G. Schoenmakers,** Department of Molecular Biology, University of Nijmegen, 6525 ED Nijmegen, The Netherlands **[229]**

**S.K.A. Sedowofia,** Department of Genetics, University of Edinburgh, Edinburgh EH9 3JN, Scotland **[239]**

**Z. Selinger,** Departments of Biological Chemistry and Physiology, The Hebrew University of Jerusalem, 91904 Jerusalem, Israel **[125]**

**Theodore W. Sery,** Department of Research, Wills Eye Hospital, Philadelphia, PA 19107 **[385,427]**

**F.C.H. Shiao,** Department of Ophthalmology, Emory University School of Medicine, Atlanta, GA 30322 **[365]**

**Toshimichi Shinohara,** Laboratory of Immunology and Section of Molecular Biology, National Eye Institute, National Institutes of Health, Bethesda, MD 20892 **[xxiii,73,385]**

**Takashi Shiono,** Department of Ophthalmology, Tohoku University School of Medicine, Sendai, Japan **[317]**

**Randall D. Shortridge,** Department of Biological Sciences, Purdue University, West Lafayette, IN 47906 **[117]**

**J-S. Si,** Laboratory of Retinal Cell and Molecular Biology, National Eye Institute, National Institutes of Health, Bethesda, MD 20892 **[93]**

**Vijay K. Singh,** Section of Molecular Biology, National Eye Institute, National Institutes of Health, Bethesda, MD 20892 **[385]**

C. Slingsby, Birkbeck College, Department of Crystallography, Laboratory of Molecular Biology, London WC1 7HX, England [419]

Bernd Sommer, Laboratory of Molecular and Developmental Biology, National Eye Institute, National Institutes of Health, Bethesda, MD 20892; present address: Institut für Säugetiergenetik, GSF, 8042 Neuherberg, Federal Republic of Germany [215]

Robert S. Sparkes, Jules Stein Eye Institute and Departments of Ophthalmology and Medical Genetics, UCLA School of Medicine, Los Angeles, CA 90024; present address: Department of Medicine/Pediatrics, UCLA School of Medicine, Los Angeles, CA 90024 [317,329]

M. Anne Spence, Jules Stein Eye Institute and Department of Ophthalmology, UCLA School of Medicine, Los Angeles, CA 90024; present address: Department of Psychiatry/Biomathematics, UCLA School of Medicine, Los Angeles, CA 90024 [329]

A. Srinivasan, Retrovirus Diseases Branch, Centers for Disease Control, Atlanta, GA 30333 [365]

Hermann Steller, Department of Biochemistry, University of California, Berkeley, CA 94720; present address: Department of Brain and Cognitive Science, Massachusetts Institute of Technology, Cambridge, MA 01239 [117]

E. Suss, Departments of Biological Chemistry and Physiology, The Hebrew University of Jerusalem, 91904 Jerusalem, Israel [125]

Masayuki Takeuchi, Department of Biophysics, Faculty of Science, Kyoto University, Kyoto 606, Japan [205]

George Thomas, Laboratory of Molecular and Developmental Biology, National Eye Institute, National Institutes of Health, Bethesda, MD 20892 [179]

J. Toffenetti, Laboratory of Retinal Cell and Molecular Biology, National Eye Institute, National Institutes of Health, Bethesda, MD 20892 [93]

M. Tsuda, Laboratory of Immunology, National Eye Institute, National Institutes of Health, Bethesda, MD 20892 [73]

Narendra Tuteja, Jules Stein Eye Institute and Department of Ophthalmology, UCLA School of Medicine, Los Angeles, CA 90024 [339]

Y. Ueda, Department of Biophysics, Faculty of Science, Kyoto University, Kyoto 606, Japan; present address: Department of Applied Biological Science, Science University of Tokyo, Noda 278, Japan [189]

P. van der Logt, Department of Molecular Biology, University of Nijmegen, 6525 ED Nijmegen, The Netherlands [229]

Lily Vardimon, Laboratory for Developmental Biology, Department of Molecular Genetics and Cell Biology, The University of Chicago, Chicago, IL 60637 [259]

Malini Vatal, Laboratory of Molecular and Developmental Biology, National Eye Institute, National Institutes of Health, Bethesda, MD 20892 [249]

**Martha Vaughan,** Laboratory of Cellular Metabolism, National Heart, Lung, and Blood Institute, National Institutes of Health, Bethesda, MD 20892 **[63]**

**Gabriel Vogeli,** Molecular Biology Research, The Upjohn Company, Kalamazoo, MI 49001 **[169]**

**Eric F. Wawrousek,** Laboratory of Molecular and Developmental Biology, National Eye Institute, National Institutes of Health, Bethesda, MD 20892 **[179, 215]**

**Richard Weleber,** Department of Ophthalmology and Medical Genetics, Oregon Health Sciences University, Portland, OR 97201 **[317]**

**Heiner Westphal,** Section on Mammalian Gene Regulation, Laboratory of Molecular Genetics, National Institute of Child Health and Human Development, National Institutes of Health, Bethesda, MD 20892 **[445]**

**H. White,** Birkbeck College, Department of Crystallography, Laboratory of Molecular Biology, London WC1 7HX, England **[419]**

**B. Wiggert,** National Eye Institute, National Institutes of Health, Bethesda, MD 20892 **[399]**

**David K. Wilcox,** Department of Ophthalmology, The Eye and Ear Institute, University of Pittsburgh, Pittsburgh, PA 15213 **[449]**

**Graeme J. Wistow,** Laboratory of Molecular and Developmental Biology, National Eye Institute, National Institutes of Health, Bethesda, MD 20892 **[139]**

**Linda Wood,** Molecular Biology Research, The Upjohn Company, Kalamazoo, MI 49001 **[169]**

**A.F. Wright,** M.R.C. Clinical and Population Cytogenetics Unit, Western General Hospital, Edinburgh EH4 2XU, Scotland **[293]**

**K. Yamaki,** Laboratory of Immunology, National Eye Institute, National Institutes of Health, Bethesda, MD 20892 **[73]**

**Kunio Yasuda,** Department of Biophysics, Faculty of Science, Kyoto University, Kyoto 606, Japan **[205]**

**R. Yuan,** Retrovirus Diseases Branch, Centers for Disease Control, Atlanta, GA 30333 **[365]**

**Song Yue,** Department of Research, Wills Eye Hospital, Philadelphia, PA 19107 **[385]**

**Peggy S. Zelenka,** Laboratory of Molecular and Developmental Biology, National Eye Institute, National Institutes of Health, Bethesda, MD 20892 **[xxiii, 249]**

**Carmelann Zintz,** Laboratory of Mechanisms of Ocular Diseases, and Clinical Branch, National Eye Institute, National Institutes of Health, Bethesda, MD 20892 **[317]**

**Charles S. Zuker,** Department of Biology, University of California, San Diego, CA 92093 **[277]**

# Preface

The National Eye Institute–UCLA Symposium held at Santa Fe, New Mexico February 6–12, 1988 brought together investigators who study various aspects of vision relative to molecular genetics. The many features of the eye have been studied in detail by different subgroups that have formed productive and scientifically exciting communities. In many of these subsets of eye research, the last few years have seen numerous inroads at the gene level. Even more important than any one discovery—and there have been many—is the fact that the common outlook and language of molecular genetics have set the scene for a new union of eye researchers. The idea behind this meeting, as its title implies, was to examine the eye from the vantage point of its genes. Thus, phototransduction and retina, lens, and ocular diseases such as cancer, retinal degenerations, cataract, viral infections, and connective tissues disorders have been brought together for the first time. The general themes of growth and development, gene expression, evolution, and gene protein structure, which are being so successfully approached today by molecular genetics, were emphasized and applied to the special problems of the eye and vision.

It is fitting that the keynote speaker, Dr. Thomas Caskey of Baylor College of Medicine, discussed the prospects of genetic engineering, and that a special lecture presented by Dr. Russell Doolittle of the University of California, San Diego, concerned protein evolution. These two topics represent well the effort to infuse general aspects of molecular genetics into the vision science community, and to unite advances in the basic and clinical sciences. The tone of both addresses was optimistic: progress is being made to treat genetic disease, and the evolution and relationships among proteins are yielding to the great deluge of sequence data.

In addition to uniting different areas of eye research, this meeting brought together scientists from around the world. We were happy to see representatives from Canada, Australia, Japan, Taiwan, China, England, Scotland, France, Germany, The Netherlands, Sweden, Israel, and of course the United States.

We owe a special debt to the National Eye Institute (USHHS grant EY7561-01) for helping to make this meeting reality, and we hope to repay their support in abundance through the enthusiasm, new directions, scientific exchange, and collaborations fostered there. Additional support for this conference was provided by The Upjohn Company. Finally, we thank Dr. Robin Yeaton and Betty Handy for encouragement and help for the organization of this conference, Dr. Robert H. Harwood for expertly overseeing the meeting and ironing out the many hitches associated with any meeting, and Mrs. Dawn Chicchirichi for invaluable secretarial support.

**Joram Piatigorsky**
**Toshimichi Shinohara**
**Peggy S. Zelenka**

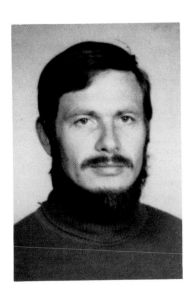

HERMANN KÜHN
1939-1988

Hermann Kühn was 49 years old when he died tragically in a mountaineering accident on March 29th, 1988. He was in the prime of his life and of his scientific career. He had begun his studies on the biochemistry of vision eighteen years earlier--work which was to greatly influence the direction of vision research and which was to bring him international recognition. Hermann addressed this symposium, "Molecular Biology of the Eye", on his most recent studies, "Proteins Involved in the Activation and Deactivation of cGMP-phosphodiesterase in Rods". It was his last talk at a scientific meeting. He did not submit a manuscript for publication in this Proceedings volume, but following this tribute to his memory we append a complete list of his scientific publications.

The son of a chemist, Hermann grew up and received his early education near Heidelberg. He was a well-rounded youth, accomplished in music and sports as well as academics. Hermann studied chemistry at the universities of Heidelberg and Munich and received his Ph.D. in 1967 for thesis work performed at the Max Planck Institut für Medizinesche Forschung at Heidelberg. He continued his research in Heidelberg until 1970 when he travelled to the U.S. with his wife Annie and their infant son, Christoph. At CalTech he studied membrane biochemistry with William Dreyer, along with three other post-doctoral fellows (David Papermaster, Paul Hargrave, and Bob Molday) working on photoreceptor membranes. It was there that Hermann observed the light-dependent phosphorylation of rhodopsin[3,5]--a finding that propelled him into vision biochemistry and shaped the direction of his scientific career. In 1972 Hermann returned to Germany to establish his own laboratory in the Institut für Neurobiologie at the KFA in Jülich. There he made a series of discoveries that have greatly influenced the work of all of us in vision and in related areas.

Hermann demonstrated that the phosphorylation and dephosphorylation of rhodopsin occured in vivo and he established the time courses for the reactions.[6] With his first postdoctoral fellow (Hugh McDowell) and his first Ph.D. student (Ursula Wilden), he painstakingly determined the characteristics of the kinase reaction and the number of sites phosphorylated on rhodopsin.[11,20] Hermann's description of the light-dependent binding of the kinase, G-protein and 48K protein to rhodopsin[12] was a key finding which assisted him and others in their purification and in understanding their roles and mechanisms of action.[13] He established many of the parameters of G-protein rhodopsin interaction in his own laboratory[17] and in collaboration with other laboratories, including that of Marc Chabre[18,23] and Peter Hofmann.[24] His most recent work showed the role of 48K protein in enhancing the "quenching" of photoexcited rhodopsin.[37]

Hermann set a high standard for himself in his work. He had a first-rate intellect and he did the right experiments. His impact on the field was enormous. It is hard to imagine a person more highly respected and admired by his colleagues. He was thoughtful, incisive and rigorous in his work. Personally he was helpful and generous. He had a gentle manner, and had no pretensions. We will fondly remember his easy laugh, his slow careful speech, and his dry humor.

It seems that everything that Hermann did, he did well. He was musically talented. He was an excellent pianist with an extensive classical music repertoire. He played the clarinet even better. Hermann's clarinet instructor had been very disappointed when Hermann did not pursue a professional career in music. Many chamber music groups from California to Germany were pleased to have him as a member, and he was a frequent soloist with the Düren symphony.

Hermann was also an outdoorsman, a hiker, rockclimber and mountaineer. He had climbed in Greenland, the Andes, Yosemite, the Alps, and in Mexico. On weekends he went rockclimbing in the Eifel mountains near his home, and for long walks with family and friends in the forests. Many of us enjoyed simliar hikes with him at meetings around the world; at Gordon Conferences in New Hampshire, FASEB meetings in Vermont or Colorado, at meetings in Greece, Mexico, the Soviet Union and France.

His last climb, a 4000 meter peak in the Alps, was to have been an easy one. Hermann was always careful, but a patch of soft snow gave way and he plunged 400 meters to his death. Funeral services were held for Hermann in Jülich on April 6th, 1988. Hermann and his wife Annie had lived in the Jülich area for 16 years and their sons Christoph, 17, and Norbert, 14, had grown up there. Hermann's legacy to them and to us is that of a kind and generous person who lived life fully and with great accomplishment. We shall miss him greatly. Our memories of him are precious.


Paul A. Hargrave


## PUBLICATIONS OF HERMANN KÜHN

1.  Kühn R, Kühn H (1966). Quarternary structure and color of crustacyanin. Angew Chem Int 5:957.
2.  Kühn R, Kühn H (1967). Crustacyanin, ein Chromoproteid aus Hummerpanzer: Beziehungen swischen Farbe und Quartarstruktur. Eur J Biochem 2:349-360.
3.  Kühn H, Dreyer WJ (1972). Light-dependent phosphorylation of rhodopsin by ATP. FEBS Lett 20:1-6.
4.  Dreyer WJ, Papermaster DS, Kühn H (1972). On the absence of ubiquitous structural protein subunits in biological membranes. Ann NY Acad Sci 195:61-74.
5.  Kühn H, Cook JH, Dreyer WJ (1973). Phosphorylation of rhodopsin in bovine photoreceptor membranes: A dark reaction after illumination. Biochem 12:2495-2502.
6.  Kühn H (1974). Light-dependent phosphorylation of rhodopsin in living frogs. Nature (London) 250:588-590.
7.  Kühn H, Bader S (1976). The rate of rhodopsin phosphorylation in isolated retinas of frog and cattle. Biochim Biophys Acta 428:13-18.
8.  Kühn H, McDowell JH (1977). Isoelectric focusing of phosphorylated cattle rhodopsin. Biophys Struct Mech 3:199-203.
9.  Kühn H, McDowell JH, Leser KH, Bader S (1977). Phosphorylation of rhodopsin as a possible mechanism of adaptation. Biophys Struct Mech 3:175-180.

10.  Krebs W, Kühn H  (1977).  Structure of isolated bovine rod outer segment membranes. Exp Eye Res  25:511-526.

11.  McDowell JH, Kühn H  (1977).  Light-induced phosphorylation of rhodopsin in cattle photoreceptor membranes:  Substrate activation and inactivation. Biochem 16:4054-4060.

12.  Kühn H  (1978).  Light-regulated binding of rhodopsin kinase and other proteins to cattle photoreceptor membranes. Biochem 17:4389-4395.

13.  Kühn H  (1980).  Light- and GTP-regulated interaction of GTPase and other proteins with bovine photoreceptor membranes. Nature (London) 283:587-589.

14.  Kühn H  (1980).  Light-induced, reversible binding of proteins to bovine photoreceptor membranes:  Influence of nucleotides. Neurochem 1:269-285.

15.  Baumeister W, Buse G, Deuticke B, Kühn H  (1981).  Membrane proteins:  Analysis of molecular and supramolecular structure. FEBS Lett 131:1-6.

16.  Kühn H  (1981).  Interactions of rod cell proteins with the disk membrane:  Influence of light, ionic strength, and nucleotides.  In Miller WH (ed): "Current Topics in Membranes and Transport," 15, 171-201.

17.  Kühn H, Hargrave PA  (1981).  Light-induced binding of GTPase to bovine photoreceptor membranes:  Effects of limited proteolysis of the membranes. Biochem 20:2410-2417.

18.  Kühn H, Bennett N. Michel-Villaz M, Chabre M  (1981). Interactions between photoexcited rhodopsin and GTP-binding protein:  Kinetic and stoichiometric analysis from light-scattering changes. Proc Natl Acad Sci USA 18:6873-6877.

19.  Kühn H, Mommertz O, Hargrave PA (1982). Light-dependent conformational change at rhodopsin's cytoplasmic surface detected by increased susceptibility to proteolysis. Biochim Biophys Acta 679:95-100.

20.  Wilden U, Kühn H  (1982).  Light-dependent phosphorylation of rhodopsin:  Number of phosphorylation sites.  Biochem 21:3014-3022.

21.  Kühn H  (1982).  Light regulated binding of proteins to photoreceptor membranes, and its use for the purification of several rod cell proteins.  In "Methods in Enzymology," Vol 81, pp 556-564.

22.  Kühn H, Wilden U  (1982).  Assay of phosphorylation of rhodopsin in vitro and in vivo.  In "Methods in Enzymology," Vol 81, pp 489-496.

23.  Bennett N, Michel-Villaz M, Kühn H  (1982).  Light-induced interaction between rhodopsin and the GTP-binding protein: Metarhodopsin II is the major photoproduct involved.  Eur J Biochem 127:97-103.

24. Emeis D, Kühn H, Reichert J, Hofmann KP (1982). Complex formation between metarhodopsin II and GTP-binding protein in bovine photoreceptor membranes leads to a shift of the photoproduct equilibrium. FEBS Lett 143:29-34.

25. Hargrave PA, McDowell JH, Siemiatkowski-Juszczak EC, Fong SL, Kühn H, Wang JK, Curtis DR, Mohana Rao JK, Argos P, Feldmann RJ (1982). The carboxyl-terminal one-third of bovine rhodopsin: Its structure and function. Vis Res 22:1429-1437.

26. Kühn H, Chabre M (1983). Light-dependent interactions between rhodopsin and photoreceptor enzymes. Biophys Struct Mech 9:231-234.

27. Pfister C, Kühn H, Chabre M (1983). Interaction between photoexcited rhodopsin and peripheral enzymes in frog retinal rods: Influence on the post-metarhodopsin II decay and phosphorylation rate of rhodopsin. Eur J Biochem 136:489-499.

28. Chabre M, Pfister C, Deterre P, Kühn H (1984). The mechanism of control of cGMP phosphodiesterase by photoexcited rhodopsin in retinal cells. Analogies with hormone-controlled systems. In Dumond JE, Nunez J (eds): "Hormones and Cell Regulation," Elsevier Science Publ, Vol 8, pp 87-97.

29. Kühn H (1984). Early steps in the activation of photoreceptor enzymes by light: Interactions between disk membrane proteins triggered by light and regulated by GTP. In Brosellino A, Cervetto L (eds): "Photoreceptors," London, New York, Plenum Press, pp 75-98.

30. Kühn H (1984). Interactions between photoexcited rhodopsin and light-activated enzymes in rods. In Osborne NN, Chader GJ (eds): "Progress in Retinal Research," Vol 3, pp 123-156.

31. Kühn H, Hall SW, Wilden U (1984). Light-induced binding of 48 kDa protein to photoreceptor membranes is highly enhanced by phosphorylation of rhodopsin. FEBS Lett 176:473-478.

32. Kühn H (1984). Early steps in the light-triggered activation of the cyclic GMP enzymatic pathway in rod photoreceptors. In Bolis CL, Helmreich EJM, Passow H (eds): "Information and Energy Transduction in Biological Membranes," pp 303-311.

33. Pfister C, Chabre M, Plouet J, Tuyen VV, DeKozak Y, Faure JP, Kühn H (1985). Retinal S-antigen identified as the 48 K protein regulating light-dependent phosphodiesterase in rods. Science 228:891-893.

34. Deterre P, Bigay J, Robert M, Pfister C, Kühn H, Chabre M (1986). Activation of retinal rod cyclic GMP-phosphodiesterase by transducin: Characterization of the complex

formed by phosphodiesterase inhibitor and transducin α-sub-
unit. Proteins – Structure, Function and Genetics 1:188-193.

35. Kühn H (1986). Proteins involved in the control of cyclic
GMP phosphodiesterase in retinal rod cells. In Luttgau C
(ed): "Membrane Control of Cellular Activity," Fortschritte
der Zoologie 33:289-297.

36. Kühn H, Hall SW, Wehner M, Wilden U (1986). Activation
and deactivation of the cyclic nucleotide enzyme cascade in
visual rod cells. In Hamprecht B, Neuhoff V (eds): "Neuro-
biochemistry," Springer-Verlag, pp 76-87.

37. Wilden U, Hall SW, Kühn H (1986). Phosphodiesterase activation by photoexcited rhodopsin is quenched when rhodopsin
is phosphorylated and binds the intrinsic 48-kDa protein of
rod outer segments. Proc Natl Acad Sci USA 83:1174-1178.

38. Wilden U, Wust E, Wyand I, Kühn H (1986). Rapid affinity
purification of retinal arrestin (48 kDa-protein) via its light-
dependent binding to phosphorylated rhodopsin. FEBS Lett
207:292-295.

39. Hall SW, Kühn H (1986). Purification and properties of
guanylate kinase from bovine retinas and rod outer segments.
Eur J Biochem 161:551-556.

40. Hargrave PA, McDowell JH, Smyk-Randal E, Siemiatkowski-
Juszczak ED, Cao T, Arendt A, Kühn H (1987). Limited
proteolysis of rhodopsin by thermolysin as a probe of protein
structure and topography. In Cohen SC (ed): "Membrane Proteins," Bio-Rad Laboratories, pp 81-93.

41. Kühn H (1987). Interactions between proteins involved in the
activation and subsequent deactivation of phosphodiesterase
in visual rod cells. In Ovchinnikov YA, Hucho F (eds): "Receptor and Ion Channels," deGruyter, pp 227-234.

42. Kühn H, Wilden U (1987). Deactivation of photoactivated
rhodopsin by rhodopsin-kinase and arrestin. J Receptor Res
7:283-289.

43. Kühn H, Wilden U (1987). Phosphorylation of rhodopsin
involved in terminating the visual response. In Konijn TM, et
al (eds): "Molecular Mechanisms of Desensitization to Signal
Molecules," Springer-Verlag, pp 241-253.

44. Kühn H, Wilden U (1987). Light-dependent activation and
ATP-dependent deactivation of cGMP-phosphodiesterase in
rod outer segments: Interactions between proteins involved.
In Hudspeth AM, et al (eds): "Discussions in Neurosciences,
Sensory Transductions, FESN," Geneva, Switzerland, pp 75-
79.

45. Pfister C, Kühn H (1987). From the photon to the cellular
response in the vertebrate retina: The rhodopsin-triggered
regulation of cGMP. Photobiochem Photobiophys Suppl 249-
259.

46. Wehner M, Kühn H (1987). The cyclic GMP enzyme cascade of vision:  Site of light activation localized by enzymatic modifications of rhodopsin. Adv Biosci 62:345-351.

47. Benovic JL, Kühn H, Weyand I, Codina J, Caron MG, Lefkowitz RJ (1987).  Functional desensitization of the isolated β-adrenergic receptor by the β-adrenergic receptor kinase:  Potential role of an analog of the retinal protein arrestin (48-kDa protein). Proc Natl Acad Sci USA 84:8879-8882.

**Molecular Biology of the Eye: Genes, Vision, and Ocular Disease, pages 1–22**
© **1988 Alan R. Liss, Inc.**

TOWARDS GENE THERAPY FOR INHERITED
OCULAR DISEASE-STUDIES OF RETROVIRALLY MEDIATED
HUMAN ADENOSINE DEAMINASE EXPRESSION IN MICE

G.R. MacGregor, F.A. Fletcher, K.A. Moore,
S.M-W. Chang[2], J.W. Belmont, and C.T. Caskey

Institute for Molecular Genetics and Howard Hughes Medical
Institute, Baylor College of Medicine, Houston, Texas 77030

ABSTRACT Somatic gene transfer offers the possibility of a new approach to the treatment of human genetic disease. Adenosine deaminase deficiency is being used as a model in which gene transfer techniques can be developed and evaluated. Multiple replication-defective retrovirus vectors were tested for their ability to transfer and express human adenosine deaminase *in vitro* and *in vivo* in a mouse bone marrow transplantation model. High titer virus production was obtained from vectors utilizing both a retrovirus long terminal repeat promoter and internal transcriptional units with human cFos and herpes virus thymidine kinase promoters. After infection of primary murine bone marrow with one of these vectors, human ADA was detected in CFU-C, CFU-S, and in the blood of reconstituted recipient animals. This system offers the opportunity to assess methods for increasing efficiency of gene transfer, for regulation of expression of foreign genes in hematopoietic progenitors, and for long term measurement of stability of expression in these cells.

[1]This work was supported by the Howard Hughes Medical Institute, NIH grant HD21452, and Cystic Fibrosis Foundation grant R004 7-03S1.
[2]Present address: Laboratory of Molecular Genetics, NINCDS, NIH, Bethesda, MD

INTRODUCTION

There exist several inherited eye disorders which may eventually be considered as candidates for a novel therapy- somatic gene transfer. The basis of this therapy concerns the introduction of a cloned functional copy of the defective gene in question into somatic tissues of the patient. Theoretically, subsequent expression of the introduced proficient cDNA copy of the gene compliments the defection endogenous gene resulting in a scenario, the spectrum of which ranges from arrest of deterioration to a complete amelioration of the patient's dysfunction. Example of inherited ocular disorders that may be considered candidates for this therapeutic approach are gyrate atrophy (associated with ornithine aminotransferase deficiency (1) and retinoblastoma. cDNA's for genes involved in both of these disorders are available (2,3) although in the case of retinoblastoma, the necessity to introduce the gene into 100% of target cells to generate an effective treatment, may preclude this disorder's candidacy. In addition, there exist several systemic diseases such as Fabry's disease, mucopolysaccharidosis IV (MSP IV), Wilson's disease and galactokinase deficiency (4) that may also be considered as targets for gene therapy, although the molecular basis for these disorders is less well understood and cDNAs exist only for $\alpha$-galactosidase A (Fabry's disease, 5).

Towards gene therapy for these disorders, we are study- ing expression of a human adenosine deaminase cDNA in hematopoietic tissues in recipient mice. This animal model for gene transfer has the advantage that conditions for *in vitro* manipulation of the target tissue - primary bone marrow - are well established

Adenosine deaminase (ADA) deficiency is a rare autosomal recessive condition which causes a form of severe combined immune deficiency (SCID, 6). It accounts for approximately 15% of all cases of SCID or one-third of autosomal recessive SCID. The pathophysiology of ADA deficiency has been inten- sively investigated and appears to involve selective toxicity of dATP for immature T cells (6-8). Alterations in methyla- tion *via* inhibition of S-adenosyl homocysteine hydrolase have also been implicated (7,8). Human ADA is encoded at a single 35kb locus composed of 12 exons on chromosome 20q13 (9-15). A full length cDNA of 1437bp has been obtained which encodes a 362 amino acid protein of 40.7kd (12), *i.e.*, cloned DNA sequences are available for gene transfer. Bone marrow forms. Within the parental pΔXT1ADA virus-producing cell line and in one of the target cell clones a minor deletion variant was detected. In addition, total cellular RNA was isolated and subjected to Northern analysis using $^{32}$P-labelled ADA cDNA as probe (Figure 2b). RNA species corresponding to the predicted transcripts from the viral LTR and the internal promoters cFos or TK were readily detected. Taken together, these results suggest that the process of selection did not engender rearranged defective viruses.

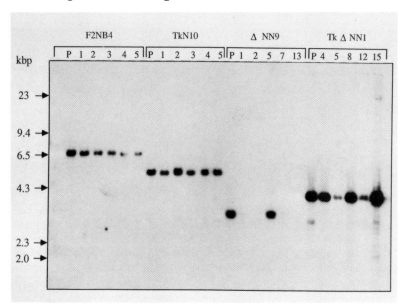

Figure 2a. Southern analysis of infected target cells. High molecular weight DNA was isolated by standard techniques from the Parental ψ2 producer cell clones (P) and from infected Rat208F clones (numbered lanes). Five μg of genomic DNA was cut with *Nhe*I, electrophoresed through a 0.7%TAE agarose gel and blot-transferred to nylon membrane (Gene Screen Plus, Dupont, Boston, MA) by the method of Southern. ADA cDNA was labeled with $^{32}$P dCTP and hybridized as described (43). Filters were washed to a final stringency of 0.1X SSC, at 65°C. The blots were exposed to Kodak XAR-5 film overnight with an intensifying screen. F2NB4 - parental cell line producing pN2Fos2ADA vector; TKN10 - pXT1ADA vector; ΔNN9 - pΔNN2ADA vector; and TKΔNN1 - pΔXT1ADA vector. ADA retroviral-specific hybridization identical to that seen in lane "P" in the ΔNN9 samples were observed in lanes 1, 2, 7,

and 13 following longer exposure of the filter (data not shown).

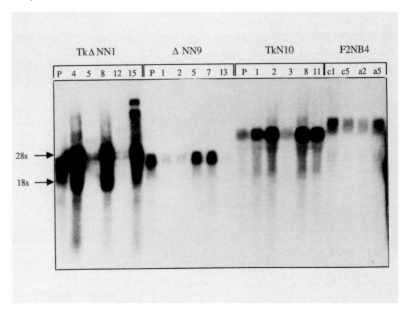

Figure 2b.  Northern analysis of infected target cells. Total cellular RNA was isolated (59) from identical cultures analyzed in Figure 2a.    Ten μg of RNA were electrophoresed through a 0.9% formaldehyde-MOPS agarose gel.    The nucleic acids were transferred, hybridized and washed as in Figure 2a.  High molecular weight species in lane 15 may indicate read-through transcription at a unique site of integration.

Because of the known propensity for gag[+]-containing vectors to recombine in the ψ2 cells, we examined these cell lines for the presence of replication competent virus.    A marker rescue assay was employed using an NIH3T3 line transfected with the defective vector SV(B) (54) as the intermediate target cell.    Supernatants from the ADA vector in ψ2 cell lines all contained helper virus capable of rescuing the defective neo-containing virus from the SV(B) line.

Infection of murine hematopoietic cells.

The four high titer viruses (N2Fos2, XT1, ΔXT1,and ΔNN2) were subsequently used to infect primary mouse bone marrow cells.    Infection was performed by 24hr co-cultivation with

irradiated virus producer lines. Infected marrow was either
plated in semisolid culture media for enumeration of G418-re-
sistant CFU-C or injected into irradiated recipients. Some
recipients received graded doses of the marrow cells so that
discrete CFU-S could be studied. Other animals received
fully reconstituting doses to allow long term studies of
human ADA expression. The results of these experiments are
summarized in Table 1. Two vectors, N2Fos2 and XT1, containing the cFos promoter and the TK promoters respectively fail

Table 1

| Vector[a] | In Vitro | | In Vivo[c] | |
|---|---|---|---|---|
| | % G418[R] CFU[b] | IEF | Southern | IEF |
| pN2Fos2ADA | 8-20% | neg | 2/35 (6%) | 0/2 |
| pXT1ADA | 1.6-8.5% | neg | 11/18 (61%) | 0/11 |
| pΔTKADA | NA | pos | 3/6 (50%) | 3/3 |
| pΔNN2ADA | NA | pos | 31/45 (69%) | 24/31 |

[a] See Figure 1 for description of vectors.
[b] Infected bone marrow cells were plated in supplemented IMDM
with 0.5% methyl cellulose as previously described (43). CFU
were counted at 10 days.
[c] Discrete (CFU-S) or whole spleens from fully reconstituted
mice were analyzed as described in Figures 3 and 4. Survival
splenectomy was performed using standard techniques (61) with
Avertin anesthesia.

to express human ADA in CFU-C or in CFU-S despite these
viruses ability to transduce ADA efficiently to tissue
culture fibroblasts and despite relatively efficient infection of CFU-C and CFU-S. (Both vectors express neo from the
LTR promoter and confer G418-resistance to between 1 and 20%
of CFU-C. However, when those colonies were picked and
assayed for human ADA expression none was found.) When
individual CFU-S or spleens from fully reconstituted animals
were studied we again failed to observe expression of human
ADA. In contrast, bone marrow cells infected with the virus
using the Moloney LTR promoter (ΔNN2) or the TK promoter and
lacking the neo gene (ΔXT1) expressed human ADA. This enzyme
activity could be detected in pooled CFU-C in the absence of

selection indicating very high infection efficiency. Likewise, when individual CFU-S were analyzed infection efficien-
cies of between 50 and 85% were observed based on Southern
analysis (Figure  3) and expression of human ADA (Figure 4).

**Southern analysis : CFU-S**
**HindIII digestion**

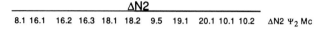

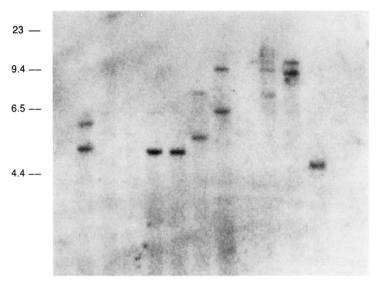

Figure 3.   Southern analysis of infected CFU-S.  Six x $10^6$
fresh bone marrow cells harvested from the tibias and femurs
of healthy 8-12wk C57Bl/6J mice (Jackson Laboratories, Bar
Harbor,  ME)  were  co-cultivated  with  6 x $10^6$  irradiated
(1500R,  Cs137  source,  Gammacell 1000,  Atomic  Energy  Ltd.
Canada) virus producer cells in Iscove's Modified Dulbecco's
Medium  (IMDM,  Gibco)  supplemented  with  BSA,  Fe-saturated
transferrin,  soybean  lipids  ( Boehringer-Mannheim  Biochemi-
cals,  Indianapolis,  IN),  10%FCS,  10%  WEHI3B(D-)  (provided by
R. Phillips) conditioned medium (interleukin3), and 10% 5637
(ATCC)  conditioned  medium  (interleukin 1$\alpha$).   After  24hr  the
nonadherent  cells  were  removed  into  petri  dishes  for  an
additional  48hr  of  culture.   With  vectors  carrying  the *neo*
gene  some  of  the  cells  were  preselected  in  1.50mg/ml  G418.
One x $10^5$ viable cells were plated into 1ml semisolid methyl-
cellulose  cultures  in  supplemented  IMDM  (43).    CFU-C  were
counted  and  picked  after  10d.   Irradiated  (1000R)  syngeneic

enable long term analysis of human ADA expression.

Two vectors, N2Fos2 and XT1 failed to express human ADA in CFU-C or CFU-S despite efficient infection of both classes of cells, (as judged by G418$^R$ CFU-C and by Southern analysis of CFU-S). In contrast, the two remaining vectors, ΔXT1 and ΔNN2 were both used with success to infect and generate high levels of expression of human ADA in CFU-C. In a first experiment, 100% of CFU-S positive for human ada DNA sequences by Southern analysis also exhibited human ADA activity by IEF.

To determine if expression of human ADA in the spleens of animals transplanted with the ΔXT1 vector-infected marrow was obtained from transcription from the LTR or the HSV tK promoter, an RNase A mapping study was performed. This strongly suggests that predominant RNA species originated in the LTR and that the HSV tK mediated transcript contributes little to production of human ADA. Southern analysis perfomed on DNA isolated from individual CFU-S indicated multiple proviral inserts with an average of 2 per cell. Since CFU-S have been shown to be clonally derived (55) this result suggests that the virus titer was not limiting but that there exist limitations as to the receptivity of certain CFU-S progenitors to infection. This can vary from experiment to experiment and suggests, as yet, uncontrolled aspects of the infection protocol which must be optimized in future experiments. In addition, we also observed large fluctuations in the expression efficiency between experiments (Table 2). This suggest that beyond the variability in the infectivity of these cells, there is also biological variation in the regulation of expression of identical vector sequences. An understanding of this variation in a prerequisite to successful application of somatic gene transfer and is the focus of present scrutiny.

At 4 weeks post-reconstitution with ΔNN2 virus infected bone marrow, 14 out of 14 recipient mice had easily detectable levels of human ADA in their blood (Table 2). The ADA enzyme from whole blood is derived almost entirely from red blood cells (RBC's) and thus, does not reflect the level of expression or the longevity of expression in the lymphocyte, granulocyte/monocyte or platelet lineages. Over time, the level of human ADA activity decreased (see Figure 6) suggesting that the cells initially expressing it originated from more mature progenitors which were infected with higher efficiency or in whom no negative regulatory effects or expression had arisen. However, 4 of the 14 animals have continued to express human ADA, although at diminished levels, up to four months post-transplant.

The average life span of a murine RBC is 45 days (56,57) so that in these animals the human ADA detected probably originates from cells whose primitive progenitors were infected with the virus. The level of human ADA observed in these mice, 10-100%, is such that in a human recipient, it would be expected to ameliorate the disease.

It is formally possible that replication competent virus introduced at the time of infection with the ADA-transducing defective virus allows spread of the defective in vivo. Indeed, serial assay serum in the ΔNN2 and ΔXT1 recipients by marker rescue assay does indicate continuing viremia with the replication-competent virus in all these animals (data not shown). However, we do not believe that in vivo spread contributes much to human ADA expression in the blood for the following reasons: (a) the orderly and consistent reduction in expression seen in all animals at around 10 wks; (b) the stability of expression observed beyond 10 wks in individual animals without apparent fluctuation; (c) the presence of replication-competent virus in animals failing to express human ADA in the blood; and (d) the lack of multiple, less than single copy insertions in individual CFU-S and in the organs of long term recipients (manuscript in preparation)

These experiments demonstrate long term expression of a human disease-related gene product in mouse hematopoietic cells. These results are consistent with previous published reports of expression of neomycin phosphotransferase in these cells (23) and extend the observations on long term stability of expression. Lim et al. (45), have recently shown that vectors which utilize the PGK promoter for ADA expression can also express in CFU-S. These results are similar to our experience with the HSVTK promoter.

These results clearly demonstrate that there is no adverse effect imposed upon expression from the Moloney LTR promoter in murine hematopoietic progenitors. This is in contrast to the poor expression from this promoter observed in embryonal carcinoma cells, early mouse embryo cells, and retrovirus transgenic animals (23-42). However, regulation of expression in the differentiated progeny of true pluripotent stem cells may be governed by the same mechanisms which restrict expression in the transgenic animals. This problem may be approached by further analysis of the types of vectors which express introduced genes in embryonal carcinoma cells compared with those that express identical genes in hematopoietic cells.

A number of technical questions remain to be addressed

before an attempt at human disease correction can be made. The long term stability and quantity of expression must be carefully studied and the origin of the expressing cells must be unequivocally related to pluripotent stem cell infection. Likewise, experiments involving humans must be performed in a strictly helper virus-free situation. Future experiments will focus on optimization of stem cell infection by enrichment using monoclonal antibodies and cell sorting and by hormonal stimulation. We are optimistic that improvements can be made that will allow exploitation of this set of methods for the therapy of a variety of human genetic diseases.

## ACKNOWLEDGEMENTS

GRM is the recipient of an Arthiritis Foundation postdoctoral fellowship; JWB is an Assistant Investigator and CTC is an Investigator in HHMI. The authors wish to thank Jenny Henkel-Tigges and Michelle Rives for technical assistance and Elsa Perez for help in preparation of the manuscript. The authors also wish to thank J. Dick, A. Bernstein, and L. Donehower for useful discussions during the completion of these studies.

## REFERENCES

1.  Inana G, Hotta Y, Zintz C, Takkio K, Kaiser-Kupfer M, Nukayasu K, Nakajima A, Shiono T (1987). Analysis of ornithine aminotransferase gene and mRNA in gyrate atrophy patients. Invet Opthalmol Vis Sci (Supp.) 28:18.
2.  Inana G, Totsuka S, Redmond M, Dougherty T, Nagle J, Shiono T, Ohura T, Kominami E, Katunuma N (1986). Molecular cloning of human ornithine human transferase mRNA. Proc Natl Acad Sci USA 83:1203.
3.  Friend SH, Bernards R, Rogelj S, Weinberg RA, Rapaport JM, Albert DA, Dryja TP (1986). A human DNA segment with properties of the gene that predisposes to retinoblastoma and osteosarcoma. Nature 323:643.
4.  Miller CA, Krachmer JH (1986). Corneal diseases. In Goldberg's Genetic and Metabolic Eye Disease. Renie WA (ed) 2nd Edition: Toronto: Little, Brown and Co. p 297.
5.  Bishop DF, Calhoun DH, Bernstein HS, Hantzopoulos P, Quinn M, Desnick RJ (1986). Human alpha galactosidase A: nucleotide sequence of a cDNA clone encoding the

mature enzyme. Proc Natl Acad Sci USA 83:4859.

6. Kredich NM, Hersfield MS (1983). Immunodeficiency Diseases Caused by Adenosine Deaminase Deficiency and Purine Nucleoside Phosphorylase Deficiency. In Stanbury JB, Wyngaarden JB, Fredrickson DS, Goldstein JL, Brown MS (eds): The Metabolic Basis of Inherited Disease, McG p 1157.

7. Hershfield MS, Kredich NM (1978). S-Adenosylhomocysteine Hydrolase Is an Adenosine Binding Protein: A target for Adenosine Toxicity. Science 202:757.

8. Hershfield M (1979). Apparent Suicide Inactivation of Human Lymphoblast S-Adenosylhomocysteine Hydrolase by 2'-Deoxyadenosine and Adenine Arabinoside. J Biol Chem 254:22.

9. Honig J, Martiniuk F, DEustachio P, Zamfirescu C, Desnick R, Hirschhorn K, Hirschhorn LR, Hirschhorn R (1984). Confirmation of the regional localization of the genes for human acid alpha-glucosidase (GAA) and adenosine deaminase (ADA) by somatic cell hybridization. Ann Hum Genet 48:49.

10. Mohandas T, Sparkes RS, Suh EJ, Hershfield MS (1984). Regional localization of the human genes for S-adenosyl-homocysteine hydrolase (cen----q131) and adenosine deaminase (q131----qter) on chromosome 20. Hum Genet 66:292.

11. Petersen MB, Tranebjaerg L, Tommerup N, Nygaard P, Edwards H (1987). New assignment of the adenosine deaminase gene locus to chromosome 20q13 X 11 by study of a patient with interstitial deletion 20q. J Med Genet 24:93.

12. Adrian GS, Wiginton DA, Hutton JJ (1984). Structure of adenosine deaminase mRNAs from normal and adenosine deaminase-deficient human cell lines. Mol Cell Biol 4:1712.

13. Wiginton DA, Kaplan DJ, States JC, Akeson AL, Perme CM, Bilyk IJ, Vaughn AJ, Lattier DL, Hutton JJ (1987). Complete sequence and structure of the gene for human adenosine deaminase. Biochemistry 88 25:8234.

14. Markert ML, Hershfield MS, Wiginton DA, States JC, Ward FE, Bigner SH, Buckley RH, Kaufman RE, Hutton JJ (1987) Identification of a deletion in the adenosine deaminase gene in a child with severe combined immunodeficiency. J Immunol 24 138:3203.

15. Akeson AL, Wiginton DA, States JC, Perme CM, Dusing MR, Hutton JJ (1987). Mutations in the human adenosine deaminase gene that affect protein structure and RNA

splicing. Proc Natl Acad Sci USA 84:5947.

16. Hirshhorn R, Roegner-Maniscalco V, Kuritsky L, Rosen F (1981). Bone Marrow Transplantation only Partially Restores Purine Metabolites to Normal In Adenosine Deaminase-deficient Patients. J Clin Invest 68:1387.

17. Fischer A, Blanche S, Veber F, LeDeist F, Gerota I, Lopez M, Durandy A, Griscelli C (1986). Correction of immune disorders by HLA matched and mismatched bone marrow transplantation. In Gale RP, Champlin R (eds): "Progress in Bone Marrow Transplantation," New York: Alan R. Liss, p 911.

18. Hershfield MS, Buckley RH, Greenberg ML, Melton AL, Schiff R, Hatem C, Kurtzberg J, Markert ML, Kobayashi RH, Kobayashi AL (1987). Treatment of adenosine deaminase deficiency with polyethylene glycol-modified adenosine deaminase. N Engl J Med 316:589.

19. Joyner A, Keller G, Phillips RA, Bernstein A (1983). Retrovirus transfer of a bacterial gene into mouse haematopoietic progenitor cells. Nature 305:556.

20. Miller AD, Eckner RJ, Jolly DJ, Friedmann T, Verma IM (1984). Expression of a Retrovirus Encoding Human HPRT in Mice. Science 225:630.

21. Williams DA, Lemischka IR, Nathan DG, Mulligan RC (1984). Introduction of new genetic material into pluripotent haematopoietic stem cells of the mouse. Nature 310:476.

22. Dick JE, Magli MC, Huszar D, Phillips RA, Bernstein A (1985). Introduction of a selectable gene into primitive stem cells capable of long-term reconstitution of the hemopoietic system of W/Wv mice. Cell 42:71.

23. Keller G, Paige C, Gilboa E, Wagner EF (1985). Expression of a foreign gene in myeloid and lymphoid cells derived from multipotent heamatopoietic precusors. Nature 318:149.

24. Eglitis MA, Kantoff P, Gilboa E, Anderson WF (1985). Gene Expression in Mice after High Efficiency Retroviral-Mediated Gene Transfer. Science 230:1395.

25. Lemischka IR, Raulet DH, Mulligan RC (1986). Developmental Potential and Dynamic Behavior of Hematopoietic Stem Cells. Cell 45:917.

26. Williams DA, Orkin SH, Mulligan RC (1986). Retrovirus-mediated transfer of human adenosine deaminase gene sequences into cells in culture and into murine hematopoietic cells in vivo. Proc Natl,Acad Sci USA 83:2566.

27. Hock RA, Miller AD (1986). Retrovirus-mediated transfer

and expression of drug resistance genes in human haematopoietic progenitor cells. Nature 320:275.

28. Kwok WW, Schuening F, Stead RB, Miller AD (1986) Retroviral transfer of genes into canine hemopoietic progenitor cells in culture: a model for human gene therapy. Proc Natl Acad Sci USA 55 83:4552.

29. Chang SM, Wager SmithK, Tsao TY, Henkel TiggesJ, Vaishnav S, Caskey CT (1987). Construction of a defective retrovirus containing the human hypoxanthine phosphoribosyltransferase cDNA and its expression in cultured cells and mouse bone marrow. Mol Cell Biol 7:854.

30. Hawley RG, Covarrubias L, Hawley T, Mintz B (1987). Handicapped retroviral vectors efficiently transduce foreign genes into hematopoietic stem cells. Proc Natl Acad Sci USA 84:2406.

31. Kantoff PW, Gillio AP, McLachlin JR, Bordignon C, Eglitis MA, Kernan NA, Moen RC, Kohn DB, Yu SF, Karson E (1987). Expression of human adenosine deaminase in nonhuman primates after retrovirus-mediated gene transfer. J Exp Med 166:219.

32. Magli M-C, Dick JE, Huszar D, Bernstein A, Phillips RA (1987). Modulation of Gene Expression in Multiple hematopoietic cell lineages following retroviral gene transfer. Proc Natl Acad Sci USA 84:789.

33. Stuhlmann H, Cone R, Mulligan RC, Jaenisch R (1984). Introduction of a selectable gene into different animal tissue by a retrovirus recombinant vector. Proc Natl Acad Sci USA 81:7151.

34. Rubenstein JL, Nicolas JF, Jacob F (1984). Construction of a retrovirus capable of transducing and expressing genes in multipotential embryonic cells. Proc Natl Acad Sci USA 81:7137.

35. Stewart CL, Vanek M, Wagner EF (1985). Expression of foreign genes from retroviral vectors in mouse teratocarcinoma chimaeras. EMBO J 4:3701.

36. Jahner D, Haase K, Mulligan R, Jaenisch R (1985). Insertion of the bacterial gpt gene into the germ line of mice by retroviral infection. Proc Natl Acad Sci USA 82:6927.

37. van derPutten H, Botteri FM, Miller AD, Rosenfeld MG, Fan H, Evans RM, Verma IM (1985). Efficient insertion of genes into the mouse germ line via retroviral vectors. Proc Natl Acad Sci USA 82:6148.

38. Wagner EF, Vanek M, Vennstrom B (1985). Transfer of genes into embryonal carcinoma cells by retrovirus infection: efficient expression from an internal

promoter. EMBO J 4:663.

39. Huszar D, Balling R, Kothary R, Magli MC, Hozumi N, Rossant J, Bernstein A (1985). Insertion of a bacterial gene into the mouse germ line using an infectious retrovirus vector. Proc Natl Acad Sci USA 82:8587.

40. Rubenstein JL, Nicolas JF, Jacob F (1986). Introduction of genes into preimplantation mouse embryos by use of a defective recombinant retrovirus. Proc Natl Acad Sci USA 83:366.

41. Soriano P, Cone RD, Mulligan RC, Jaenisch R (1986). Tissue-specific and ectopic expression of genes introduced into transgenic mice by retroviruses. Science 234:1409.

42. Bonnerot C, Rocancourt O, Briand P, Grimber A, Nicolas J-F (1987). A β-galactosidase hybrid protein targeted to nuclei as a marker for developmental studies. Proc Natl Acad Sci USA 84:6795.

43. Belmont JW, Henkel TiggesJ, Chang SM, Wager SmithK, Kellems RE, Dick JE, Magli MC, Phillips RA, Bernstein A, Caskey CT (1986). Expression of human adenosine deaminase in murine haematopoietic progenitor cells following retroviral transfer. Nature 322:385.

44. Belmont JW, Henkel-Tigges J, Wager-Smith K, Chang SM-W, Caskey CT (1987). Transfer and Expression of Human Adenosine Deaminase Gene in Murine Bone Marrow Cells. In Gale RP, Champlin R (eds): "Progress in Bone Marrow Transplantation," New York: Alan R. Liss, p 963

45. Lim B, Williams DA, Orkin SH (1987). Retrovirus-Mediated Gene Transfer of Human Adenosine Deaminase: Expression of Functional Enzyme in Murine Hematopoietic Stem Cells In Vivo. Mol Cell Biol 7:3459.

46. Miller AD, Buttimore C (1986). Redesign of retrovirus packaging cell lines to avoid recombination leading to helper virus production. Mol Cell Biol 6:2895.

47. Mann R, Mulligan RC, Baltimore D (1983). Construction of a retrovirus packaging mutant and its use to produce helper-free defective retrovirus. Cell 33:153.

48. Miller AD, Trauber DR, Buttimore C (1986). Factors involved in the production of helper virus-free retrovirus vectors. Somat Cell Mol Genet 12:175.

49. Bender MA, Palmer TD, Gelinas RE, Miller AD (1987). Evidence that the packaging signal of Moloney murine leukemia virus extends into the gag region. J Virol 61:1639.

50. Armentano D, Yu S.-F., Kantoff PW, Von Runden T, Anderson WF, Gilboa E (1987). Effect of internal viral

sequences on the utility of retroviral vectors. J Virol 61:1647.

51. Yee JK, Moores JC, Jolly DJ, Wolff JA, Respess JG, Friedmann T (1987). Gene expression from transcription- ally disabled retroviral vectors. Proc Natl Acad Sci USA 84:5197.

52. Yu S.-F, von Ruden T, Kantoff PW, Garber C, Seiberg M, Ruther U, Anderson WF, Wagner EF, Gilboa E (1986). Self-inactivating retroviral vectors designed for transfer of whole genes into mammalian cells. Proc Natl Acad Sci USA 83:3194.

53. Kriegler M, Perez CF, Hardy C, Botchan M (1984). Trans- formation mediated by the SV40 T antigens: separation of the overlapping SV40 early genes with a retroviral vector. Cell 38:483.

54. Cepko CL, Roberts BE, Mulligan RC (1984). Construction and applications of a highly transmissible murine retrovirus shuttle vector. Cell 37:1053.

55. Till JE, McCulloch EA (1961). A direct measure of the radiation sensitivity of normal mouse marrow cells. Radiat Res 14:213.

56. Bannerman RM (1983). Hematology. In Foster HL, Small JD, Fox JG (eds): "The Mouse in Biomedical Research:Volume III, New York: Academic Press, p 293.

57. Vacha J (1983). Red cell life span. In Agar NS, Board PG (eds): "Red Blood Cells of Domestic Mammals," New York: Elsevier Science Publishers B.V., p 67.

58. Deschamps J, Meijlink F, Verma I (1985). Identification of a transcriptional enhancer element upstream from the proto oncogen fos. Science 230:1174.

59. Chirgwin JM, Przybyla AE, MacDonald RJ, Rutter, WJ (1979). Isolation of biologically active ribonucleic acid from sources enriched in ribonuclease. J Bio Chem 18:5294.

60. Gibbs RA and Caskey CT (1987). Identification and localization of mutations at the Lesch-Nyhan locus by ribonuclease A cleavage. Science 236:303.

61. Hogan B, Constantini F, Lacy E. In "Manipulating the Mouse Embryo". New York: Coldspring Harbor Laboratory Press.

Molecular Biology of the Eye: Genes, Vision,
and Ocular Disease, pages 23–34
© 1988 Alan R. Liss, Inc.

# SITE-SPECIFIC MUTAGENESIS OF BOVINE RHODOPSIN[1]

Sadashiva S. Karnik, Thomas P. Sakmar,
Roland R. Franke, Barry E. Knox,
Daniel D. Oprian[2], Hai-Bao Chen[3],
and H. Gobind Khorana

Departments of Biology and Chemistry,
Massachusetts Institute of Technology
Cambridge, Massachusetts 02139

ABSTRACT  We have expressed a synthetic gene
for bovine opsin in monkey kidney cells
(COS-1) to the level of 0.3% of cell
protein. After *in vivo* reconstitution with
exogenous 11-*cis*-retinal, the COS-1 cell
rhodopsin was purified by immunoaffinity
adsorption.  Purified COS-1 cell rhodopsin
had a visible absorption spectrum similar to
that of rod outer segment (ROS) rhodopsin.
The COS-1 cell rhodopsin stimulated the
GTPase activity of transducin in a light-
dependent manner with the same specific
activity as ROS rhodopsin. We now report on
structure-function studies of rhodopsin by
site-specific mutagenesis. Three classes of
mutants were prepared as follows:    1).
Cysteine residues in different domains of
rhodopsin  were  replaced  with  serines.
Cysteine  replacements  in  the  carboxyl-

[1]This  work  was  supported  in  part  by  the
National Institutes of Health and the Office of
Naval Research.
[2]Present address:  Graduate Department of Biochemistry, Brandeis University, Waltham, MA  02254.
[3]Present address:  Shanghai Institute of Organic Chemistry, Academia Sinica, Shanghai, China.

terminal region (Cys[316,322,323]), or in the membrane-embedded region (Cys[140,167,222,264]), did not interfere with chromophore regeneration. The intradiscal cysteines (Cys[110,185,187]), however, appeared to be required for generation of a "folded" protein. 2). To investigate rhodopsin-transducin interactions, mutants were prepared in which charged amino acid residues in the loop linking putative transmembrane helices E and F were replaced by neutral residues. The mutants displayed wild-type absorption spectra. Whereas mutants EF1 (Glu[239]--Gln) and EF3 (Glu[247]--Gln, Lys[248]--Leu, Glu[249]--Gln) stimulated transducin GTPase activity in a light-dependent fashion, mutant EF2 (Lys[248]--Leu) failed to activate transducin. 3). To elucidate the role of rhodopsin phosphorylation in visual transduction, five mutants in which carboxyl-terminal domain serine or threonine residues are replaced by alanine were constructed. Characterization of these phosphorylation-site mutants is underway.


## INTRODUCTION

Rhodopsin is the major photoreceptor pigment in the disc membrane. It is an integral membrane protein which appears to consist of seven transmembrane segments. The chromophore is 11-*cis*-retinal attached covalently to a membrane-buried lysine forming a Schiff's base with an absorbance maximum of 500 nm. Absorption of light causes iso-merization of 11-*cis*-retinal to the all-*trans* form which produces a series of transient intermediates. Transducin binds to photoexcited rhodopsin and exchanges bound GDP for GTP. This leads to dissociation of the transducin $\alpha$-subunit (T$\alpha$) from T$\beta\gamma$. T$\alpha$–GTP then activates the cyclic GMP phospho-diesterase. This activation process ultimately leads to the reduction of cation conductance across the plasma membrane of rod cells, which results in the generation of a neuronal signal. The cation channel is regulated by cGMP concentration in the rod cell which is modulated by the phospho-diesterase.

Clearly, phototransduction involves a series of protein-protein interactions resulting from conformational changes in protein structure. The primary event is the light-induced conformational change in rhodopsin which causes a catalytic activation of transducin. To understand the events involved in signal transduction across the biological membrane, we are studying the structure-function relationships of rhodospin in detail. Our approach is to carry out amino acid replacements in rhodopsin and measure the effect on function in a purified reconstituted system. We employ techniques of recombinant DNA to prepare mutant proteins. To facilitate structure-function studies by site-specific mutagenesis we have synthesized a gene for rhodopsin (1). High level expression of this gene in mammalian cells was reported (2). Opsin expressed in mammalian cells was shown to reconstitute with exogenous, 11-*cis* -retinal. A single-step immunoaffinity purification procedure was developed to obtain a homogeneous preparation of rhodopsin in a detergent solubilized form. The visual absorption spectrum and specific activities of transducin activation by this preparation were nearly identical to rhodopsin from rod outer segment.

Using the system described above, we now report on three classes of rhodopsin mutants which were prepared to evaluate: 1). the role of cysteine residues in rhodopsin, 2). the interaction of transducin with the cytoplasmic loop between putative helices E and F, and 3). the role of phosphorylation of rhodopsin.


## RESULTS AND DISCUSSION

Expression of the Rhodopsin Gene.

Expression of rhodopsin in mammalian cells. The synthetic rhodopsin gene was introduced into mammalian expression vectors, p91023(B) or pMT2 (2,3). This placed the gene under the control of the adenovirus major late promoter. The vector was transfected into a monkey kidney derived cell line (COS-1). Detergent solubilized cell extracts prepared 48-72 hours after transfection of COS-1 cells were examined by immunoblotting. As shown in figure 1, only the cells transfected with the vector containing the rhodopsin gene produced immunoreactive material. The major band of opsin produced in COS-1 cells migrated slightly slower than ROS opsin in gel electrophoresis. In separate experiments, we have shown that COS-1 rhodopsin binds concanavalin A, and migrates to the cytoplasmic membrane. The yield of protein expressed in COS-1 cells is estimated to be about 5 ug/$10^7$ cells.

1 2 3 4

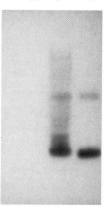

FIGURE 1. Immunoblot analysis of COS-1 cell extract to detect rhodopsin expressed in cells transfected with the synthetic rhodopsin gene. Detergent solubilized extracts from mock transfected cells (lane 1), cells transfected with vector (lane 2), and with vector containing the opsin gene (lane 3) were compared to ROS rhodopsin (lane 4) run on the same gel. Rhodopsin from COS-1 cells has a slower mobility than ROS rhodopsin due to glycosylation differences.

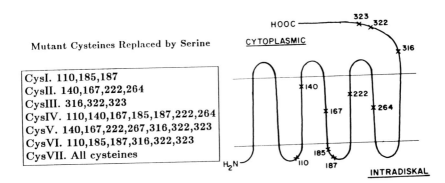

Mutant Cysteines Replaced by Serine

CysI. 110,185,187
CysII. 140,167,222,264
CysIII. 316,322,323
CysIV. 110,140,167,185,187,222,264
CysV. 140,167,222,267,316,322,323
CysVI. 110,185,187,316,322,323
CysVII. All cysteines

FIGURE 5. Disposition of cysteines in bovine rhodopsin and the alteration each mutant contains. In each case, the cysteines located in the intradiscal, membrane-embedded, or cytoplasmic region were replaced with serine.

Mutant CysVII had all ten cysteine residues replaced.
The cysteine mutants showed differences in level of expression, glycosylation, and chromophore regeneration. Upon expression in COS-1 cells, mutants CysII and CysIII were produced at wild-type levels, mutants CysIV and CysVII were produced at low levels, and mutants CysI, CysV, and CysVI were not stably produced. Rhodopsin cysteine mutants which were stably produced showed two glycosylation patterns as follows: 1). mutants CysII and CysIII were normal, and 2). mutants CysIV and CysVII were incompletely glycosylated. Of the mutants stably produced, only mutants CysII and CysIII folded correctly so as to regenerate a normal chromophore with 11-*cis*-retinal. The results obtained showed that replacement of cysteines in the cytoplasmic and membrane-embedded region of rhodopsin did not interfere with its ability to produce native chromophore. Mutants which carry the replacement of intradiscal cysteines did not yield native chromophore and in some cases stable protein was not produced. This indicates a structural role for intradiscal cysteines and might suggest the involvement of a disulphide bond stabilizing

rhodopsin secondary structure. Similar results were obtained by Dixon *et al.* (9) in which substitution of the cysteine on the β-adrenergic receptor corresponding to $Cys^{110}$ of rhodopsin drastically altered agonist binding properties.

TABLE 1

CHARACTERIZATION OF RHODOPSIN CYSTEINE MUTANTS

| Mutant | Mutated Domain | Express. Levels | Glycos- ylation | Chromo- phore |
|--------|----------------|-----------------|-----------------|---------------|
| CysI | Intradiscal ($Cys^{110,185,187}$) | low | n.d.[1] | n.d. |
| CysII | Membrane ($Cys^{140,167,222,264}$) | w.t.[2] | w.t. | w.t. |
| CysIII | Cytoplasmic ($Cys^{316,322,323}$) | w.t. | w.t. | w.t. |
| CysVII | All | low | 3 bands | n.d. |

[1]Not detectable in the present assay.
[2]Wild-type.


Mutants Affecting the Interaction with Transducin.

To probe the structural domains of rhodopsin which interact with transducin, a number of rhodopsin mutants were prepared. Three mutants, EF1, EF2, and EF3 have been characterized in some detail. All three mutants gave rise to absorption spectra similar to wild-type. While EF1 and EF3 were fully active in stimulating transducin, mutant EF2 ($Lys^{248}$--Leu) was defective. The mutation involves the most conserved charged residue in a region shown to be important for interaction with transducin (see Franke *et al.* in this volume for more details). A number of other deletion and point mutants have been generated in the cytoplasmic domain of rhodopsin.

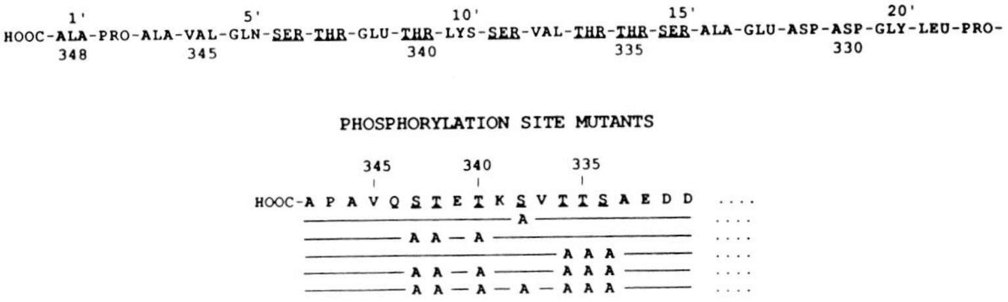
1' 5' 10' 15' 20'
HOOC-ALA-PRO-ALA-VAL-GLN-SER-THR-GLU-THR-LYS-SER-VAL-THR-THR-SER-ALA-GLU-ASP-ASP-GLY-LEU-PRO-
348 345 340 335 330
PHOSPHORYLATION SITE MUTANTS
345 340 335
HOOC-A P A V Q S T E T K S V T T S A E D D ....
A
A A — A
A A A
A A — A A A A
A A — A — A — A A A

FIGURE 6. Site-specific mutants to evaluate the role of serine and threonine phosphorylation.

Mutants Affecting Rhodopsin Phosphorylation.

Rhodopsin has been shown to undergo phosphorylation at multiple sites (up to 9 residues) located close to the carboxyl-terminus (10). We intend to evaluate this process in light adaptation of rhodopsin. A cluster of mutants have been constructed (figure 6) to ask: 1). is phosphorylation at multiple sites required, and 2). is there an order in the residues phosphorylated and can this order be modified? These mutants have been expressed in COS-1 cells and characterization is underway.

ACKNOWLEDGEMENTS

TPS was supported by a National Institutes of Health NRSA (GM11305). RRF was supported by Deutscher Akademischer Austauschdienst. BEK was supported by a National Institutes of Health NRSA (EY05316).

REFERENCES

1. Ferretti L, Karnik SS, Khorana HG, Nassal M, Oprian DD (1986). Proc. Natl. Acad. Sci. USA 83:599.
2. Oprian DD, Molday RS, Kaufman RJ, Khorana HG (1987). Proc. Natl. Acad. Sci. USA 84:8874.

3.  Franke RR, Sakmar TP, Oprian DD, Khorana HG (1988). J. Biol. Chem. 263: 2119.
4.  DeGrip WJ, Damen FJM (1982). Methods Enzym. 82:223.
5.  Al-Saleh S, Gore M, Akhtar M (1987). Biochem. J. 246:131.
6.  Findlay JPC, Pappin DJC (1986). Biochem. J. 238:625.
7.  Applebury ML, Hargrave PA (1986). Vision Res. 26:1881.
8.  Dratz EA, Hargrave PA (1983). Trends Biochem. Sci. 8:128.
9.  Dixon RAF, Sigal IS, Candelore MR, Register RB, Scattergood W, Rands E, Strader CD (1987). Embo J. 6:3269.
10. Wilden U, Kuhn H (1982) Biochemistry 21:3014.

Lolley (34). Inclusion of inhibitors of proteolysis in the extraction buffer minimizes formation of the $M_r$ 52,000 species which we believe to be a proteolysis fragment of the native enzyme.

Rhodopsin kinase has a decided preference for ATP as substrate ($V_{max}/K_m = 5 \times 10^5 \, s^{-1} M^{-1}$) as compared to GTP ($V_{max}/K_m = 10 \, s^{-1} M^{-1}$). Its preference for the adenine ring is absolute; adenosine, AMP and ADP are all excellent inhibitors with $K_I$ values in the micromolar range, whereas no other bases can effectively substitute. Rhodopsin kinase requires most elements of the ribose moiety. Only the 3' OH group can be removed without significant effect on function (32). The ATP-binding requirements seem to be more specific than those for other kinases.

$Mg^{++}$ is invariably important for activity of kinases due to the formation of the substrate $Mg^{++}ATP$ complex. For rhodopsin kinase, however, $Mg^{++}$ appears to exhibit additional effects, activating the enzyme directly. There is an optimal $[Mg^{++}]$ for any particular [ATP], and a narrow range of $[Mg^{++}]$ for which maximum kinase activity is observed. Above this concentration, additional $Mg^{++}$ causes kinase inhibition. This is probably due to formation of a $Mg^{++}_2ATP$ complex which reduces the concentration of the $Mg^{++}ATP$ needed for activity (10).

## What is the Basis of the Substrate Specificity of Rhodopsin Kinase for its Protein Substrate?

Rhodopsin kinase, as mentioned above, is very selective for the nucleotide it will accept as a substrate. It is also highly selective for its protein substrate. It will phosphorylate photoactivated rhodopsin, R*. It will also phosphorylate a homologous receptor protein, the ligand-bound form of the β-adrenergic receptor, but only to a very limited extent (35). It fails to phosphorylate another related receptor protein, the muscarinic acetylcholine receptor (M. Schimerlik, personal communication). How can we explore the molecular basis for this observed substrate specificity?

Many protein kinases not only phosphorylate their substrate as the intact protein, but will phosphorylate a peptide containing the sequence of the protein phosphorylation site. By using synthetic peptides based upon the native sequence of the phosphorylation site, it is possible to determine what characteristics are required in order to be a substrate for phosphorylation. We are using this approach to determine the protein substrate requirements for rhodopsin kinase (10).

Peptides from rhodopsin's two regions which become phosphorylated in the native protein (it's carboxyl-terminal region and it s third cytoplasmic loop region) serve as substrates for rhodopsin kinase. Both peptides 337-348 and 231-252 incorporate $^{32}$P from $[\gamma-^{32}]$P-ATP over a period of hours, but their $K_m$ values are too high for accurate measurement ($> 30$ mM). Increasing the length of the carboxyl-terminal peptide to 25 amino acids improves the $K_m$ value to 8 mM. This, in conjunction with a $V_{max}$ of 5 nmol/min/mg, gives sufficient phosphate incorporation to allow reasonable comparison of the effects of amino acid sequence substitution on the extent of phosphorylation. In preliminary experiments we find that a substitution of serines for threonines in the carboxyl-terminal sequence of bovine rhodopsin makes the peptide a better substrate by improving its $V_{max}$.

Although peptides from the rhodopsin sequence will serve as substrates for the kinase, the $K_m$ values for the peptides are higher by a factor of $\sim 4 \times 10^3$. The $K_m$'s for peptide substrates for other kinases are higher than that for the protein substrate, but generally by a much smaller amount. This suggests to us that there must be more involved in the kinase recognition of rhodopsin as a substrate than just simple recognition at the level of the protein sequence.


How Does Rhodopsin Kinase Recognize Rhodopsin as its Substrate?

Protein phosphorylation is a common method for regulation of cellular metabolic processes. In order to be effective it must operate under control. A kinase must act specifically on a defined substrate under appropriate conditions. It is therefore of interest to learn what factors control the specificity of rhodopsin kinase for rhodopsin.

It seems clear that light has no effect on the activity of the kinase (14,36). The effect of light on the phosphorylation reaction is due to its action on rhodopsin. Rhodopsin kinase is one of only three proteins which binds to freshly light-exposed rhodopsin-containing membranes (25). Presumably this is due to the recognition of a new binding site made available on the surface of photolyzed rhodopsin--a binding site not present on the protein surface prior to exposure of light. Four segments of the rhodopsin polypeptide chain comprise its cytoplasmic surface; three helix-connecting loops and a $\sim 40$-amino acid carboxyl-terminal sequence (37). It is reasonable to suppose that a protein/protein binding site would be comprised of amino acids contributed from more than one portion of the rhodopsin polypeptide chain.

In order to test what types of amino acids might be involved in kinase/rhodopsin recognition we prepared some chemically modified rhodopsins (10). Modification of the two cysteines available on rhodopsin's cytoplasmic surface (with N-ethyl maleimide) had no effect on rhodopsin phosphorylation. The nine cytoplasmic surface lysines could be reductively methylated (which maintains lysine's positive charge) or acetylated (which forms an uncharged side chain) also, without inhibiting the ability of rhodopsin kinase to phosphorylate rhodopsin. We conclude that neither the cysteines nor the lysines make any substantial contribution to recognition of rhodopsin by its kinase.

By another approach we sought to determine which of the four regions of rhodopsin's surface sequence might be involved in kinase recognition. Peptides from each of the regions were added to a kinase assay system, containing rhodopsin and rhodopsin kinase, to see whether any of the peptides inhibited the ability of the kinase to phosphorylate rhodopsin (10). We observed ~80% inhibition of the phosphorylation of rhodopsin in the presence of two peptides; 337-348, which is part of the carboxyl-terminal sequence, and 231-252 which represents the third cytoplasmic loop. Very little inhibition was observed for other peptides tested. Since the peptides were examined under conditions in which they are poor substrates, we tentatively conclude that they were interfering with the phosphorylation of rhodopsin by mimicking the binding sites for rhodopsin kinase on the surface of rhodopsin. Thus these two regions of the rhodopsin sequence are suspected of being binding sites for the kinase as well as containing sites for phosphorylation by the kinase.

## ACKNOWLEDGEMENTS

The authors express their appreciation to Ms. Peggy Franklin for her technical assistance and to Ms. Mabel Wilson for her expert assistance with manuscript preparation.

## REFERENCES

1.  Kühn H, Hargrave PA (1981). Light-induced binding of guanosinetriphosphatase to bovine photoreceptor membranes: Effect of limited proteolysis of the membrane. Biochem 20:2410-2417.
2.  Stryer L (1986). Cyclic GMP cascade of vision. Ann Rev Neurosci 9:87-119.
3.  Fung BK (1987). Transducin: Structure, function and role in phototransduction. In Osborne N, Chader G (eds): "Progress in Retinal Research", Vol. 6, Oxford: Pergamon Press, p 151-177.

4.  Wilden U, Hall SW, Kühn H (1986). Phosphodiesterase activation by photoexcited rhodopsin is quenched when rhodopsin is phosphorylated and binds the intrinsic 48 kDa protein of rod outer segments. Proc Natl Acad Sci USA 83:1174-1178.

5.  Miller JL, Fox DA, Litman BJ (1986). Amplification of phosphodiesterase activation is greatly reduced by rhodopsin phosphorylation. Biochem 25:4983-4988.

6.  Dohlman HG, Caron MG, Lefkowitz RJ (1987). A family of receptors coupled to guanine nucleotide regulatory proteins. Biochem 26:2657-2664.

7.  Kühn H (1974). Light-dependent phosphorylation of rhodopsin in living frogs. Nature 250:588-590.

8.  Kühn H, Bader S (1976). The rate of rhodopsin phosphorylation in isolated retinas of frog and cattle. Biochim Biophys Acta 428:13-18.

9.  Wilden U, Kühn H (1982). Light-dependent phosphorylation of rhodopsin: Number of phosphorylation sites. Biochem 21:3014-3022.

10. Palczewski K, McDowell JH, Hargrave PA (1988). Rhodopsin kinase: Substrate specificity and factors that influence activity. Biochem 27, in press.

11. Shichi H, Somers RL (1978). Light-dependent phosphorylation of rhodopsin. J Biol Chem 253:7040-7046.

12. Yamamoto K, Shichi H (1983). Rhodopsin phosphorylation occurs at Metarhodopsin II level. Biophys Struct Mech 9:259-267.

13. Kühn H, Mommertz O, Hargrave PA (1982). Light-dependent conformational change at rhodopsin's cytoplasmic surface detected by increased susceptibility to proteolysis. Biochim Biophys Acta 679:95-100.

14. McDowell JH, Kühn H (1977). Light-induced phosphorylation of rhodopsin in cattle photoreceptor membranes: Substrate activation and inactivation. Biochem 16:4054-4060.

15. Miller JA, Paulsen R, Bownds MD (1977). Control of light-activated phosphorylation in frog photoreceptor membranes. Biochem 16:2633-2639.

16. Miller JA, Paulsen R (1975). Phosphorylation and dephosphorylation of frog rod outer segment membranes as part of the visual process. J Biol Chem 250:4427-4432.

17. Aton BR, Litman BJ, Jackson ML (1984). Isolation and identification of the phosphorylated species of rhodopsin. Biochem 23:1737-1741.

18. Hargrave PA, Fong SL, McDowell JH, Mas MT, Curtis DR, Wang JK, Juszczak E, Smith DP (1980). The partial primary structure of bovine rhodopsin and its topography in the retinal rod cell disc membrane. Neurochem 1:231-244.

11-*cis* -retinal which was added to the cells *in vivo* . The COS-1 cell rhodopsin was purified by immunoaffinity adsorption. The purified rhodopsin had a visible absorption spectrum indistin-guishable from rhodopsin purified from retinas. The COS-1 cell rhodopsin stimulated the GTPase activity of transducin with the same specific activity as ROS rhodopsin (2).

According to currently accepted models of rhodopsin secondary structure and topography (3), the amino terminal tail is located on the intradiscal surface of the disc membrane, seven

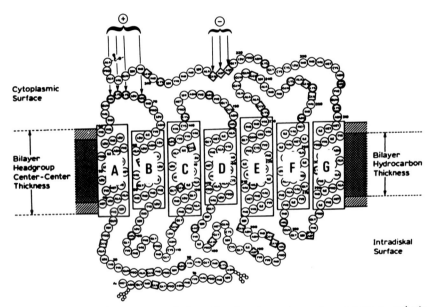

FIGURE 1. A model of rhodopsin structure with respect to the disc membrane according to Dratz and Hargrave (3). The seven putative transmem-brane helical segments are labeled A-G. A series of rhodopsin mutants was prepared to identify domains on the cytoplasmic surface responsible for GTPase activation. Table 1 lists loop EF mutants. Table 2 lists loop AB and carboxyl tail (CT) mutants. As indicated, loop AB has a cluster of positively charged amino acids whereas the carboxyl tail contains three consecutive acidic residues.

helices (A-G) span the membrane bilayer, and the carboxyl terminal tail is on the cytoplasmic surface as shown in figure 1. Three classes of mutant rhodopsin genes are described in which the cytoplasmic domain had been altered: 1). loop EF mutants, 2). loop AB mutants, and 3). cytoplasmic tail (CT) mutants. To date three of the mutants have been characterized as to their ability to activate transducin: mutant EF1, $Glu^{239}$--Gln; mutant EF2, $Lys^{248}$--Leu; and mutant EF3, $Glu^{247}$--Gln, $Lys^{248}$--Leu, and $Glu^{249}$--Gln. Mutants EF1 and EF3 activated transducin similarly to wild-type rhodopsin, whereas mutant EF2 failed to activate transducin (4).

## RESULTS AND DISCUSSION

Expression of a Synthetic Rhodopsin Gene in COS-1 Cells.

Our goal has been to develop a system in which techniques of molecular biology can be applied to structure-function studies of the proteins of the visual cascade. We aim to reconstitute purified proteins containing specific mutations and perform a number of *in vitro* functional assays. Toward this goal, a synthetic gene for bovine rhodopsin was synthesized (1). The gene was expressed in COS-1 cells. After addition of 11-*cis*-retinal *in vivo*, rhodopsin was purified by an immunoaffinity procedure in which detergent solubilized cells were incubated with an anti-rhodopsin monoclonal antibody. Bound protein was then eluted with a synthetic peptide corresponding to the epitope of the antibody. The COS-1 cell rhodopsin was compared to ROS rhodopsin. Electrophoretic mobility of the COS-1 cell rhodopsin was slightly less than that of ROS rhodopsin due to different extents of glycosylation. The visible absorption spectra and specific activities of GTPase activation were nearly identical (2).

Characterization of Rhodopsin Mutants.

Using this system, we have prepared a number of mutants designed to answer the question, what

Molecular Biology of the Eye: Genes, Vision,
and Ocular Disease, pages 53–61
© 1988 Alan R. Liss, Inc.

Transducins in human rod and cone photoreceptors and their
relationships to other G-proteins

Connie Lerea[1], Carol Raport[1], Beverley Dere[1], Ann Bunt-
Milam[2] and James B. Hurley[1].

[1]Department of Biochemistry and the Howard Hughes Medical
Institute and [2]Department of Ophthalmology, University of
Washington, Seattle, WA 98195

ABSTRACT    cDNA clones encoding human rod and cone
photoreceptor transducin α subunits have been
characterized. Antibodies were raised that
specifically bind either to red/green or to blue cone
outer segments. These antibodies were used for double
label immunocytochemistry together with antibodies
that label the human cone transducin α subunit to
demonstrate that all three types of cones express
either the same transducin gene or related genes that
encode nearly identical proteins. In addition, a
possible evolutionary history of transducins and other
G-proteins was determined by estimating the number of
third base substitutions between pairs of cDNA
sequences that encode G-protein subunits.

INTRODUCTION

Light activates a G-protein mediated enzymatic cascade
present in vertebrate rod and cone photoreceptor cells (1).
This cascade stimulates cyclic GMP phosphodiesterase
activity which ultimately hyperpolarizes the cell. G-
proteins that mediate this process are referred to as
transducins.

Both rod and cone photoreceptor cells hyperpolarize
when exposed to light, but the kinetics and sensitivities of
their responses are quite different. Primate rods respond
with slow kinetics and are very sensitive to light. Primate
cones respond more quickly than rods but are much less
sensitive to light (2). The enzymes of the cyclic GMP

cascade in rods and cones are similar but many of them are the products of different genes. For example, two different forms of cyclic GMP phosphodiesterase are expressed differentially in rods and cones and these isozymes have been isolated from bovine retinas and characterized (3). The genes encoding opsins from human rod cells as well as from human red, green and blue cone cells have been cloned and characterized (4). Finally, two different cDNA clones that encode rod and cone specific forms of bovine transducin have been characterized (5). The rod and cone transducins are the products of different genes. Here we describe human rod and cone transducins and present a model for the evolution of transducin and other G-protein genes.

RESULTS AND DISCUSSION

Human rod and cone transducins

There are three types of cones in human retinas and each has a characteristic spectral sensitivity. Three different cone opsin genes are present in the human genome (4) and each is expressed exclusively in either red, green or blue sensitive cones. The experiments reported here were designed to determine whether the three types of cones also express different forms of transducin.

Clones were isolated from a human retina cDNA library (provided by J. Nathans) using bovine rod and cone transducin α subunit cDNAs as probes. The human cDNA's encode human rod transducin α subunit ($T_\alpha r$), which is 98% identical to bovine $T_\alpha r$, and human cone transducin α subunit ($T_\alpha c$) which is 93% identical to bovine $T_\alpha c$. In order to localize these polypeptides in human retinas, rabbit polyclonal antibodies were raised against synthetic peptides having sequences derived from unique regions of the human $T_\alpha r$ and $T_\alpha c$ sequences:

Human $T_\alpha r$ peptide:     LERLVTPGYVPT  (peptide HR1)
Human $T_\alpha c$ peptide:     LERITDPEYLPS  (peptide HC1)

These antibodies were used to localize these proteins in sections of human retina (see ref. 5 for methods). In agreement with previous results using bovine retinas (5), rod transducin localized specifically to human rod photoreceptors whereas cone transducin localized specifically to human cone photoreceptor cells.

In order to determine whether different cone types each express the same or different transducins, it was necessary to develop reagents that identify each type of cone in human retinas. Red and green opsins are sufficiently different from blue opsin that they can be distinguished immunologically using anti-peptide antibodies (4). Rabbit polyclonal antibodies were raised against synthetic peptides with amino acid sequences derived from the carboxy terminus of red and green opsin and from the amino terminus of blue opsin:

Red/green opsin:        LQLFGKKVDDGSELSSAS  (peptide HRGO)

Blue opsin            CMRKMSEEEFYLFKNISSV (peptide HBO)

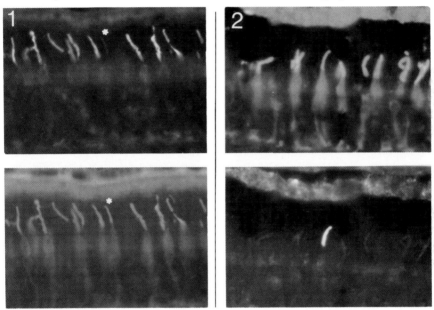

Fig. 1 (left). Top: Human retina section treated with rabbit anti-red/green opsin followed by FITC labelled goat anti-rabbit IgG. Bottom: Rhodamine labelling of guinea pig anti-cone transducin in the same section. Arrow identifies a blue cone. Fig. 2 (right). Top: Human retina section in which transducin is labelled with rhodamine. Bottom: same section in which blue opsin is labelled with fluorescein.

Antibodies raised against these peptides distinguish red and green cones from blue cones when used for immunocytochemical analysis of frozen and LR-white thin sections of human retinas. Human retina sections were treated with guinea pig anti-[human cone transducin $\alpha$ subunit] antibodies and with either rabbit anti-[red and green opsin] or rabbit anti-[blue opsin] antibodies. Cone transducin reactivity was then localized using rhodamine labelled goat anti-[guinea pig IgG] and opsin reactivities were localized using fluorescein labeled goat anti-[rabbit IgG]. The results are shown in Fig. 1 and Fig. 2. Cone transducin $\alpha$ subunits having the amino acid sequence of the HCl peptide are present in both red and green cones and also in blue cones. These results have been further confirmed using antibodies against peptides having sequences derived from the amino terminal portion of the human cone transducin $\alpha$ subunit (results not shown).

## Evolutionary history of G-protein subunits

The rod and cone transducins are just two members of the family of related proteins referred to as G-proteins (6). This family includes transducins, $G_s$'s which activate adenylyl cyclase, $G_o$, which regulates $Ca^{++}$ channels (7), and three different forms of $G_i$. The roles of $G_{i1}$, $G_{i2}$ and $G_{i3}$ are uncertain, but there is evidence that they may inhibit adenylyl cyclase as well as regulate $K^+$ channels and phospholipase C (6). The genes that encode each of these proteins appear to be derived from a common ancestral gene. In order to determine the ancestry of these genes we estimated the number of nucleotide substitutions that have occurred between pairs of G-protein sequences using a method reported by Kimura (8).

An example of this type of analysis is shown in Table 1. Comparisons of the $\alpha$ subunit of $G_{i2}$ (9,10) with the $\alpha$ subunits of human $T_r$ and human $G_{i3}$ (9,10) are shown. At the amino acid level, $G_{i2}$ is 20% more identical to $G_{i3}$ than to $T_r$. Yet, the number of third base substitutions that have occurred between $G_{i2}$ and $G_{i3}$ is about twice the number that occurred between $G_{i2}$ and $T_r$. On the basis of the assumption that nucleotide substitutions occur at a relatively constant rate for most genes, this indicates that $G_{i2}$ diverged from $T_r$ significantly more recently than it diverged from $G_{i3}$. The selective pressures on the $G_{i2}$ and $G_{i3}$ polypeptides

TABLE 1

Example of how third base substitution analysis suggests that $G_{i2}$ is more closely related to $G_{rod}$ than to $G_{i3}$.

| Sequences compared (human) | % amino acid identity | 3rd base substitutions |
|---|---|---|
| $G_{i2}$ vs. $G_{rod}$ | 67% | 0.67 +/- 0.07 |
| $G_{i2}$ vs. $G_{i3}$ | 87% | 1.33 +/- 0.28 |

DNA SEQUENCE ALIGNMENT (human) corresponding to conserved amino acids 34-56

```
Gi2   ...GTG AAG TTG CTG CTG TTG GGT GCT GGG GAG TCA GGG AAG AGC ACC ATC GTC AAG CAG ATG AAG ATC ATC...
              1       3   1   3   3                                                               3

Grod  ...GTG AAG CTG CTG CTT CTG GGT GCC GGT GAG TCC GGG AAG AGC ACC ATC GTC AAG CAG ATG AAG ATT ATC...

(34)  ...  V   K   L   L   L   L   G   A   G   E   S   G   K   S   I   I   V   K   Q   M   K   I   I  ... (56)

Gi2   ...GTG AAG TTG CTG CTG TTG GGT GCT GGG GAG TCA GGG AAG AGC ACC ATC GTC AAG CAG ATG AAG ATC ATC...
              1       3   1 3               3   3   3                       3   3               3   3

Gi3   ...GTG AAG CTG CTG CTA CTC GGT GCT GGA GAA TCT GGT AAA AGC ACC ATT GTG AAA CAG ATG AAA ATC ATT...
```

appear to have been strong enough to maintain 87% amino acid
sequence identity. Such selective pressures may have
included interactions with specific receptors, effectors and
G-protein $\beta$ and $\gamma$ subunits.

Analyses of cDNA sequences of a variety of mammalian
G-protein $\alpha$ subunits and two G-protein $\beta$ subunits are shown
in Fig. 3.

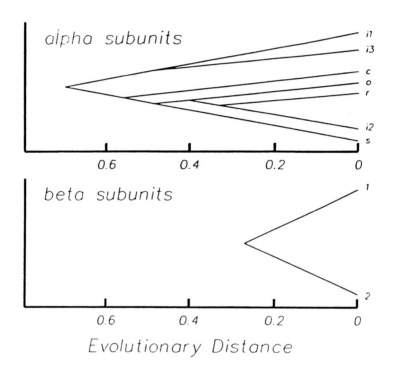

Fig. 3        A likely evolutionary history of G-protein
subunit genes. The abscissa values are numbers of nucleotide
substitutions that are estimated to have occurred between
pairs of sequences (8). i1,i2 and i3 designate the $\alpha$
subunits of $G_{i1}$, $G_{i2}$, and $G_{i3}$ respectively, r and c
designate rod and cone transducin $\alpha$ subunits, and o and s
designate the alpha subunits of $G_o$ and $G_s$.

According to this analysis, the cone transducin $\alpha$ subunit diverged from an ancestor that became $T_r$, $G_o$, $G_{i2}$ and $G_s$. An analysis using two Drosophila G-protein subunit sequences suggests that the cone transducin diverged from this line at about the same time as vertebrates diverged from invertebrates approximately 500 million years ago (15) ($\sim$0.5 in Fig. 3).

Exon/intron structure of G-protein $\alpha$ subunit genes

In the course of studying Drosophila and mouse G-protein genes, we determined the exon/intron structures of the mouse rod transducin $\alpha$ subunit gene (11) and of a Drosophila $G_i$ $\alpha$ subunit gene (12). A comparison of these genes is shown in Fig. 4. Three intron splice sites are located in exactly the same positions in these two genes. The locations of these splice sites within the amino acid sequences of the corresponding $\alpha$ subunits is particularly intriguing. The first intron occurs after the first base in the codon for amino acid 36 in $T_r\alpha$. This is a very highly conserved sequence in G-proteins that binds phosphoryl

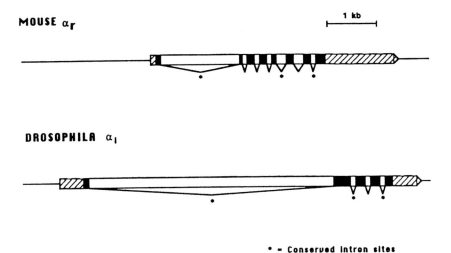

Fig. 4    Exon/intron structure of the mouse rod transducin $\alpha$ subunit gene and of an embryonically expressed Drosophila $G_i$ $\alpha$ subunit gene.

groups within the guanyl nucleotide binding site (13,14).
The second Drosophila intron and the fifth mouse intron also
occur after the second base in the codon for amino acid 193
in $T_r\alpha$. This region also binds a phosphoryl group within the
nucleotide binding site. The last conserved intron (at amino
acid 288) is in a region that has not been implicated in a
specific function.

Why might these splice sites be conserved? One current
model suggests that introns were incorporated into
primordial genes as those genes were pieced together from
preexisting genes (15). Introns were then gradually lost as
the genes evolved into their present day forms. The
mechanisms by which introns are lost during evolution is not
understood. However, if this mechanism were not accurate,
loss of an intron might alter the amino acid sequence
encoded across the original splice site. This could explain
conservation of introns such as the ones described above.
Loss of an intron in the critical phosphoryl binding regions
may not regenerate the original amino acid sequences so that
non-functional proteins would be produced. These types of
introns might therefore be referred to as "trapped" introns.
This hypothesis can be more completely tested as more $\alpha$
subunit gene sequences are determined and as the mechanism
by which introns are lost from genes becomes better
understood.

### ACKNOWLEDGEMENTS

We wish to thank Nicole Provost, Roger Perlmutter and Chan
Beals for stimulating discussions and Feridah Dahlan and
Ingrid Klock for expert technical assistance This work was
supported by the Howard Hughes Medical Institute and grants
EYO 6641 and 1133 from the National Institutes of Health.

### REFERENCES

1.      Hurley, J.B. (1987) Molecular Properties of the cGMP
        cascade of Vision. Ann. Rev. Physiol. 49:793.

2.      Baylor, D.A. (1987) Photoreceptor signals and vision.
        Inv. Opthal. and Vis. Sci. 28:34.

3.      Gillespie, P.G. and Beavo, J.A. (1988)

Characterization of a bovine cone photoreceptor phosphodiesterase purified by cyclic GMP sepharose chromatography J. Biol. Chem. in press

4. Nathans, J., Thomas, D. and Hogness, D.S. (1986) Molecular genetics of human color vision: the genes encoding blue, green and red pigments. Science 232:193

5. Lerea, C.L., Somers, D.E., Hurley, J.B., Klock, I.B. and Bunt-Milam, A.H. (1986) Identification of specific transducin $\alpha$ subunits in retinal rod and cone photoreceptors. Science 234:77

6. Gilman, A.G. (1987) G proteins: transducers of receptor-generated signals. Ann. Rev. Biochem. 56:615

7. Heschler, J., Rosenthal, W., Trautwein, W. and Schultz, G. (1987) The GTP-binding protein, $G_o$, regulates neuronal calcium channels. Nature 325:445

8. Kimura, M. (1981) Estimation of evolutionary distances between homologous nucleotide sequences. Proc. Natl. Acad. Sci. USA 78:454.

9. Jones, D.T. and Reed, R.R. (1987) Molecular cloning of five GTP binding protein cDNA species from rat olfactory neuroepithelium. J. Biol. Chem. 262:14241.

10. Beals, C.R., Wilson, C.B. and Perlmutter, R.M. A small multigene family encodes $G_i$ signal transduction proteins. Proc. Natl. Acad Sci. USA 84 in press.

11. C. Raport and B. Dere, unpublished results.

12. N. Provost, personal communication.

13. Jurnak, F. (1985) Structure of the GDP domain of EF-Tu and location of the amino acids homologous to *ras* oncogene proteins. Science 230:32.

14. Masters, S.B. Stroud, R.M., Bourne, H.R. (1986) Protein Eng. 1:47.

15. Gilbert, W., Marchionni, M. and Mcknight, G. (1986) On the antiquity of introns. Cell 46:151.

12. Burns DL, Moss J, Vaughan M (1982). Choleragen-stimulated release of guanyl nucleotides from turkey erythrocyte membranes. J Biol Chem 257:32.
13. Kahn RA, Gilman AG (1984). ADP-ribosylation of $G_s$ promotes the dissociation of its α and β subunits. J Biol Chem 259:6235.
14. Pinkett MO, Anderson WB (1982). Plasma membrane-associated component(s) that confer(s) cholera toxin sensitivity to adenylate cyclase. Biochim Biophys Acta 714:337.
15. Le Vine H III, Cuatrecasas P (1981). Activation of pigeon erythrocyte adenylate cyclase by cholera toxin. Partial purification of an essential macromolecular factor from horse erythrocyte cytosol. Biochim Biophys Acta 672:248.
16. Gill DM, Meren R (1983). A second guanyl nucleotide-binding site associated with adenylate cyclase. Distinct nucleotides activate adenylate cyclase and permit ADP-ribosylation by cholera toxin. J Biol Chem 258:11908.
17. Kahn RA, Gilman AG (1984). Purification of a protein cofactor required for ADP-ribosylation of the stimulatory regulatory component of adenylate cyclase by cholera toxin. J Biol Chem 259:6228.
18. Kahn RA, Gilman AG (1986). The protein cofactor necessary for ADP-ribosylation of $G_s$ by cholera toxin is itself a GTP binding protein. J Biol Chem 261:7906.
19. Tsai S-C, Noda M, Adamik R, Moss J, Vaughan M (1987) Enhancement of choleragen ADP-ribosyltransferase activities by guanyl nucleotides and a 19 kDa membrane protein. Proc Natl Acad Sci USA 84:5139.
20. Tsai S-C, Noda M, Adamik R, Chang PP, Chen H-C, Moss J, Vaughan M (1988). Stimulation of choleragen enzymatic activity by GTP and two soluble proteins purified from bovine brain. J Biol Chem, in press.
21. Noda M, Tsai S-C, Adamik R, Moss J, Vaughan M (1988). Effects of detergents on activation of cholera toxin by 19 kDa membrane and soluble brain proteins (ADP-ribosylation factors). Fed Proc, in press.

Molecular Biology of the Eye: Genes, Vision,
and Ocular Disease, pages 73–82
© 1988 Alan R. Liss, Inc.

# STRUCTURAL AND FUNCTIONAL ELUCIDATION OF S-ANTIGEN

T. Shinohara, K. Yamaki, M. Tsuda,
L. A. Donoso[1] and B. Amaladoss

Laboratory of Immunology, National Eye Institute,
NIH, Bethesda, MD 20892
[1]Wills Eye Hospital, Philadelphia, PA 19107

## ABSTRACT

Complete amino acid sequences of retinal S-antigen from human, bovine and mouse have been determined. S-antigen do not have over all sequence homology with any other known protein, but regional homology was found between S-antigen and $\alpha$ subunit of Transducin including putative phosphoryl binding sites and putative rhodopsin binding sites.

These results are consistent with the previous observation that S-antigen is bound to phosphorylated rhodopsin and quenches the amplified phototransduction cascade.

## INTRODUCTION

The eye has a remarkable property that it can function efficiently over a very wide range of illuminations from single photon to bright sun. This process is called light adaptation. The light adaptation is controlled in part by the pupillary aperature, but mostly by the participation of different types of cells. The rod cells which have photosensitive rhodopsin are more sensitive to dim light and dark-adapts to increase their sensitivity. However, the rod cells cease their phototransduction in bright light, the cone cells are in contrast operative in bright light. This phototransduction mechanism has been studied for over 100 years.

Photopigments, rhodopsin (1,2), color pigments (3), transducin (4), 3'5' cyclic guanosine monophosphate phosphodiesterase (PDE) (4), rhodopsin kinase (4) and S-antigen (S-Ag) (48kd- protein) (4-6) have been identified as important photoreceptor cell proteins which participate in this process. Although significant recent advances in our understanding of this process include the structure of photopigments (2,3), transducin (7), and G proteins (8) and the role of the cGMP in the transduction of light to photocurrent (9), its mechanism is still far from our understanding.

Previously, S-Ag has been found to reversibly bind to photo-activated and phosphorylated rhodopsin (R*-P) and quench the activation of PDE (10). An alternative hypothesis suggests that S-Ag in the presence of ATP directly inhibits the PDE to achieve rapid turnoff of the cascade (11). In either case it is obvious that S-Ag plays a regulatory role in the phototransduction cascade of the rod cells.

S-Ag is also present in mammalian pineal gland in which it has no or minute amounts of rhodopsin (12). It is possible to speculate that S-Ag has a rhodopsin independent regulatory function. Moreover, the phototransduction cascade has striking similarities to the adenyl cyclase system for the hormone-receptor complex (13). It is possible that the adenyl cyclase system also has a protein analogous to S-Ag, playing a similar role in negative regulation.

In this article, we present the structures of S-Ag, its mRNA and gene, and further discuss a functional role of this protein in the rod cells phototransduction cascade.

## 1. GENE AND mRNA STRUCTURE

Both the human and mouse (BALB/c) S-Ag genes have been isolated. The mouse gene contains multiple large introns, the largest being approximately 15 kb in length. The smallest exon examined to date is 11 nucleotides long and codes for three amino acids. Using a S-Ag cDNA probe we identified similar mRNAs (1700 ± 200 nucleotides) in retinal and pineal tissue indicating that S-Ag from these two organs is similar.

Immunol 61:357.

19. Gregerson DS and Putterman GJ (1984). Preparation, isolation and immunochemical studies of the cyanogen bromide peptides from a retinal photoreceptor cell autoantigen, S-antigen. J Immunol 133:843.

20. Kalsow CM and Wacker WB (1977). Pineal reactivity of anti-retina sera. Invest Ophthalmol Vis Sci 16:181.

21. van Veen T, Elofsson R, Hartwig H-G, Gery I, Mochizuki M, Ceña V and Klein DC (1986). Retinal S-antigen: Immunocytochemical and immunochemical studies on distribution in animal photoreceptors and pineal organs. Exp Biol 45:15.

22. Korf HW, Moller M, Gery I, Zigler JS land Klein DC (1985). Immunocytochemical demonstration of retinal S-antigen in the pineal organ of four mammalian species. Cell Tissue Res 239:81.

23. Mirshahi M, Faure JP, Brisson P, Falcon J, Guerlotte J and Collin JP (1984). S-antigen immunoreactivity in retinal rods and cones and pineal photosensitive cells. Biol Cell 52:195.

24. Dever TE, Glynias MJ, Merrick (1987). GTP-binding domain: Three consensus sequence elements with distinct spacing. Proc Natl Acad Sci USA 84:1814.

25. Feig LA, Pan BT, Roberts TM and Cooper GM (1986). Isolation of ras GTP-binding mutants using an in situ colony-binding assay. Proc Natl Acad Sci USA 83:4607.

26. Clanton DJ, Hattori S, Shih TY (1986). Mutations of the ras gene product p21 that abolish guanine nucleotide binding. Proc Natl Acad Sci USA 83:5076.

27. Van Dop C, Yamanaka G, Steinberg F, Sekura RD, Manclark CR, Stryer L and Bourne HR (1984). ADP- ribosylation of transducin by pertussis toxin blocks the light-stimulated hydrolysis of GTP and cGMP in retinal photoreceptors. J Biol Chem 259:23.

28. Kühn H (1978). Light-regulated binding of rhodopsin kinase and other proteins to cattle photoreceptor membranes. Biochemistry 17:4389.

29. Takemoto DJ, Takemoto LJ, Hansen J and Morrison D (1985). Regulation of retinal transducin by C-terminal peptides of rhodopsin. Biochem J 232:669.

30. Kühn H and Hargrave PA (1981). Light-induced binding of

guanosine triphosphate to bovine photoreceptor membranes: effect of limited proteolysis of the membranes. Biochemistry 20:2410.

31. Wilden U and Kühn H (1982). Light-dependent phosphorylation of rhodopsin: Number of phsophorylation sites. Biochemistry 21:3014.

32. Rodrigues M, Hackett J, Gaskins R, Wiggert B, Lee L, Redmond T and Chader G (1986). Interphotoreceptor retinoid-binding protein in retinal rod cells and pineal gland. Invest Ophthalmol Vis Sci 27:844.

33. Somers RL and Klein DC (1984). Rhodopsin kinase activity in the mammalian pineal gland and other tissues. Science 226:182.

34. Korf HW, Oksche A, Ekstrom P, Gery I, Zigler S, Jr. and Klein DC (1986). Pinealocyte projection into the mammalian brain revealed with S-antigen antiserum. Science 231:735.

35. Craft CM, Morgan WW, Jones DJ and Reiter RJ (1985). Hamster and rat pineal gland β-adrenoceptor characterization with iodocyanopindolol and the effect of decreased catecholamine synthesis on the receptor. J Pineal Res 2:51.

36. Dixon RAF, Kobilka BK, Strader DJ, Benovic JL, Dohlman HE, Frielle T, Bolanowski MA, Bennett CD, Rands E, Diehl RE, Mumford RA, Slater EE, Sigal IS, Caron MG, Lefkowitz RJ and Strader CD (1986). Cloning of the gene and cDNA for mammalion β-adrenergic receptor and homology with rhodopsin. Nature 321:75.

37. Benovic JL, Strasser RH, Caron MG and Lefkowitz RJ (1986). β-adrenergic receptor kinase: Identification of a novel protein kinase that phosphorylates the agonist-occupied form of the receptor. Proc Natl Acad Sci USA 83:2797.

38. Benovic JL, Kühn H, Weyand I, Codina J, Caron MG and Lefkowitz RJ (1987). Functional desensitization of the isolated β-adrenergic receptor kinase: Potential role of an analog of the retinal protein arrestin (48-kDa protein). Proc Natl Acad Sci USA 84:8879.

**Molecular Biology of the Eye: Genes, Vision, and Ocular Disease, pages 83–92**
© **1988 Alan R. Liss, Inc.**

# MOLECULAR INTERACTION OF FIBROBLAST GROWTH FACTOR, LIGHT-ACTIVATED RHODOPSIN, AND S-ANTIGEN[1]

Jean Plouet[2]

U 86 INSERM - Centre Biomedical des Cordeliers-
75006 - PARIS

## ABSTRACT

Molecular weight of the component of rod outer segment [ROS] to which fibroblast growth factor [FGF] binds upon illumination was determined by covalent cross-linking and by gel filtration high-pressure liquid chromatography. Both techniques have shown that the molecular weight [$M_r$] of 35-40 kDa is consistent with that of photolysed rhodopsin. Acidic and basic fibroblast growth factor [aFGF, bFGF] can bind with an apparent dissociation constant of $1.6 \times 10^{-9}$ M and $6 \times 10^{-9}$ M, respectively. The maximal binding of aFGF was in agreement with the level of biological activity found in isolated ROS. Both FGF forms interact with the same membrane binding site. S-antigen [SAg] strongly inhibits the binding of FGF to rhodopsin, but has only a minimal effect on FGF's binding to cell surface receptors.

## INTRODUCTION

Retina, like virtually all neuronal tissues, is known to be a source of mitogens for a wide variety of cells. This growth promoting activator, also

[1]This work was supported by a Grant from Association de la Recherche sur le Cancer.
[2]Present address: Cancer Research Institute, M-1282, University of California Medical Center, San Francisco, CA 94143

known as eye-derived growth factor [EDGF] [1], was purified and shown to be identical to acidic and basic growth factors [aFGF, bFGF] [2,3]. The retina rod outer segment [ROS] displayed a higher specific activity than all other parts [4]. This bioactivity is mainly due to aFGF. Since FGF binds to purified ROS membranes in a light-dependent fashion [5], identification of its binding entity was made. Moreover, as the binding of endogenous FGF is modulated by GTP and ATP the possible interference of transducin [6] and the 48 kDa protein [7], which is also known as S-antigen [SAg] or arrestin] [8] were assessed.

## MATERIALS AND METHODS

### 1. Protein and membrane purification procedures.

Acidic and basic FGF were purified [as in Ref.8]. Transducin and SAg were prepared as in References 6 and 10, respectively, and further purified by HPLC on a $TSK^{125}$ column preequilibrated in hepes 10 mM buffer containing 2 mM $MgCl_2$ and 150 mM NaCl, and checked for the absence of mitogenicity. ROS were prepared from dark adapted bovine retinas by centrifugation on a continuous sucrose gradient. ROS membranes were further purified as previously described [5]. Bovine hamster kidney cells were grown and membranes were prepared as described[11].

### 2. Cross-linking Experiments

Iodinated acidic FGF and 50 ug of ROS membranes were mixed under dim red light in 0.2 ml of hepes/gelatin buffer  Binding was achieved under agitation , either in dim red light or in the light [700 lux] within 10 minutes. Samples were centrifuged at $4^{o}C$, the pellet washed with 1 ml of cold buffer and cross-linking was performed with 0.2 mM disuccinidyl suberate as described [11]. Samples were  analyzed on a straight 10% polyacrylamide $NaDodSO_4$ slab gel After electrophoresis, gels were stained, dried and processed for autoradiography.

### 3.  Gel Filtration on high-pressure liquid chromatography.

ROS membranes were dissolved in the dark in a 10 mM hepes buffer, pH 7.4, containing 2 mM $MgCl_2$, 150 mM NaCl and 0.5% octylglucoside at $37^{o}C$ for 1 hour, and then ultracentrifuged for 1 hour at 100,000g. 2 ng of iodinated acidic FGF mixed with 50 ug of membrane proteins in the hepes buffer containing 0.1% octylglucoside in the absence or presence of a 100 molar excess of unlabelled aFGF, and was illuminated as above. The sample was further analyzed by high-pressure liquid chromatography on a TSK[125] column at a flow rate of 0.5 ml/minute. The effluent was collected every minute, and [125]I counted.

4. Binding of acidic [125]I-FGF to ROS membranes.

5 ug of ROS membranes were mixed in the dark with desired concentrations of acidic or basic [125]I-FGF. The reaction was initiated by illumination and occurred during a 10 minute period. Non-specific binding was determined in the presence of 1 ug of unlabelled acidic or basic FGF, without illumination. Radioreceptor assays were performed as described [12], using 15 ug of either BHK or ROS membranes and 0.5 ng of [125]I-aFGF.

RESULTS

FGF binds to a 35-40 kDa component.

As shown in Figure 1, the membrane binding sites for FGF in ROS membranes were characterized by affinity cross-linking techniques. In these experiments, [125]I-FGF specifically bound to membranes was covalently linked to its binding sites by using the homobifunctional cross-linker, disuccinimidyl-suberate. The first set of experiments [Fig.1A] shows that decreasing concentrations of [125]I-labelled aFGF are cross-linked to a species of molecular weight ranging from 50 to 55 kDa. Due to the molecular weight of FGF [15 kDa], the binding site would have a $M_r$ of about 37 kDa. This is consistent with the molecular weight of rhodopsin, which usually migrates in SDS PAGE electrophoresis as a smear. That might explain the poor resolution of the complex seen on the autoradiograms. The band seen at 30 kDa likely represents the dimer of FGF. The cross-linking of [125]I-FGF to macromolecular species was inhibited as a function of the concentrations of unlabelled aFGF [Figure 1B, lanes 1-4], or bFGF [lanes 5-6]. No cross-linking was seen if experiments were conducted in the dark [lanes 7-12], indicating that only photolysed ROS membranes display a binding site for FGF. Similar results were obtained if labelled bFGF was used instead of labelled aFGF.

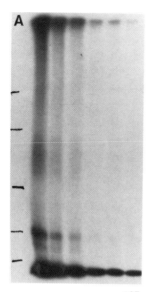

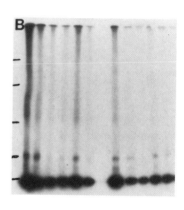

FIGURE 1. Cross-linking of $^{125}$I-aFGF to ROS membrane.
A- Decreasing concentrations of $^{125}$I-aFGF [Lane 1   20ng/ml; Lane 2   10 ng/ml; Lane 3   5 ng/ml;  Lane 4   2.5 ng/ml; Lane 5   1.25 ng/ml; Lane 6   0.62 ng/ml].

B - Competition of 10 ng/ml $^{125}$I-aFGF with unlabelled aFGF [ Lanes 1 and 7 0 ng/ml; Lanes 2 and 8  10 ng/ml;  Lanes 3 and 9   100ng/ml; and Lanes 4 and 10 1000 ng/ml]; or bFGF [Lanes 5 and 11   50 ng/ml;  Lanes 6 and 12   1000 ng/ml]. [Lanes 1-6   after illumination; Lanes 7-12   in the dark.]  Bars represent molecular weight markers: 92 kDa, 66 kDa, 43 kDa, 30 kDa, 20 kDa, 14.4 kDa.

The molecular weight of the complex formed between FGF and its binding site was assessed directly without any cross-linking by HPLC. As shown in Figure 2, there are three peaks of radioactivity at molecular weights 55 kDa, 15 kDa, and 1 kDa. These last two peaks correspond to free-FGF and iodide, respectively. When an excess of acidic FGF was present, the first peak decreased [maximum 8,000 cpm versus 15,000 cpm], and the peak of free-FGF increased, indicating that FGF binding is specific and involves a molecular species with $M_r$ 40 kDa. Approximately 30% of the total cpm was recovered in  fractions 24-26, which correspond to the rhodopsin-FGF complex, but no significant radioactivity was recovered in the 140-160 kDa fractions corresponding to FGF-receptor complexes as seen in numerous cells [reviewed in 13].

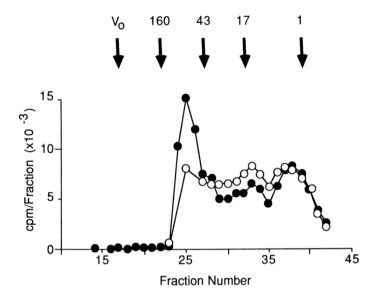

FIGURE 2. Gel filtration high-pressure liquid chromatography of solubilized $^{125}I$-aFGF/ROS membrane complex incubated with [m m] or without [1 1] an excess of unlabelled aFGF.

aFGF and bFGF bind to the same ROS membrane component.

The binding of both aFGF and bFGF was analyzed as a function of concentration. Apparent saturation occurs at 12 ng/ml and 18 ng/ml for aFGF and bFGF, respectively. Non-specific binding was rather high [40%], in contrast to that obtained with BHK membranes at 18-20% [12]. Scatchard analysis of the binding process is shown in an insert to Figure 3. The Scatchard plot indicates that a single class of binding sites is most likely over the concentration range of aFGF and bFGF studied, and the apparent dissociation constants are $1.6 \times 10^{-9}M$ and $6 \times 10^{-9}M$. However, a discrete sigmoidicity was observed with aFGF. Approximately 180 ng and 55 ng could be bound per mg of membranes.

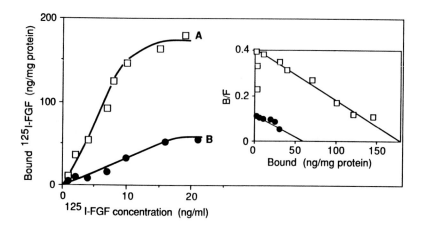

FIGURE 3.   Binding of aFGF [ ❑ ❑ ] or bFGF [ ● ● ] to ROS membranes.
Insert: Scatchard plot.

        To test whether basic FGF can compete with acidic FGF for rhodopsin
binding as they compete for their common receptors on numerous cells [12], the
ability of increasing concentrations of native aFGF and bFGF to displace [125]I-
aFGF bound to membranes was analyzed.  As shown in Figure 4, the concentration
of native aFGF and bFGF required to displace  50% of the total [125]I-aFGF bound
to membranes were 20 and 150 ng/ml.  These concentrations are higher than
those required to displace 50% of  [125]I-aFGF from BHK membranes,
respectively 8 and 1.5 ng/ml, due to the higher non-specific binding rate in ROS
membranes.

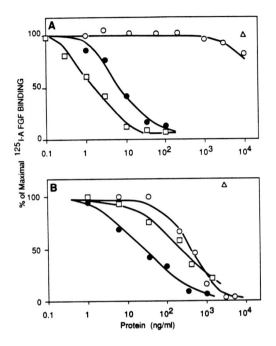

FIGURE 4. Radioreceptor assay for [125]I-aFGF on BHK-21 membranes, A and ROS membranes, B. [ ☐ ☐ ]aFGF; [ ● ● ]bFGF; [ ○ ○ ]SAg.

SAg competition of [125]I-aFGF binding to ROS membranes.

    Since the binding of endogenous FGF to ROS membranes was shown to be light-dependent and modulated by GTP and ATP, the influence of other light-induced bound proteins, such as S Ag and transducin was explored. SAg displaced the binding or [125]I-aFGF from ROS membranes [providing a 50% displacement at a concentration of 400 ng/ml, or 20 times higher than purified aFGF]. Due to their respective molecular weights, 3 molecules of SAg would compete with one molecule of aFGF. In contrast, transducin slightly enhanced the binding of aFGF [at a 10-20% level]. Conversely, transducin does not compete with aFGF toward FGF receptors of BHK membranes, and SAg only weakly [2000 times the level of aFGF].

## DISCUSSION

The process of FGF binding to ROS membranes raises the question of the identification of the component to which it binds. The more likely FGF binding site in these membranes, which are formed by invagination of plasmic membranes, was the FGF receptor [asdescribed for other cells as two entities of 125 kDa and 145 kDa]. However, since the FGF binding process is light-dependent, photolysed rhodopsin was also considered a possible binding site. In order to establish the receptor species, a technique was developed to cross-link membrane-bound [125]I-labelled ligands to membrane components. This technique has been used to characterize specific receptors for many growth factors, and most recently, for similar identification of receptors for insulin-like growth factor I on ROS membranes [14]. These results show that the species has a molecular weight consistent with rhodopsin's, and is seen only upon illumination. Gel filtration was also used to analyze the molecular weight of the complex, and produced similar results. In both cases, no binding was seen in the 140-160 kDa range, suggesting the absence of FGF receptors.

It is not possible, however, to rule out the presence of FGF receptors in ROS membranes, since attempts to visualize cross-linking of labelled FGF to purified BHK cell membranes were inconclusive [data not shown]. Moreover, the maximal apparent binding capacity of these membranes is roughly 20 times lower than that of ROS membranes. At such low levels of activity, the presence of FGF receptor complexes could be difficult to detect. The data on saturation [180 ng of aFGF/mg protein] is in agreement with that obtained by direct assessment of bioactivity of FGF content in ROS [300 u/mg of protein]. In addition, bFGF's binding capacity is lower than aFGF's, paralleling the relative abundance of aFGF to bFGF as demonstrated by specific radio-immunoassays yielding 4 molecules of aFGF for 1 molecule of bFGF. The sigmoidicity observed in Scatchard plot for [125]I-aFGF binding might represent positive cooperative interactions with oligomeric rhodopsin, as it was shown for transducin [15]. This hypothesis remains to be determined by the use of purified rhodopsin reconstituted into vesicles.

The radioreceptor assay confirms that both aFGF and bFGF interact in ROS binding as they do toward cell membrane receptors. More striking was the strong inhibition of binding to ROS membranes triggered by SAg. SAg also interferes with aFGF and bFGF, competing not only in the cell receptor binding process, but also acting as an inhibitor of their mitogenic activity [data not shown]. This competition might be due to conformational homologies between either the FGF receptor and rhodopsin or FGF and SAg. At present, nothing is known about FGF receptor structure, but it seems unlikely that it could be involved in ATP modulation of FGF binding [5], since it is not phosphorylated [11,16]. Conversely, a sequence homology exists between amino acids 118-129 of SAg and 27-37 of aFGF. The binding of SAg to phosphorylated rhodopsin triggers the quenching of cyclic GMP-dependent phosphodiesterase. It was this triggering process that indicated further examination of this molecular

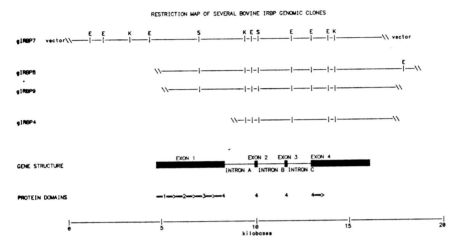

FIGURE 1. Restriction map of several bovine IRBP genomic clones, IRBP gene structure, and IRBP protein domains.

We determined the complete sequence of λgIRBP7 and parts of the other gene clones. All sequences from the other bovine gene clones are identical to that of λgIRBP7. We determined the protein sequence of several tryptic and cyanogen bromide fragments and the N-terminal end of the purified IRBP protein. We have localized all 30 of these fragments in the predicted protein sequence of the gene. The deduced protein sequence contains a putative signal sequence and a short 5 amino acid sequence positioned between the signal sequence and the authentic N-terminus of the secreted extracellular IRBP (Fig. 2). Among the many possibilities, the sequence may represent a pro-polypeptide extension or may represent a part of the signal sequence. This extra 5 amino acid sequence is found attached to monkey and human IRBP after secretion in 40-50% of the protein, but has not been identified in secreted bovine IRBP (19). The existence of the 5 extra amino acids raises questions about the processing of the primary translation product, and about the possible functions of this short extension.

```
Monkey  "N"                              FQPSLVLDMAKVLLDNY...
Monkey  "N+5"                     GPTHLFQPSLVLDMAKVLLDNY...

Human   "N"                              FQPSLVLDMAKVLLDNY...
Human   "N+5"                     GPTHLFQPSLVLDMAKVLLD

Bovine                                   FQPSLVLEMAQVLLDNY...
Bovine Gene     MVRKWALLLPMLLCGLTGPAHLFQPSLVLEMAQVLLDNY...
                ++ooooooooo  o  oo !

                  ^signal peptide  ^pro^
                   (putative)       peptide?
```

FIGURE 2. Amino-Terminal Sequences of IRBP. Monkey, human and bovine protein sequences are compared showing the conserved nature of the N-terminal sequences. The putative signal peptide obtained from the bovine gene sequence is shown. The signal sequence displays many of the characteristics common to signal sequences including basic amino acids near the beginning (+) and hydrophobic sequences in the middle (o). The leucine (!) is rare as the last residue of a signal sequence (see 18).

There is a four-fold repeat structure to the protein sequence with about 30-35% sequence identity between any two of the four protein domains (Fig. 3). There are many conservative substitutions as well. Each domain is about 300 amino acids long. The first two domains are slightly more similar to each other and the third and fourth are slightly more similar than to the other domains.

We have identified 5 sequences that match the N-linked carbohydrate attachment site consensus sequence NX(T/S). Three of the CHO attachment sites are located in equivalant positions (shifted by not more than 1 amino acid residue) within their respective domains. There appear to be about 15 potential phosphorylation sites (RXY(Z)(S/T)). The gene contains three introns resulting in exons of 3135, 190, 144, and 2300 bp. The fourth exon contains mostly 3' untranslated sequence. All three introns (2233, 1961 and 1500 bp in length) fall in the fourth protein domain. This pattern raises questions about the evolution of the four major protein domains and the evolution of the IRBP gene structure.

Near the 3' end of the IRBP mRNA is a sequence of (AC) repeated 14 times. Similar sequences of alternating purines and pyrimidines are involved in enhancement of selected viral promoters, and may convert to a Z-DNA conformation (20).

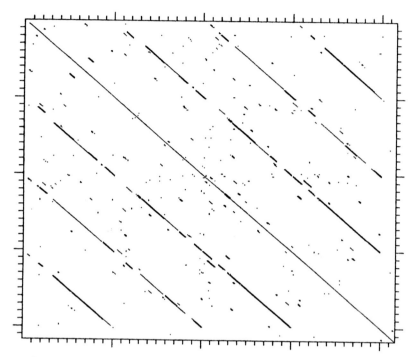

FIGURE 3. Dot matrix comparison of the bovine IRBP protein sequence to itself. Evidence for a four-fold repeat is indicated by four diagonal lines along any column. The mutation data matrix allowed for conservative and semiconservative substitutions to be accepted.

We have obtained a human genomic clone for IRBP in order to begin the characterization of its structural features. We screened a human chromosome 10 library (chosen on the basis of the localization of the IRBP gene which is described later), and we obtained several independent isolates. However, they all contained only one 2.0 kb insert. One of these clones, λgIRBP16, was characterized further by DNA sequence analysis. Part of the sequence is shown in Fig. 4.

```
BOVINE cDNA (mRNA)                    ....TGTCGACATGAG
BOVINE GENE    ....TTCTGCCCCTTAGTGGGCAACTTTTCCCTTCCTTCAG  GTTCAACATCGGTGGCCCCACCTCCTCCATCTCTGCCCTGTGCTCC
               :: ::::::: :   :::            :::::  :::::::::  :::::::::::::::::::::::  :::::::  : : :  : :::::::::
HUMAN GENE     ....CTCAGCCCCTGAACAGGCTCTGCTTCCCATCCTTCAG  GTTCAACATCGGTGGCCCCACATCCTCCATTCCCATCTTGTGCTCC
                 || ||   ||||            |||||| |||| ||| |
                 CTGAC    CTGAC          YYYYYYYYYYYNYAG  G   CONSENSUS SPLICE ACCEPTOR SITE

          LARIAT SPLICE SIGNALS?                     INTRON | EXON


                                                                                    BOVINE cDNA
TACTTTTTCGACGAAGCCCCACCTATTCTGCTGGACAAAATCTACAACCGGCCCAACAACTCTGTCAGTGAGCTCTGGACCC...   BOVINE GENE
::::::  :: ::  ::::::::: :: :::::::::::::: :::::::  ::::::  : ::::::::::::::: ::::: :: :
TACTTCTTTGATGAAGGCCCTCCAGTTCTGCTGGACAAGATCTACAGCCGGCCTGATGACTCTGTCAGTGAACTCTGCACAC...   HUMAN GENE
```

FIGURE 4. Partial sequence analysis of the human IRBP genomic clone, λgIRBP16. Alignment with bovine IRBP mRNA sequence and gene sequence, showing the consensus splice acceptor site in the bovine and human genes and possible lariat signal sequences.

The human IRBP gene sequence is very similar to the bovine cDNA and gene sequences. The similarity includes a match of 106 out of 128 nucleotides between the human gene and bovine cDNA sequences. Part of the human gene sequence is identical to the human cDNA sequence of Liou et al. (21). The sequences are identical for 128 nucleotides, and then diverge at a splice acceptor site (22) found only in the gene sequence. Two possible lariat signal sequences (23) are just upstream from the putative splice site. This suggests that the boundary of an intron and exon had been crossed and indicates that the human IRBP gene, like the bovine gene, has at least one intron in it. This splice acceptor site shown in Fig. 4 is located in an identical position in the bovine gene. At the other end of the 2.0 kb Hind III fragment, there is sequence similarity to the bovine second intron, and the sequences are about 55% identical (data not shown). Thus, this gene fragment, 2.0 kb in size, contains parts of one exon and one intron of the human IRBP gene.

The human exonic sequence has been translated into protein and is compared to the corresponding bovine protein in Fig. 5.

```
                            CHO
                             |
RFNIGGPTSSISALCSYFFDEGPPILLDKIYNRPNDSVSELWTLS..     BOVINE
::::::::::::   ::::::::::::  ::::::  :: :::::: :
RFNIGGPTSSIPILCSYFFDEGPPVLLDKIYSRPDDSVSELCTRQ..     HUMAN
```

FIGURE 5. Sequence similarity between bovine and human IRBP at the protein level.

The similarity of these sequences is great. 37 out of 43 amino acids are identical and 4 are conservative substitutions. There is one change to note, however. The putative N-linked carbohydrate site in the bovine sequence (NDS) has been lost in the human sequnce (DDS). This might account for some of the difference in the molecular weights between bovine and human IRBP (24). The bovine protein sequence shown in Fig. 5 is contained in a cyanogen bromide fragment (CB58) of IRBP that has been shown to cause experimental uveitis (25 and Redmond et al., this volume). Thus, it is possible that some of the human sequences that could cause experimental uveitis may have been identified. Experiments to demonstrate this are in progress.

CHROMOSOMAL LOCALIZATIONS

We have used the bovine gene to probe for the chromosomal location of IRBP in both human and canine species (26). Fig. 6 shows the localization in dogs to chromosome 4 and in humans to chromosome 10.

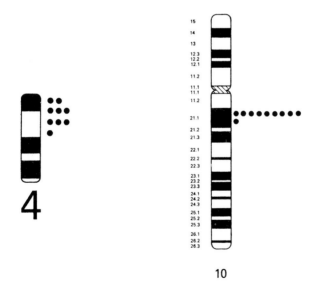

FIGURE 6. In situ hybridization of λgIRBP7 to chromosome preparations of dog and human chromosomes. Left, an idiogram of dog chromosome 4. Right, an idiogram of human chromosome 10.

These specific signals indicate conservation between the

bovine IRBP gene, which was used as the probe, and the human and canine genes. In human, close inspection of ten chromosome splashes showed that the grains were localized to the boundary of 10q11.2 and 10q21.1. Human chromosome 10 has 23 markers, and only 8 of these have been mapped to a subchromosomal region, and only 4 to the level of 1 or 2 bands (27). Thus, the addition of the IRBP locus is important for filling in the human cytogenetic map. Our localization of IRBP in humans to 10q11.2-10q21.1 is in agreement with and slightly refines a recent report by Liou et al. (21). They also have localized IRBP on chromosome 10 near the centromere using a human IRBP cDNA probe. Simpson et al. (28) have linked IRBP with the anonymous probe D10S5 and MEN2A on chromosome 10 by multipoint linkage analysis.

We confirmed the presence of an IRBP gene on human chromosome 10 by isolating a genomic clone (λgIRBP16, described above) from a chromosome 10-specific library. Discordance analyses have been performed (21,29).

This localization is important for linkage studies, interspecies synteny, and the examination of gross cytogenetic alterations. The possibility exists that a defect in the IRBP gene results in retinal degeneration. Of particular interest are the dog models of retinal degeneration (reviewed in 30). Inbred strains (breeds) are available and detailed pedigrees frequently exist. A few studies have addressed the domestic dog genome (31-33) and the closely related wolves (34,35). The assignment of the IRBP gene to chromosome 4 of the dog provides a start towards the cytogenetic mapping of the genes for ocular proteins that might be of importance in well-defined canine models of retinal degeneration. It also raises the possibility of synteny between the long arm of human chromosome 10 and dog chromosome 4. This possibility could be tested by the use of other nearby human chromosome 10 markers that, like IRBP, also might cross-hybridize.

## IRBP mRNA LOCATION AND SIZE VARIATION

IRBP mRNA is found in the outer nuclear layer of the retina (6). This implies that IRBP protein is synthesized and secreted by the photoreceptor and that the gene is transcribed actively in the photoreceptor. We have examined IRBP mRNA in retinas from several species and in bovine pineals by northern blot analysis. The results are shown in Fig. 7.

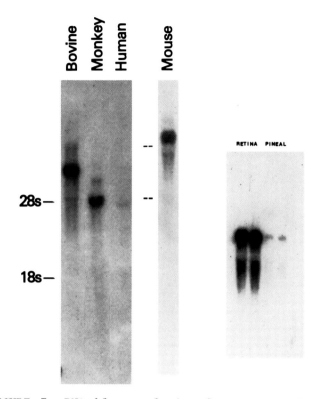

FIGURE 7. RNA blot analysis of IRBP mRNA from several species.    LEFT.  Size variation in IRBP mRNAs.    Total RNA from bovine, monkey, and mouse retinas and RNA from human Y-79 retinoblastoma cells were probed with a 900 bp fragment of an IRBP cDNA (pIRBP10-2000) from the translated portion of the mRNA. Note the shift upwards in the position of the 28S and 18S RNA markers on the mouse lane. RIGHT. Comparison of bovine retina and pineal RNAs.    The retina and pineal RNAs were probed with pIRBP10-2000.

While the IRBP mRNAs are all very large, there is variability in size ranging from 4.8 to 7.4 kb (36). Perhaps this size variation reflects differences in the size of the untranslated parts of the mRNAs. There are no apparent differences in IRBP mRNAs isolated from bovine retina and pineal.    In certain species, rat in particular, a second larger band is present (36).

## SUMMARY

In conclusion, studies on the structure and expression of the IRBP gene by sequence analysis, blot analysis and cytogenetics provide clues about the normal function of IRBP and its possible role in retinal dysfunction.

## ACKNOWLEDGEMENTS

We wish to thank Drs. D. Capon, J. Nathans, D. Oprian, M.A. Van Dilla, and M. Young for providing their cDNA and genomic libraries.

## REFERENCES

1.  Bunt-Milam A, and Saari J (1983) Immunocytochemical localization of two retinoid-binding proteins in the vertebrate retina. J Cell Biol 97:703.
2.  Wiggert B, Bergsma DR, Lewis M, and Chader GJ (1977) Vitamin A receptors: Retinol binding in neural retina and pigment epithelium. J Neurochem 29:947.
3.  Bazan NG, Reddy TS, Redmond TM, Wiggert B, and Chader GJ (1985) Endogenous fatty acids are covalently and non-covalently bound to interphotoreceptor retinoid-binding protein in the monkey. J Biol Chem 260:13677.
4.  Pfeffer B, Wiggert B, Lee L, Zonnenberg B, Newsome D, and Chader GJ (1983) The presence of a soluble interphotoreceptor retinoid-binding protein (IRBP) in the retinal interphotoreceptor space. J Cell Physiol 117: 331.
5.  Chader G, Wiggert B, Lai Y-L and Fletcher, R (1983) Interphotoreceptor retinoid-binding protein: a possible role in retinoid transport to the retina. Prog Ret Res 2:163.
6.  Van Veen T, Katial A, Shinohara T, Barrett DJ, Wiggert B, Chader GJ, and Nickerson JM (1986) Retinal photoreceptor neurons and pinealocytes accumulate mRNA for interphotoreceptor retinoid-binding protein. FEBS Lett 208:133.
7.  Wiggert B, Lee L, Hirose Y, Sanyal S, Chader G, and Van Veen T (1987) Interphotoreceptor retinoid-binding protein (IRBP) in rds mutant mice. Invest Ophthal Vis Sci (Suppl) 28:252.

Molecular Biology of the Eye: Genes, Vision,
and Ocular Disease, pages 107–116
© 1988 Alan R. Liss, Inc.

# STRUCTURAL STUDIES OF CELLULAR RETINALDEHYDE-BINDING PROTEIN FROM HUMAN AND BOVINE RETINA

John W. Crabb, Steven Goldflam, Charles M. Johnson,
Steven A. Carr+ Steven E. Harris, Lyman G. Armes,
John C. Saari++

W. Alton Jones Cell Science Center, Inc. Lake Placid, NY
12946 +SmithKline and French Laboratories, Swedeland, PA
19479,++University of Washington, Seattle, WA 98195

**ABSTRACT** The complete primary structure of the cellular retinaldehyde-binding protein (CRALBP) from bovine retina ($M_r$, 36,377) has been determined by direct microanalysis of the protein. Fast atom bombardment and tandem mass spectrometry identified the amino-terminal blocking group as an acetyl moiety. Concomitant with protein sequence analysis, cDNA encoding CRALBP was cloned from a bovine retinal cDNA expression library. The amino acid sequence deduced from the cDNA corresponds exactly to that determined by direct analysis of bovine CRALBP. Nick-translated bovine cDNA was then used to clone the cDNA encoding human CRALBP. Bovine and human CRALBP are 91% identical in sequence and not related to any other proteins in the Protein Identification Resource data base.

## INTRODUCTION

Cellular retinaldehyde-binding protein (CRALBP) of retina may be a functional component of the visual cycle, perhaps acting as a substrate carrier protein and/or stereoselective agent. The endogenous ligands bound by CRALBP are 11-*cis*-retinol or 11-*cis*-retinaldehyde, retinoids that are only known to function in the visual process (1). CRALBP is known to interact specifically

[1]This work was supported in part by USPHS grants EY-02317, EY-06603 and CA37589 and by RJR Nabisco.

with a visual cycle enzyme since 11-*cis*-retinol dehydrogenase of retinal pigment epitheliam (RPE) readily reduces 11-*cis*-retinaldehyde bound to CRALBP even though water soluble reducing agents are without effect (2). Retinyl ester synthase of RPE, another visual cycle enzyme, esterifies 11-*cis*-retinol bound to CRALBP, resulting in dissociation of the retinoid (3). Finally, CRALBP is able to select 11-*cis*-retinaldehyde from a mixture of steroisomers, suggesting a role for the protein in the generation of 11-*cis*-retinoids (4). As part of our continuing study of the role of CRALBP in the physiology of the retina we have directly determined the amino acid sequence of CRALBP from bovine retina and concomitantly cloned and sequenced bovine and human cDNA encoding CRALBP. In the present communication the amino acid and nucleotide sequences corresponding to human and bovine CRALBP are presented and discussed. The experimental details of the sequence determinations will be presented elsewhere.

## MATERIALS AND METHODS

Direct Sequence Analysis of Bovine CRALBP

Bovine CRALBP was purified from frozen cattle retinas (Hormel) (5). Sulfhydryl groups were either pyridylethylated (6) or carboxymethylated (7). Selective proteolytic and chemical fragmentations of bovine CRALBP were performed and peptide digests fractionated by reverse phase high performance liquid chromatography. Amino acid compositions were determined by phenylthiocarbamyl (PTC) amino acid analysis (7). Automatic Edman degradations were performed with an Applied Biosystems gas phase sequencer with an on line phenylthiohydantoin (PTH)-analyzer (7). Carboxyterminal sequence analysis was performed by carboxypeptidase Y digestion (8).

Characterization of the amino-terminal blocking group of bovine CRALBP was performed by a combination of fast atom bombardment (FAB-MS) and tandem mass spectrometry (MS/MS) (7). Conventional FAB-MS were obtained with a VG ZAB 1F-HF instrument and MS/MS was performed with a VG ZAB SE-4F four sector magnetic deflection instrument.

Homology with other proteins was sought by searching the Protein Identification Resource (PIR) data base (4721 sequences composed of 1,181,447 amino acids). Hydropathy profiles were predicted according to Kyte and Doolittle (9)

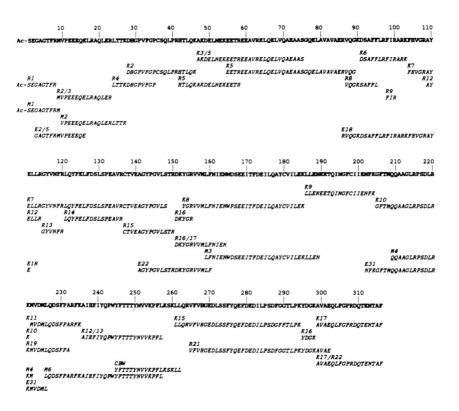

Figure 1. <u>Summary of the proof of the sequence of bovine CRALBP.</u> The determined sequences of specific peptides (in italics) are given in one-letter code below the summary sequence. Prefixes K, R, E and M denote peptides generated by cleavage at lysyl, arginyl, glutamyl and methionyl residues, respectively; prefix CBW denotes a cyanogen bromide peptide generated by cleavage at a tryptophanyl residue. Peptides are numbered sequentially from the amino terminus except where an uncleaved residue gives an overlap (e.g. K3/5). All peptide sequences were proven by Edman degradation except R1 and M1 where tandem mass spectrometry was used. Ac denotes an acetyl group that was identified as the N-terminal blocking group by FAB-MS.

and Hopp and Woods (10) using GENEPRO Software (River-side Scientific Enterprises). Secondary structure was predicted according to Chou and Fasman (11) using the PIR.

## Characterization of Bovine and Human CRALBP cDNA

A bovine retinal cDNA expression library in λgt11, generously provided by D. Oprian, was screened with anti-CRALBP polyclonal and monoclonal antibodies (12). CRALBP cDNA inserts were subcloned into pTZ19R (Pharmacia) and a resulting EcoR1 fragment was sequenced by the chain termination method (13). Portions of bovine CRALBP cDNA were also sequenced using the Maxam-Gilbert method (14).

A human retinal cDNA library in λgt10, generously provided by J. Nathans, was screened with nick-translated bovine CRALBP cDNA probes. A full length human CRALBP cDNA insert was subcloned into pSK (Stratagene) and sequenced entirely by the Sanger method using the same oligonucleotide primers synthesized for analysis of the bovine cDNA.

## RESULTS

## Protein Sequence Analysis of Bovine CRALBP

The complete amino acid sequence of CRALBP determined by direct analysis of the protein from bovine retina is shown in Figure 1. The single, amino terminally blocked polypeptide chain contains 316 amino acids, and exhibits a molecular weight of 36,377. The CRALBP sequence is consistent with the amino acid composition and molecular weight determined previously (15).

The sequence of bovine CRALBP was determined largely by Edman degradation of overlapping peptides generated by cleavage of lysyl, arginyl, methionyl and glutamyl residues (Fig.1). One tryptophanyl peptide generated during cyanogen bromide cleavage was also utilized in establishing an overlap. The chemical nature of the N-terminal blocking group was established to be an acetyl group by FAB-MS and amino acid analysis of the N-terminal arginyl and methionyl peptides. The blocked arginyl and methionyl peptides each were sequenced by MS/MS and the N-terminal sequence determined to be Acetyl-Ser-Glu-Gly-Ala-Gly-Thr-Phe-Arg-Met. The carboxy-terminal sequence was identified by carboxy-peptidase Y digestion to be ...Thr-Ala-Phe-COOH.

```
                          CGA CGA AGT GGG CTC CTT CTT TGT TTG CAG CAC TCA CAG TCT TCC ACA GAC AGC ATG
                                                                                                    57

                  10                      20                      30
Ac-Ser Glu Gly Ala Gly Thr Phe Arg Met Val Pro Glu Glu Gln Glu Glu Leu Arg Ala Ala Lys Asp His Thr Lys Leu Arg Gly Val Phe Gly Pro
   TCA GAG GGG GCG GGC ACG TTC CGC ATG GTC CCT GAA GAG CAA GAG GAG CTC CGT GCC GCC AAA GAC CAT ACC AAG CTT AGG GGT GTT TTT GGC CCG

          40                      50                      60                      70
Cys Ser Gln Leu Pro Arg His Thr Leu Gln Leu Asn Glu Lys Ala Asp Glu Lys Glu Glu Val Arg Glu Glu Thr Arg Ala Val Glu Glu Leu Gln Glu Leu Val Gln
TGC AGC CAG CTG CCC CGC CAC ACC CTG CAG CTG AAT GAG AAG GCC GAC GAG AAG GAG GAG GTG CGG GAG GAG ACC CGG GCA GTG GAG GAG CTA CAG GAG CTG GTG CAG

                   80                      90                     100
Ala Glu Ala Ala Ser Gly Val Arg Tyr Val Arg Gly Leu Leu Ile Glu Arg Tyr Asn Phe Tyr Pro Glu Leu Tyr Asp Lys Arg Asp Ser Ile Leu Asn Ile Glu Asn
GCG GAG GCC GCG TCG GGG GTG AGG TAC GTG AGG GGC CTC CTC ATA GAG CGG TAC AAC TTC CGG GAC CTG TAC GAC AAG CGG GAC AGC ATT CTC AAC ATT GAG AAT

           110                     120                     130                     140
Val Gly Arg Arg Ala Ala Tyr Gly Tyr Val Leu Glu Leu Leu Arg Asn Phe Tyr Leu Gln Tyr Pro Glu Ser Leu Phe Asp Glu Val Ala Lys Arg Cys Thr Val Glu His
GTG GGG CGC CGC GCC GCC TAC GGC TAC GTG CTC CTC AGA GGC CTG CTG CGG AAC TTC TAC CTG CAG TAC CCA GAG TCC CTG TTC GAC GAG GTC GCT GTC ACC GTT CAC

                  150                     160                     170
Ala Gly Tyr Pro Gly Val Leu Ser Ser Thr Asp Lys Asp Arg Asn Ile Ile Phe Leu Met Val Val Glu Glu Glu Ile Thr Phe Asp Glu Ile
GCT GGC TAC CCT GGT GTC CTC TCC ACG GAC AAG GAC CGA CGG AAT ATT ATT TTC CTC ATG GTC GTG GAG GAA GAG TCT GAG GAA TTT GAT GAG ATC

           180                     190                     200                     210
Leu Gln Ala Tyr Cys Val Ile Leu Glu Leu Leu Glu Asn Asn Tyr Gly Ile Ile Gly Thr Gln Lys Ile Asn Gly Phe Cys Ile Phe Ser Gly Phe Met Thr Thr Gln
TTG CAG GCA TAC TGC GTC ATC CTG GAG CTA CTG GAG AAT AAT TAC GGC ATT ATT GGG ACT CAA AAG ATT AAT GGC TTT TGC ATC TTC AGC GGC TTC ATG ACC ACC CAG

                  220                     230                     240
Ala Ala Gly Leu Arg Pro Ser Asp Leu Lys Arg Met Val Asp Met Ser Phe Pro Ala Arg Phe Lys Ala Ile His Phe Ile Tyr Gln Pro Trp Tyr
GCT GCC GGA CTT CGG CCT TCC GAT CTC AGA AAG ATG GTG GAC ATG TCC TTC CCA GCT CGG TTC AAA GCC ATC CAC TTC ATC TAC CAG CCC TGG TAC

           250                     260                     270                     280
Phe Thr Thr Asn Tyr Asn Val Val Lys Pro Phe Leu Lys Ser Leu Gln Leu Arg Gln Val His Val Phe Gly Ser Ser Tyr Gln Glu Gln Phe Glu Thr Glu Asn Thr Asp
TTC ACC ACC AAC TAC AAC GTG GTC AAG CCC TTC TTG AAG AGC CTC TTG CAG CTC AGG CAG GTA TTT GTC CAT GGA GAA TCC AGC TAC CAG GAG CAG TTT GAG ACT GAC

                  290                     300                     310
Glu Asp Ile Leu Pro Ser Asp Phe Gly Gly Thr Leu Pro Lys Tyr Asp Gly Lys Ala Val Ala Glu Gln Leu Phe Gly Pro Arg Asp Gln Thr Glu Asn Thr Ala
GAG GAC ATC CTG CCC TCC GAC TTT GGG GGT ACA CTG CCA AAG TAT GAT GGG AAG GCC GTT GCT GAG CAG CTG TTT GGT CCT CGG GAC CAA ACA GAG AAC ACA GCC

316
Phe End
Phe End
TTC TGA GAA CAT CTC CTG CCA TCT GAC CTG TAG TTA GCA TCC TTA GGC CTC TCC TCA ACT GCC CTG GAC CCA GAA TGC TGT GAA AAA GGG CTT CCT GGG GTG ACT
1005                                                                                                                            1173

GTG GTT CCT CTG AAC CAT CTG CTG AAC TCT TCT AAG TTT GGG CAA ACT CAG ATG TCA TTC TCC TCC CAA GCT GGG GGG
                                                                                                    1173
```

Figure 2. Bovine CRALBP nucleotide and amino acid sequences. The nucleotides are numbered 1-1173 below the cDNA sequence and the amino acids are numbered 1-316 above the deduced protein sequences.

CGG AAG AGA ACT TGA ACC CAG GTC CAA CTT TTG CGC CAC AGC AGG CTG CCT GAC AGG AAG TCA CAA CTT

GGC CCT GAC TTC CTA TCC TAG GGA AGG GGC CGG CTG GAG AGG CCA CAG AGA AAG CAG ATC TCT TTT TCC AAG GAC TCT GTG TCT ATA GGC AAC ATG
186

```
                10                          20                          30
Ac-Ser Glu Gly Val Gly Thr Phe Arg Met Val Pro Glu Gln Glu Gln Glu Leu Gln Leu Gln Leu Lys Thr Thr Lys Asp His Gly Pro Val Phe Gly Pro
TCA GAA GGG GTG GGC ATG GTC GTA CCT GAA GAG GAG CTC CGT GCC CAA CAG CAG CTC ACA ACC AAG GAC CAT GGA CCT GTC TTT GGC CCG
```

```
        40                          50                          60                      70
Cys Ser Gln Leu Pro Arg His Thr Leu Gln Glu Lys Asp Glu Leu Asn Glu Arg Glu Glu Thr Arg Glu Glu Ala Val Arg Glu Glu Met Val Gln
TGC AGC CAG CTG CCC CGC CAC ACC TTG CAG GAG AAG GCC AAG GAG AAC GAG AGA GAG GAG ACC CGG GAG GCA GTG CGA ATG GAG GTG CAG
```

```
                80                          90                          100
Ala Gln Ala Ala Ser Gly Glu Glu Leu Ala Val Ala Val Glu Val Gln Arg Val Gln Lys Asp Val Gly Pro Phe Phe Ile Arg Ala Arg Lys Phe Asn
GCG CAG GCG GCC TCG GGG GAG GAG CTG GCG GTG GCC GTG GAG GTG CAA AGG GTG CAA AAG GAC GAC GTG GGC TTC TTC ATC CGC GCA CGG AAG TTC AAC
```

```
        110                         120                         130                         140
Val Gly Arg Ala Tyr Tyr Glu Leu Leu Arg Gly Tyr Val Asn Pro Glu Leu Phe Arg Ser Leu Phe Asp Ser Pro Glu Leu Ala Val Arg Cys Thr Ile Glu
GTG GGC CGT GCA TAT TAC GAG CTG CTC AGA GGC TAT GTG AAT CCG GAG CTC TTT CGG AGC CTC TTT GAC AGC CCA GAG CTG GCA GCT GTC CGC TGC ACC ATT GAA
```

```
            150                         160                         170
Ala Gly Tyr Pro Gly Val Leu Ser Ser Arg Asp Lys Tyr Gly Arg Val Val Met Leu Phe Asn Ile Leu Asn Ile Glu Ser Trp Gln Ser Ile Ile Thr Asp Glu Ile
GCT GGC TAC CCT GGT GTC CTC TCT AGT CGG GAC AAG TAT GGC CGA GTG GTC ATG CTC TTC AAC ATT CTC AAC ATT GAG AGT CAA GAA ATC ATC ACC TTT GAT GAG ATC
```

```
        180                         190                         200                         210
Leu Gln Ala Tyr Cys Phe Ile Leu Glu Lys Leu Leu Gln Asn Glu Glu Thr Gln Ile Asn Gly Phe Cys Ile Ile Glu Asn Phe Lys Gly Phe Thr Met Gln Gln
TTG CAG GCA TAT TGC TTC ATC CTG GAG AAG CTG CTG CAG AAC GAG GAG ACT CAA ATC AAT GGC TTC TGC ATC ATT GAG AAC TTC AAA GGC TTT ACC ATG CAG CAG
```

```
            220                         230                         240
Ala Ala Ser Leu Arg Thr Ser Asp Leu Lys Met Val Asp Met Leu Gln Asn Ala Arg Phe Lys Ala Ala Ile His Ile His His Gln Ile Gln Pro Trp Tyr Tyr
GCT GCT AGT CTC CGG ACT TCA GAT CTC AAG ATG GTG GAC ATG CTC CAG AAC GCC CGG TTC AAA GCC ATC CAC ATC CAC CAC CAG ATC CAG CCA TGG TAC TAC
```

```
        250                         260                         270                         280
Phe Thr Thr Thr Asn Val Val Lys Pro Ser Leu Lys Leu Leu Arg Val Phe His Val Asp Gly Ser Leu Phe Gln Asp Tyr Gln Glu Ile Asp
TTC ACC ACC ACC AAT GTG GTC AAG CCC TTC TTG AAG AGC CTG CTT GAG CTT GTC CAC GTT GAT GGG AGC CTT TCT GGT TTC TAC CAG GAG ATC GAT
```

```
                290                         300                         310
Glu Asn Ile Leu Pro Ser Asp Phe Gly Gly Thr Leu Pro Lys Tyr Leu Asp Gly Tyr Lys Lys Ala Ile Ala Val Ala Glu Gln Leu Phe Gly Pro Gln Ala Glu Ala Thr Ala
GAG AAC ATC CTG CCC TCT GAC TTC GGG GGC ACG CTG CCC AAG TAT CTG GAT GGC TAT AAG AAG GCC GTT GCT GCC GTT GCT GAA CAG CTG TTT GGC CCA CAG GCT GAG GCT AAC ACA GCC
```

```
316
Phe End
TTC TGA AAA CAT CTC CTG CCA GCT GAA TCT CTG TAG TTA GAA TCT CTG GGC CTC TCA ACT GTC CTG GAC AGG AAG GGC TGC TTG AGA TGA CTG TGG
1134
```

TCC CCC CTT AGA CTC CCT AAG CCC GAG TGA GCT CAG GTG TCA CCC TGT TCT CAA GTT GGG GGA TGG GGA ATA AAG GAG GGG
1317

Figure 3. Human CRALBP nucleotide and amino acid sequences. The nucleotides are numbered 1-1317 below the cDNA sequence and the amino acids are numbered 1-316 above the deduced protein sequence. A potential polyadenylation signal in the 3' untranslated region is underlined.

## Cloning and Sequencing Bovine CRALBP cDNA

A primary screen of about $10^6$ recombinant phage using a polyclonal anti-CRALBP antibody yielded 33 positive signals. Each positive signal was rescreened utilizing both the polyclonal antibody and a monoclonal antibody recognizing an apparent N-terminal CRALBP epitope. Three clones recognized by both the polyclonal and monoclonal antibodies were purified and found to contain EcoR1 inserts of about 1.2 Kb. One of the clones was further characterized and found by sequence analysis to contain a 1173 bp insert composed of an open reading frame encoding the 316 amino acid CRALBP plus 57 nucleotides from the 5' and 168 nucleotides from the 3' flanking regions (Fig. 2). No polyadenylation sites were apparent in the 3' untranslated region. The protein sequence deduced from the cDNA sequence corresponds exactly to that determined by direct analysis of bovine CRALBP.

## Cloning and Sequencing Human CRALBP cDNA

Forty positive signals were obtained from about $1.5 \times 10^6$ recombinant phage screened with the nick-translated full-length bovine CRALBP cDNA. Fifteen of the positive clones were rescreened with oligonucleotide probes for 5' and 3' specific regions of the bovine CRALBP cDNA. One of the five clones which hybridized to both probes was subcloned and found by dideoxy sequence analysis to contain a 1317 bp EcoR1 insert composed of the CRALBP coding region and 186 and 183 nucleotides, respectively of 5' and 3' flanking regions (Fig. 3). A potential polyadenylation site AATAAA was found 13 bases from the 3' end.

## DISCUSSION

Proof of the amino acid sequence of bovine CRALBP was derived from both direct Edman analysis of overlapping peptides covering the entire polypeptide chain as well as by cloning and sequencing a full-length cDNA encoding the protein. FAB-MS and MS/MS provided the data necessary to assign the first 9 amino acid residues and to determine that bovine CRALBP is $N^\alpha$-acetyl blocked. The complete primary structure of human CRALBP was deduced from cDNA. Bovine and human CRALBPs are 91% identical in sequence but are not related to any other known protein sequence in the

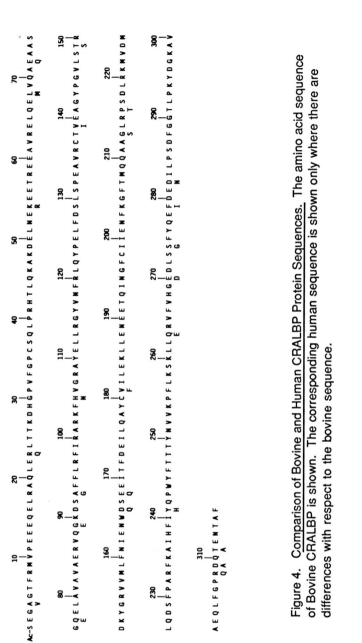

Figure 4.   Comparison of Bovine and Human CRALBP Protein Sequences.   The amino acid sequence of Bovine CRALBP is shown.  The corresponding human sequence is shown only where there are differences with respect to the bovine sequence.

the photoreceptor begins to take place.

One of the norpA mutants isolated, norpA^H52, was found to be reversibly temperature-sensitive (9). At permissive temperatures ($\sim 17^\circ$C) the electroretinogram (ERG) of this mutant is nearly normal. However, raising the temperature above $\sim 35^\circ$ instantly abolishes the ERG. One can recover the ERG by lowering the temperature once again, providing that the fly is not exposed to the restrictive temperature too long. Results such as these suggested that the norpA gene encodes a protein directly involved in the generation of the receptor potential. Although the identity of the protein remained unknown, it was shown not to be rhodopsin (10). The temperature-sensitive norpA mutant, for example, was found to contain nearly normal amounts of rhodopsin at either permissive or restrictive temperatures. In addition, norpA mutations seemed to have no direct effect on the amplitude and time course of quantum bumps (the elementary units of the receptor potential), suggesting that the mutations do not directly affect the properties of ion channels. Thus, it was proposed that the norpA gene product is involved in an intermediate step of phototransduction.

Recently, several lines of evidence have fueled speculation that the norpA gene product might be a phospholipase C (PLC). For example, injection of inositol 1,4,5-trisphosphate (IP$_3$) and related compounds into Limulus ventral photoreceptors was found to mimic the effects of light (11, 12). These and related experiments have led to the proposal that the transduction cascade in invertebrate photoreceptors involves G-protein coupled activation of PLC, which in turn hydrolyzes phosphatidylinositol 4,5-bisphosphate (PIP$_2$) to produce diacylglycerol (DG) and IP$_3$ (13, 14). Subsequently, Devary et al. (15) presented evidence that, in isolated fly photoreceptor membranes, photo-excitation of rhodopsin is coupled to the hydrolysis of inositol phospholipid through a G-protein. Meanwhile, in a related development, Yoshioka et al. (16) reported that the PLC activity is highly concentrated in the Drosophila eye and is greatly reduced in norpA mutants. In fact, in several norpA alleles tested, the degree of reduction in PLC activity was found to be correlated with behavioral and electrophysiological deficits (1). Perhaps the strongest evidence, to this point, that the norpA gene encodes the enzyme PLC was the work reported by Dr. Zvi Selinger in the previous talk that in the temperature-sensitive norpA mutant, norpA^H52, the PLC activity is blocked at restrictive temperatures but is normal at permissive temperatures.

A growing body of evidence suggests that inositol phosphates are used as second messengers in transmembrane signaling mechanisms of a wide variety of tissues in a wide range of species (17). However, little was known about the molecular nature of the enzyme PLC involved in any of these pathways. It thus seemed important to clone and study the norpA gene.

Our attempt to clone the gene actually began a number of years ago -- before most of the above evidence had been obtained. The first step in this attempt was to localize the gene as accurately as possible. The work consisted of isolating deficiencies that uncover norpA mutations and defining the deficiencies cytogenetically. This work was carried out as a collaboration between the Pak laboratory and the James Boyd laboratory at the University of California, Davis (18). Two deficiencies, Df(1)rb41, isolated in the Pak laboratory, and Df(1)biD2, isolated in the Boyd laboratory, were particularly useful in localizing the norpA gene. The distal breakpoints of these deficiencies are cytogenetically indistinguishable: they both break in the interband region between 4B6 and 4C1. Yet, rb41 deletes the norpA function while biD2 leaves it intact. Thus, the entire norpA gene is outside the biD2 deficiency, but at least a portion of the gene is within the rb41 deficiency.

H. Steller and C. Montell in G. Rubin's laboratory at the University of California, Berkeley, isolated two cosmids containing DNA from the region of the breakpoints in chromosome walking. The two overlapping inserts contained in these cosmids define a genomic region of approximately 50 kb in length. In situ hybridizations of the insert DNA to larval salivary polytene chromosomes of rb41 and biD2 deficiency stocks showed that the entire 50-kb region is contained between the distal breakpoints of these two deficiencies. Moreover, Northern hybridizations of head and body polyA RNA probed with genomic DNA from the 50-kb region revealed that a putative message of approximately seven kb in length is transcribed in the adult head but not in the body. These results strongly suggested, but did not prove, that at least a portion of the norpA gene had been cloned in the cosmids.

To obtain more definitive evidence that the norpA gene had been cloned, attempts were made to rescue a norpA mutant by P-factor mediated germ line transformation (19) using the entire genomic DNA contained in one of the cosmids. The attempts were unsuccessful possibly because the DNA used in the transformation experiments did not contain the entire

norpA gene. As an alternative approach, hybrid dysgenic
crosses were performed to induce mutations in the norpA gene
by mobilization of transposons in the germ line. A class of
transposons known as hobo was used for this purpose (20).
The objective was to generate and identify norpA mutants
resulting from the insertion of a hobo element into the
norpA gene in this reshuffling of hobo elements in the germ
line. A norpA mutant, resulting from such an event, indeed,
was recovered from these experiments. Southern hybridizations of genomic DNA of the dysgenically induced norpA
mutant with probes from the head-specific region of the
cloned DNA showed an increase in the size of the hybridizing
fragments by approximately 3 kb, consistent with a hobo
insertion in this region (20). Furthermore, in situ
hybridizations of hobo DNA to larval salivary chromosomes of
the dysgenically induced mutant showed a label in the
4B6-4C1 region of the X chromosome, previously determined
to be the location of the norpA gene. Not only did these
experiments provide strong evidence that at least a portion
of the norpA gene had been cloned but also did allow one to
localize the norpA gene in the genomic DNA clones from the
site of hobo insertion.

Over 200 cDNAs were isolated by screening four different libraries using genomic fragments corresponding to the
region of hobo insertion and the regions surrounding the
insertion site as probes. Sequence analysis of several
representative classes of cDNAs is currently under way. One
of the cDNAs that have been sequenced to date is a 1.9-kb
cDNA that overlaps the region of DNA containing the hobo
insertion site in the hobo-induced norpA mutant. This particular cDNA contains a long open reading frame that would
encode a polypeptide of 580 residues. The cDNA, however, is
not full-length, and the norpA gene product is almost certain to be much larger. No sequence information had been
reported for any phospholipase C of any eukaryotes at the
time of the meeting, and a search of databanks produced no
known proteins with any reliable sequence similarity with
the polypeptide deduced from the cDNA. Recently, however,
the deduced amino acid sequence of a bovine brain phospholipase C has been reported (21). Even though only a portion
of the norpA sequence is available, extensive similarity
between the amino acid sequence of the bovine PLC and that
of the norpA cDNA suggests that the norpA gene does encode a
PLC. Since strong norpA mutations abolish the receptor
potential, it follows that phospholipase C, indeed, is an
integral component of the transduction pathway in Drosophila

photoreceptors.


ACKNOWLEDGMENTS

We thank M. Floreani, L. L. Randall, and K. Phillips
for their isolation of the hobo-induced norpA allele.


REFERENCES

1.  Inoue H, Yoshioka T, Hotta Y (1985). A genetic study of
    inositol trisphosphate involvement in phototransduction
    using Drosophila mutants. Biochem Biophys Res Comm
    132:513-519.
2.  Pak, WL (1979). Study of photoreceptor function using
    Drosophila mutants. In Breakefield XO (ed):
    "Neurogenetics: Genetic Approaches to the Nervous
    System," New York: Elsevier North Holland, p 67.
3.  Scavarda NJ, O'Tousa J, Pak WL (1983). Drosophila locus
    with gene-dosage effects on rhodopsin. Proc Natl Acad
    Sci USA 80:4441.
4.  O'Tousa JE, Baehr W, Martin RL, Hirsh J, Pak WL,
    Applebury ML (1985). The Drosophila ninaE gene encodes
    an opsin. Cell 40:839.
5.  Zuker CS, Cowman AF, Rubin GM (1985). Isolation and
    structure of a rhodopsin gene from D. melanogaster.
    Cell 40:851.
6.  Pak WL, Grossfield J, Arnold K (1970). Mutants of the
    visual pathway of Drosophila melanogaster. Nature
    227:518.
7.  Hotta Y, Benzer S (1970). Genetic dissection of the
    Drosophila nervous system by means of mosaics. Proc
    Natl Acad Sci USA 67:1156.
8.  Meyertholen EP, Stein PJ, Williams MA, Ostroy SE (1987).
    Studies of the Drosophila norpA phototransduction
    mutant, II. Photoreceptor degeneration and rhodopsin
    maintenance. J Comp Physiol A 161:793.
9.  Deland MC, Pak WL (1973). Reversibly temperature
    sensitive phototransduction mutant of Drosophila
    melanogaster. Nature New Biol 244:184.
10. Pak WL, Ostroy SE, Deland MC, Wu CF (1976).
    Photoreceptor mutant of Drosophila: Is protein involved
    in intermediate steps of phototransduction? Science
    194:956.
11. Fein A, Payne R, Corson DW, Berridge MJ, Irvine RF

ion of InsP$_2$, thus further supporting the relevance of
light-dependent phosphoinositide hydrolysis to the phototransduction process in the fly receptor cell.

Several transduction mechanisms, including phosphoinositide hydrolysis, are mediated by a guanine nucleotide binding protein (G-protein) which is active in the GTP bound form
and reverses to the inactive state upon hydrolysis of the
bound GTP to GDP (Cassel *et al.*, 1977; Fung and Stryer, 1980;
Cockroft and Gomperts, 1985). Since omitting GTP from the
incubation system of *Musca* eye membranes had little, if any,
effect, the role of a G-protein in phosphoinositide hydrolysis was tested by the addition of GTPγS or GDPβS hydrolysis
resistant analogs of GTP and GDP, respectively (Eckstein *et
al.*, 1979).

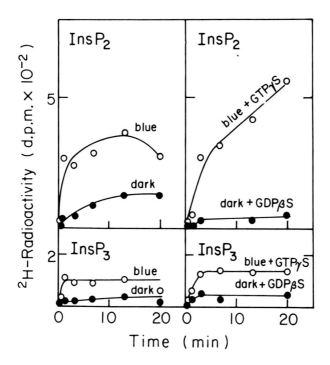

Figure 3. Effect of GTPγS and GDPβS on inositol phosphate
production in *Musca* eye membranes. Incubation conditions
were as described in Fig. 1. Where indicated the concentrations of GTPγS were 10 μM and GDPβS 100 μM.

In the control systems incubated in the absence of
GTPγS and GDPβS (Fig. 3, left panel) illumination with blue
light considerably increased the hydrolysis of phosphoinositides resulting in burst of InsP$_3$ production which levelled
off after 1 minute and longer and greater extent of accumulation of InsP$_2$. With the aid of 2,3 diphosphoglycerate
which competitively inhibits the hydrolysis of InsP$_3$ we
have shown that this kinetic of inositol phosphates accumulation is due to production of InsP$_3$ and its further conversion to InsP$_2$ by specific phosphomoesterase (Devary et al.,
1987). In the presence of GDPβS there is a marked decrease
in the accumulation of InsP$_2$ in the dark whereas in presence
of GTPγS light further increases both the length and the
extent of InsP$_3$ and InsP$_2$ accumulation (Fig. 3, left panel).
These results indicate that the light dependent phosphoinositide hydrolysis in the fly eye membrane is under a
stringent control of a G-protein which is inactive when it
contains bound GDPβS and is persistently active when the
bound nucleotide is the hydrolysis resistent analog GTPγS.

Two criteria of an internal second messenger are:
(i) introduction of the putative messenger into the cell
should reproduce the physiological response; and (ii) agents
that inhibit the inactivation of the messenger should aug-
ment the effect of the physiological stimulus. These criteria were tested for by light-induced introduction of InsP$_3$
+ DPG and of 8-Br-cGMP into the *Musca* photoreceptor cells.

Continuous illuminations with dim red lights of increasing intensity show correspondingly increased depolarization
with larger noise. Likewise, introduction of increasing
amounts of InsP$_3$ + DPG by application of lights of corresponding greater intensity results in a progressively
increased depolarization and noise (Fig. 4). Power spectrum
analysis, reveals that light and InsP$_3$ + DPG produce similar
effects both causing an increased variance density throughout the whole range of frequencies (Fig. 4). After application
of DPG alone and its introduction into the cell there is not
much change in the dark noise but DPG does potentiate the
effect of dim light suggesting an endogenous production of
InsP$_3$ during illumination (not shown). Both the excitation
of the photoreceptor cells by InsP$_3$ which closely resembles
the effect of light and the potentiation of the effect of
dim light by DPG are consistent with a second messenger role
for InsP$_3$ in fly phototransduction.

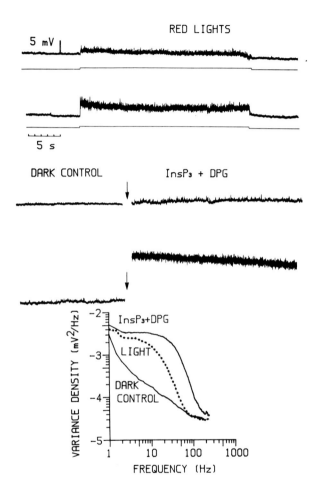

Figure 4. Excitation of *Musca* photoreceptors by inositol 1,4,5 trisphosphate ($InsP_3$) + 2,3, diphosphoglycerate (DPG). Intracellular recording from single photoreceptor. Upper two traces are responses to dim red-orange light (OG-590 edge filter Schott maximal intensity 14mWcm$^{-2}$) attenuated by 5 and 3 log units by neutral density filters for the upper and second traces respectively. The third and fourth traces show effect of injection of $InsP_3$ 1 mM + DPG 50 mM diluted about 10 fold in the retinal extracellular space. The left

half of the lower two traces shows the noise in the dark 60
sec after short orange flash (150-J photographic flash in
conjunction with Schott OG 570 nm edge filter), third trace;
and 1 sec maximal intensity white light, fourth trace. The
same illumination were applied after injection of $InsP_3$ +
DPG indicated by arrows. The bottom graph shows power
spectra calculated as previously described (Devary et al.,
1987). Dark, control; third trace, $InsP_3$ + DPG; fourth
trace, and light; dim illumination of red light attenuated by
4 log units (not shown).

---

Injection of 8-Br-cyclic GMP into the Musca fly retina
and its introduction into the photoreceptor cells by light
potentiated the effect of subsequent dim red light and
caused noisy depolarization in the dark after the light had
been turned off (fig. 5). These effects were specific to the
cyclic guanine nucleotide analog since 8-Br-cyclic AMP had
no effect. Power spectrum analysis of the noise during the
dark period, after introduction of the nucleotide by intense
light, revealed however, that the large increase in variance
density caused by 8-Br-cyclic GMP was confined to low frequencies (fig. 5, left). It was thus different from the effect
of light or of $InsP_3$ + DPG which increased the variance
density also at high frequencies (cf. Fig. 4 and 5).

Biochemical assays of guanylate cyclase (both the soluble and the membrane bound enzyme) and cyclic GMP phosphodiesterase did not show any effect of light on the enzymes'
activities. Furthermore, the specific activity of the membrane bound guanylate cyclase in the fly eye membranes was
similar to the specific activity of this enzyme in membranes
prepared from the fly brain. This is in contrast to the
enzymes of phosphoinositides metabolism which are greatly
enriched (about ten fold) in the eye membranes over the
activities of these enzymes in the brain membranes (not
shown).

A powerful approach to identification of the intermediate steps in complex biochemical pathways,including phototransduction,is the use of genetic mutants (Pak, 1979). It is
preferable to use conditional mutants as in this case one
can avoid some ambiguities that may arise from different
genetic backgrounds in fly stocks which are kept in culture
for long periods. A suitable mutant for this purpose is the
norp A$^{H52}$ which is a reversible temperature sensitive phototransduction mutant of Drosophila melanogaster (Deland and
Pak, 1973). It should be pointed out that in contrast to

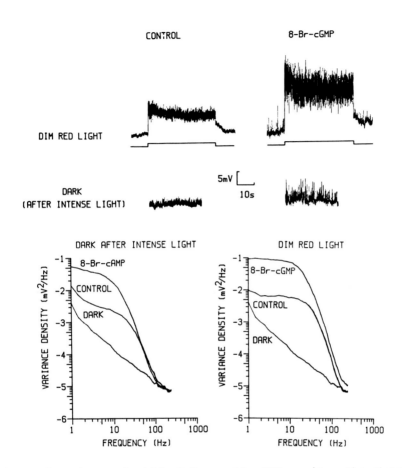

Figure 5. The nucleotide 8-Br-cyclic GMP excites the *Musca* photoreceptors in the dark and enhances the excitation during illumination by dim light. The upper left trace shows response to orange-red light attenuated by 4 log units. The second left trace shows dark noise recorded 1 min after 5 sec maximal intensity white light pulse. The corresponding right traces show records of the effect of the same stimuli in the same cell after extrocellular injection of 1 mM 8-Br-cyclic GMP and its introduction into the photoreceptors by 1 min maximal intensity white illumination. Power spectra were calculated as in fig. 4.

many *Drosophila* mutants which are developmentally temperature sensitive revealing their characteristic phenotype only if grown at the restrictive temperature throughout their life cycle. The norp $A^{H52}$ fly promptly loses its light-induced photoreceptor potential upon transfer to the restrictive temperature even if it has been grown in permissive temperature.

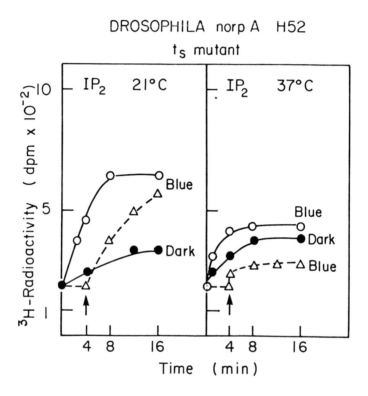

Figure 6. Light dependent phosphoinositide hydrolysis by *Drosophila* norp $A^{H52}$ eye membranes incubated at permissive and restrictive temperatures. *Drosophila* norp $A^{H52}$ temperature sensitive mutant flies (Deland and Pak, 1973) up to 5 days old were used. Incorporation of [³H]-inositol and preparation of crude *Drosophila* eye membranes were carried out as previously described (Devary *et al.*, 1987). The reaction was initiated by addition of membranes to reaction media pre-equilibrated at the indicated temperatures and processed as described in fig. 1. Systems depicted in dotted lines were preincubated for 4 min at the indicated temperatures in

medium lacking ATP and regeneration system and these latter components were subsequently added (arrow) to initiate the reaction.

---

Assays of light dependent polyphosphoinositide hydrolysis, monitoring the accumulation of $InsP_2$ in membrane preparations incubated in the dark or preilluminated with blue light reveal that the phospholipase C activity is greatly reduced at the restrictive temperature of 37°C (Fig. 6). This effect is greatly enhanced in membranes which had been preincubated for 4 min at the restrictive temperature. In contrast, phospholipase C activity in membranes prepared from wild type flies is not decreased at the restrictive temperature (not shown). These results are consistent with previous studies (Yoshioka et al., 1984; Inoue et al., 1985) reporting that diglyceride kinase and phospholipase C activities,assayed in the dark,are absent from membrane preparations of several norp A alleles. Since diglyceride kinase activity is a turn-off mechanism for protein kinase C, it was not clear from these studies which enzyme is primarily affected by the mutation.

CONCLUSIONS

Our biochemical,electrophysiological and genetic studies suggest that the flow of information in the fly phototransduction cascade is from photoexcited rhodopsin to G-protein and from G-protein to phospholipase C and that inositol trisphosphate fulfills the criteria of a second messenger in phototransduction. Cyclic GMP seems to interact with the phototransduction cascade but its site of action and mode of interaction remains to be elucidated by future studies.

REFERENCES

Berridge MJ, Dawson MC, Downes CP, Heslop JP, Irvine RF (1983). Changes in the levels of inositol phosphates after agonist-dependent hydrolysis of membrane phosphoinositides. Biochem. J. 212:473-482.

Blumenfeld A, Erusalimsky J, Heichal O, Selinger Z, Minke B (1985). Light-activated guanosine triphosphatase in *Musca* eye membranes resembles the prolonged depolarizing afterpotential in photoreceptor cells. Proc. Natl. Acad. Sci. USA 82:7116-7120.

Brown, JE, Rubin LJ, Ghalayini AJ, Tarver AP, Irvine RF, Berridge MJ, Anderson RE (1984). Myo-inositol polyphosphate may be a messenger for visual excitation in *Limulus* photoreceptors. Nature 311:160-163.

Cassel D, Levkovitz H, Selinger Z (1977). The regulatory GTPase cycle of turkey erythrocyte adenylate cyclase. J. Cycl. Nucl. Res. 3:393-406.

Cockroft S, Gomperts BD (1985). Role of guanine nucleotide binding protein in the activation of polyphosphoinositide phosphodiesterase. Nature 314:534-536.

Deland MC, Pak Wl (1973). Reversible temperature sensitive phototransduction mutant of *Drosophila melanogaster*. Nature New Biol. 244:184-186.

Devary O, Heichal O, Blumenfeld A, Cassel D, Suss E, Barash S, Rubinstein CT, Minke B, Selinger Z (1987). Coupling of photoexcited rhodopsin to inositol phospholipid hydrolysis in fly photoreceptors. Proc. Natl. Acad. Sci. USA 84: 6939-6943.

Eckstein F, Cassel D, Levkovitz H, Lowe M, Selinger Z (1979). Guanosine 5'-0-(2-thiodiphosphate): An inhibitor of adenylate cyclase stimulation by guanine nucleotides and fluoride ions. J. Biol. Chem. 254:9829-9834.

Fein A, Payne R, Corson DW, Berridge MJ, Irvine R (1984). Photoreceptor excitation and adaptation by inositol 1,4,5-trisphosphate. Nature 311:157-160.

Fung BKK, Stryer L (1980). Photolysed rhodopsin catalyzes the exchange of GTP for GDP in rod outer segment membranes. Proc. Natl. Acad. Sci. USA 77:2500-2504.

Hillman P, Hochstein S, Minke B (1983). Transduction in invertebrate photoreceptors: The role of pigment bistability. Physiol. Rev. 63:668-772.

Inoue H, Yoshioka T, Hotta Y (1985). A genetic study of inositol trisphosphate involvement in phototransduction using *Drosophila* mutants. Biochem. Biophys. Res. Commun. 132:513-519.

Johnson EC, Robinson PR, Lisman JE (1986). Cyclic GMP is involved in the excitation of invertebrate photoreceptors. Nature 324:468-470.

Minke B (1986). Photopigment-dependent adaptation in invertebrates: Implication for vertebrate. *In* "The Molecular Mechanism of Photoreception" (H Stieve, ed), Dahlem Konferenzen, Springer-Verlag, Berlin, pp. 241-265.

Pak WL (1979). Study of photoreceptor function using *Drosophila* mutants in neurogenetics: Genetic approaches to the nervous system (X Breakefield, ed) Elsevier North Holland, New York, pp. 67-99.

Pugh EN, Cobbs WH (1986). The visual transduction in vertebrates rods and cones: A tale of two transmitters, calcium and cyclic GMP. Vision Res. 26:1613-1643.

Saibil HR, Michel-Villaz M (1984). Squid rhodopsin and GTP-binding protein crossreact with vertebrate photoreceptor enzymes. Proc. Natl. Acad. Sci. USA 81:5111-5115.

Saibil HR (1984). A light-stimulated increase of cyclic GMP in squid photoreceptors. FEBS Lett. 168:213-216.

Stryer L (1986). Cyclic GMP cascade of vision. Ann. Rev. Neurosci. 9:87-119.

Szuts EZ, Wood SF, Reid MS, Fein A (1986). Light stimulates the rapid formation of inositol trisphosphate in squid retinas. Biochem. J. 240:929-932.

Vanderberg CA, Montal M (1984). Light-regulated phosphorylation of rhodopsin and phosphoinositides in squid photoreceptor membranes. Biochemistry 23:2347-2352.

Yoshioka T, Inoue H, Hotta Y (1984). Absence of diglyceride kinase activity in the photoreceptor cells of *Drosophila* mutants. Biochem. Biophys. Res. Commun. 119:389-395.

view it is interesting to speculate that the kinds of
proteins that have become crystallins tell us something
about the developmental origins of the lens itself. Several
crystallins are, or are related to, proteins prominently
expresed in a variety of proliferating cell types (1,21).
Conceivably the development of the lens fiber cell results
from a failure to complete a stage that many cells pass
through in normal growth and development.

## REFERENCES

1.    Wistow G, Piatigorsky J (1988). Lens Crystallins:
      Evolution and Expression of Proteins for a Highly
      Specialized Tissue Ann Rev Biochem 57:479-504
2.    Bloemendal H. (ed) (1981). Molecular and Cellular
      Biology of the Eye Lens. New York:Wiley-Interscience.
3.    Harding JJ, Crabbe MJC (1984). The Lens: Development,
      Proteins, Metabolism and Cataract. The Eye pp207-492
      New York:Academic Press.
4.    Chiesa R, Gawinowicz-Kolks MA, Spector A (1987). The
      phosphorylation of the primary gene products of
      $\alpha$-crystallin. J Biol Chem 262:1438-41.
5.    Chiesa R, Gawinowicz-Kolks MA, Kleiman NJ, Spector A
      (1987). The phosphorylation sites of the B2 chain of
      bovine $\alpha$-crystallin. Biochem Biophys Res Commun
      144:1340-7.
6.    King CR, Piatigorsky J (1983). Alternative RNA splicing
      of the murine $\alpha$A-crystallin gene: protein-coding
      information within an intron. Cell 32:707-12
7.    Ingolia TD, Craig EA (1982). Four small Drosophila heat
      shock proteins are related to each other to mammalian
      $\alpha$-crystallin. Proc Natl Acad Sci USA 79:2360-4.
8.    Nene V, Dunne DW, Johnson KS, Taylor DW, Cordingley JS
      (1986). Sequence and expression of a major egg antigen
      from Schistosoma mansoni. Homologies to heat shock
      proteins and $\alpha$-crystallins. Mol Biochem Parasitol
      21:179-88.
9.    Wistow G (1985). Domain structure and evolution in
      $\alpha$-crystallins and small heat-shock proteins. FEBS Lett
      181:1-6.
10.   Sharma KK, Olesen PR, Ortwerth BJ (1987). The binding
      and inhibition of trypsin by $\alpha$-crystallin. Biochim
      Biophys Acta 915:284-91.
11.   Driessen HP, Herbrink P, Bloemendal H, de Jong WW
      (1980). The $\beta$-crystallin Bp chain is internally

duplicated and homologous to γ-crystallin. Exp Eye Res 31:243-6.

12. Blundell T, Lindley P, Miller L, Moss D, Slingsby C, Tickle I, Turnell B, Wistow, G (1981). The molecular structure and stability of the eye lens: x-ray analysis of γ-crystallin II. Nature 289:771-7.

13. Wistow G, Slingsby C, Blundell T, Driessen H, De Jong W, Bloemendal H (1981). Eye-lens proteins: the three-dimensional structure of β-crystallin predicted from monomeric γ-crystallin. FEBS Lett 133:9-16.

14. Wistow G, Turnell B, Summers L, Slingsby C, Moss D, Miller L, Lindley P, Blundell T (1983). X-ray analysis of the eye lens protein γ-II crystallin at 1.9 A resolution. J Mol Biol 170:175-202.

15. Wistow G, Summers L, Blundell T (1985). Myxococcus xanthus spore coat protein S may have a similar structure vertebrate lens β γ-crystallins. Nature 315:771-3.

16.  Tomarev SI, Krayev AS, Skryabin KG, Bayev AA, Gause GG, Jr (1982). The nucleotide sequence of a cloned cDNA corresponding to one of th γ-crystallins from the eye lens of the frog Rana temporaria. FEBS Lett 146:314-8.

17. Crabbe MJ (1985). Partial sequence homologies between cytoskeletal proteins, c-myc, Rous sarcoma virus and adenovirus proteins, transducin, and β- and γ-crystallins. Biosci Rep 5:167-74.

18. Crabbe MJ (1985). Partial sequence homology of human myc oncogene protein to β- and γ-crystallins. FEBS Lett 181:157-9.

19. Wistow GJ, Mulders JW, de Jong WW (1987). The enzyme lactate dehydrogenase as a structural protein in avian and crocodilian lenses. Nature 326:622-4.

20. Grau UM, Trommer WE, Rossmann MG (1981). Structure of the active ternary complex of pig heart lactate dehydrogenase with S-lac-NAD at 2.7A resolution. J Mol Biol 151:289-307.

21. Wistow G, Piatigorsky J (1987). Recruitment of enzymes as lens structural proteins. Science 236:1554-6.

22. Piatigorsky J, Norman B, Jones R (1987). Conservation of δ-crystallin gene structure in ducks and chickens. J. Mol. Evol. 25:308-317.

23. Piatigorsky J, O'Brien WE, Norman BL, Kalumuk K, Wistow GJ, Borras T, Nickerson J, Wawrousek EF (1988). Gene Sharing by δ-crystallin and Argininosuccinate lyase. Proc Natl Acad Sci USA:in press.

24. Williams LA, Ding L, Horwitz J, Piatigorsky J (1985). τ-Crystallin from the turtle lens: purification and partial characterization. Exp Eye Res 40:741-9.

25. Stapel SO, de Jong WW (1983). Lamprey 48-kDa lens protein represents a novel class of crystallins FEBS Lett 162:305-9.

26. Carper D, Nishimura C, Shinohara T, Dietzschold B, Wistow G, Craft C, Kador P, Kinoshita JH (1987). Aldose reductase and rho-crystallin belongto the same protein superfamily as aldehyde reductase. FEBS Lett 220:209-13.

27. Siezen RJ, Shaw DC (1982). Physicochemical characterization of lens proteins of the squid Nototodarus gouldi and comparison with vertebrate crystallins. Biochim Biophys Acta 704:304-20.

28. Sanger F, Coulson AR, Barrel BG, Smith AJ, Roe BA (1980). Cloning in single-stranded bacteriophage as an aid to rapid DNA sequencing. J Mol Biol 143:161-178.

29. Giallongo A, Feo S, Moore R, Croce CM, Showe LC (1986). Molecular Cloning and Nucleotide Sequence of a Full-length cDNA for Human α Enolase. Proc Natl Acad Sci USA 83:6741.

Molecular Biology of the Eye: Genes, Vision,
and Ocular Disease, pages 149–158
© 1988 Alan R. Liss, Inc.

MOLECULAR EVOLUTION OF α-CRYSTALLIN
IN QUEST OF A FUNCTION[1]

W.W. de Jong, J.A.M. Leunissen, W. Hendriks, and H. Bloemendal

Department of Biochemistry, University of Nijmegen,
PO Box 9101, 6500 HB Nijmegen, The Netherlands

ABSTRACT  An analysis of the evolutionary origin and
changes of α-crystallin may shed some light on the as
yet unknown functional features of this ubiquitous and
abundant lens protein. The relationship with the small
heat-shock proteins suggests that α-crystallin perhaps
functions as a constitutive stress protein in the lens
fiber cells.  The slow rate of evolution of α-crystallin
is accelerated in higher primates, perhaps because of
positive selection, and in the blind mole rat, as a
result of loss of functional constraints. Notable is the
extreme avoidance of changes in charge during the evolution of α-crystallin.


WHAT, IF ANYTHING, ARE CRYSTALLINS?

The designation of crystallins as lens-specific proteins
has become obsolete after the recent findings that most "crystallins" are in fact closely related or even identical to a
variety of enzymes (1).  However, the crystallins can opera-
tionally still be defined as those proteins that are abundant
in the cytoplasm of lens fiber cells. In the lens they probably serve mainly a structural role, to maintain the tran-
sparancy and proper refraction of this organ. But if such
diverse proteins as lactate dehydrogenase and argininosuccinate lyase can function as crystallins in different
species, what then are the structural and functional proper-

---

[1]This work was supported by the Netherlands Foundation
for Chemical Research (SON) and the Netherlands Organization for Scientific Research (NWO).

ties required for this role? Is there any advantage for
herons to have 23% LDH-B4 (ε-crystallin) in their lenses and
for  the huge amount of active argininosuccinate lyase (δ-
crystallin) in duck lenses?  Would any protein that has sufficient structural stability and can be closely packed at
high concentrations be suitable as a lens protein? Or are
there additional, more subtle, structural or biological properties required? The search for such properties will here be
illustrated in the case of α-crystallin.

## INTRODUCING α-CRYSTALLIN

α-Crystallin is, together with the β-crystallins, the
most ubiquitous vertebrate lens protein (for reviews see refs
2-4).  It only seems to be lacking in many bony fishes.  It
is most abundant in mammalian lenses, where it reaches levels
of up to 50% of total lens protein in certain species.

α-Crystallin forms aggregates of 300-800 kDa (varying
between species), which are composed of two types of polypeptides, αA and αB, which are partially phosphorylated (5).
Both are approximately 175 residues in length and have about
58% sequence homology.  The αA and αB subunits are encoded by
single-copy genes which, in man, are located on different
chromosomes. The gene structures of αA and αB, and the regulation of their expression, are well-characterized in several
species (6).  Rodents (7) and some other mammals (8) have a
minor αA chain ($\alpha A^{ins}$) that is identical to normal αA with an
insertion of 23 residues. This is the result of alternative
splicing of the primary αA gene transcript (7).

The primary structures of αA, and to a lesser extent αB,
have been determined in many vertebrate species, which has
provided much information about their evolutionary history
(9). α-Crystallin is mainly composed of β-pleated sheet
structure, but the tertiary structure is not known (10). The
quaternary structure is obviously complex, and a matter of
continuing debate (11, 12).

α-Crystallin is related to the ubiquitous eukaryotic
small heat-shock proteins (HSPs) (13). It has been proposed
that α-crystallin might therefore share high thermodynamic
stability with the HSPs, a favorable property in the lens en-
vironment (14).  Alternatively, α-crystallin might have, like
the HSPs, a homeostatic, protective role against the many
forms of stress during the lifetime of the lens. α-Crystallin
not only has the tendency for self-association but does also
bind to actin (15) and to the plasma membrane (16).  Such as-

Molecular Biology of the Eye: Genes, Vision,
and Ocular Disease, pages 159–168
© 1988 Alan R. Liss, Inc.

# HUMAN INTERSTITIAL RETINOL-BINDING PROTEIN: CLONING, STRUCTURE, EVOLUTION AND MOLECULAR GENETICS[1]

C. David Bridges and Shao-Ling Fong

Department of Biological Sciences, Purdue University, West Lafayette, Indiana 47907

ABSTRACT   This report discusses and describes the properties, distribution, biosynthesis, expression, cloning, primary and predicted secondary structure, chromosomal location and molecular genetics of human interstitial retinol-binding protein (IRBP).

## INTRODUCTION

IRBP is the most abundant protein constituent of the interphotoreceptor matrix, and its discovery has prompted an enormous surge of interest in this area (1-10).   IRBP has been purified and characterized from human, bovine, monkey, rat and frog eyes.   Bovine IRBP has an apparent molecular mass of 140-144k on SDS poly-acrylamide gels.   The molecule appears to be elongated, with an axial ratio of about 8:1 (1,2,8).   It consists of a single polypeptide chain that binds two molecules of 11-<u>cis</u> or all-<u>trans</u> retinol.   Bovine IRBP is a glycoprotein containing 8.4% of carbohydrate, the N-linked oligosaccharide chains consisting of 40% mono-sialylated hybrid-type, the remaining 60% being

---
[1]Supported by the Retina Research Foundation of Houston, Knights Templar Eye Foundation and the National Eye Institute (National Institutes of Health).

di-, tri- and tetrasialylated complex biantennary structures (3,11).

IRBP has been identified in all vertebrate classes (9). With the exception of the teleosts, its average $M_r$ is 134.2k. In the teleosts the $M_r$ of IRBP is half this value, namely 67.6k. IRBP-like proteins that cross-react with anti-frog IRBP antibodies and have an average $M_r$ of 132.4k have been observed in six species of cephalopods (12).

IRBP is synthesized and secreted by the photoreceptors (6,10,13). During retinal development in mice, rats and humans it is first detected during differentiation of the inner segments (6,10,14). IRBP and IRBP mRNA transcripts have been demonstrated in retinoblastoma tumors and in a number of established retinoblastoma cell lines (15-17). The protein also appears to be expressed in the mammalian pineal (18-20), and possibly in other parts of the brain (20).

IRBP may be involved in the transport of a number of hydrophobic compounds through the inter-photoreceptor matrix. Fatty acids are one example (21). However, because its endogenous ligands are 11-_cis_ retinal, 11-_cis_ retinol and all-_trans_ retinol, it is likely that IRBP serves as an important link between retinol isomerase in the pigment epithelium (22-24) and the visual pigments in the photoreceptors. In darkness, frog IRBP contains the 11-_cis_ isomers of retinal and retinol together with a trace of all-_trans_ retinol. In the early stages of strong light-adaptation, there is an increase in the proportion of all-_trans_ retinol coupled with a drop in the 11-_cis_ retinal (25). These observations are consistent with the idea that during the visual cycle IRBP delivers 11-_cis_ retinal for rhodopsin regeneration, and transports all-_trans_ retinol from bleached rod outer segments to the pigment epithelium.

Because of the importance of IRBP in the physiological process of light- and dark-adaptation, and because of its possible role in the transport of compounds other than retinoids through the interphotoreceptor matrix, we wish to understand the structure of its molecule and the regulation of its gene.

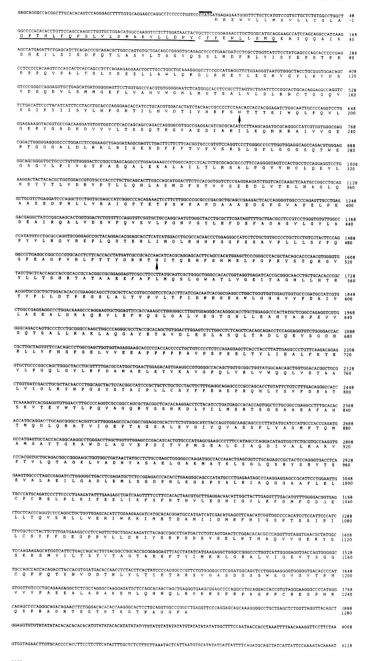

Fig 1   cDNA and amino acid sequence of human IRBP.

### AMINO ACID SEQUENCE OF HUMAN IRBP
### FROM ITS FULL-LENGTH CLONED cDNA

We first isolated a bovine cDNA probe using antibody screening of a retina cDNA library in the expression vector lambda gt11 (26). The bovine probe was then used to obtain a 2,184bp human IRBP cDNA (H.4 IRBP) from a human retina library in lambda gt10 (27). This work was made possible by generous gifts of retina cDNA libraries from Drs Gobind Khorana, Daniel Oprian and Jeremy Nathans.

The probe H.4 IRBP enabled us to isolate 5 overlapping clones encoding the full sequence of human IRBP. A 17kb genomic DNA clone encompassing the full coding region and putative regulatory sequences upstream from the transcription initiation site has also been obtained with this probe.

The 4,223-base human IRBP cDNA sequence is displayed in Fig 1. The 3' untranslated sequence extends for 295 nucleotides, but does not contain a poly(A) tract. It is likely that there is an extensive 3' untranslated segment as reported for bovine IRBP cDNA (26). An open reading frame encodes the N-terminal sequence of human IRBP (underlined), and predicts a protein of 1,262 amino acids with an $M_r$ of 136,600. Two putative N-linked glycosylation sites are arrowed. The sequence can be aligned with 87% identity with the amino acid sequences of 31 tryptic peptides from bovine IRBP. The translated sequence predicts a 16-residue signal peptide rich in Leu and Val and with a high alpha-helix probability.

### EVIDENCE FOR GENE DUPLICATION IN THE
### EVOLUTION OF HUMAN IRBP

As shown in Fig 2, the protein sequence of human IRBP contains four duplicated segments (302-310 amino acids long) with 33-38% identity. From the similarity of the bovine and human sequences, which diverged about 80mya, it is probable that IRBP evolved by several gene duplications that occurred 600 - 800mya, before emergence of the vertebrates. In conformity with this suggestion,

```
              +                               +   + +
     GPTHLFQPSLVLDMAKVLLDNYCFPENLLGMQEAIQQAIKSHEILSISDPQTLASVLTAGVQSSL
308  ALPGVVHCLQEVLKDYYT     LVDRVPTLLQHLASMDFSTVVSEEDLVTKLNAGLQAAS
618  SLGALVEGTGHLLEAHYARPEVVGQTSALLRAKLAQGAYRTAVDLESLASQLTADLQEVS
919  KVPTVLQTAGKLVADNYASAELGAKMATKLSG  LQSRYSRVTSEVALAEILGADLEMLS


      +   +                                         ++     +
66   NDPRLVISYEPSTPEPP              PQVPALTSLSEEELLAWLQRGLRHEVLEGNVG
364  EDPRLLVRAIGPTETPSWPAPDAAAEDSPGVAPELPEDEAIRQALVDSVFQVSVLPGNVG
678  GDHRLLVFHSPGELVVEEAPP          PPPAVPSPEELTYLIEAL    FKTEVLPGQLG
977  GDPHLKGSPYALRIAQGGAAF          LELCPCRSLPLKIFEELIKFSFHTNVLEDNIG


     +++ ++                          +    + +  +      +  ++
115  YLRVDSVPGQEVLSMMGEFLVAHVWGNLMGTSALVLDLRHCTGGQVSGIPYIISYLH PG
424  YLRFDSFADASVLGVLAPYVLRQVREPLQDTEHLIMDLRHNPGGPSSAVPLLLSYFQGPE
728  YLRFDAMAELETVKAVGPQLVRLVWQQLVDTAALVIDLRYNPGSYSTAIPLLCSYFFEAE
1030 YLRFDMFGDGELLTQVSRLLVEHIWKKIMHTDAMIIDMRFNIGGPTSSIPILCSYFFDEG


         +         +       + ++      + +      ++
174  NTILHVDTIYNRPSNTTTEIWQLPQVLGERYGADKDVVVLTSSQTRGVAEDIAHILKQMR
484  AGPVHLFTTYDRRTNITQEHFSHMELPGPRYSTQRGVYLLTSHRTATAAEEFAFLMQSLG
788  P RQHLYSVFDRATSKVTEVWTLPQVAGQRYGSHKDLYILMSHTSGSAAEAFAHTMQDLQ
1090 P PVLLDKIYSRPDDSVSELWTHAQVVGERYGSKKSMVILTSTVTAGTAEEFTYIMKRLG


      +   ++   + +  +
234  RAIVVGERTGGGALDLRKLRIGESDFFFTVPVSRSLGPLGGGSQTWEGSGVLPCVGTPAE
544  WATLVGEITAGNLLHHTRTVPLLDTPEGSLALTVPVLTFIDNHGEAWLGGGVVPDAIVLAE
847  RATVIGEPTAGGALSVGIYQVASSPL   YASMPTQMAMSATTGKAWDLAGVEPDITVPMS
1149 RALVIGEVTSGGCQPPQTYHVDDTNL   YLTIPTARSVGASDGSSWEGVGVTPHVVVPAE


      ++  +
294  QALEKALAILTLRS
604  EALDKAQEVLEFHQ
905  EALSIAQDIVALRA
1207 EALARAKEMLQHNQLRVKRSPRPAGPPCREGPHRQSPRADRTSGTHTKGTPAGGPA
```

Fig 2  Internal homology of human IRBP protein, demonstrated by optimal alignment of the protein sequences corresponding to the four homology domains. The first residue is the N-terminal of the mature protein.

we have recently described IRBP-like proteins in the eyes of cephalopods (12).

## PREDICTED SECONDARY STRUCTURE OF HUMAN IRBP

We have identified several hydrophobic regions near the centers of the four homology domains. They may form folding structures that create two retinol-binding clefts (27). The secondary structure analysis predicts 39% alpha-helix, 41% beta-sheet, 8% reverse turn, and 13% random coil. The beginning of each homology domain has a high alpha-helix probability.

## IRBP mRNA AND SIZE OF IN VITRO TRANSLATED PROTEIN

On Northern blots, IRBP cDNA probes hybridize with a 5.2kb polyadenylated RNA from human retina and to a 6.3kb polyadenylated RNA from bovine retina (Fig 3; 27). A large segment of this RNA seems to be untranslated. When bovine retina polyadenylated RNA is translated using a rabbit reticulocyte lysate system, a protein is formed that is immunoprecipitable with antibovine IRBP antibodies and is similar in size to non-glycosylated, mature IRBP (26).

## RESTRICTION FRAGMENT LENGTH POLYMORPHISMS RECOGNIZED BY THE cDNA PROBE H.4 IRBP

The restriction enzyme Bgl II (AGATCT) identifies a 2-allele polymorphism with bands at 6.3 and 4.3 kb (Fig 4). The frequency of the 6.3kb allele is 0.85 (28). Polymorphisms are also detected with StyI (CCA$^T_A$TGG; 2.3, 1.95kb) and MspI (CCGG; 3.15, 2.7kb; ref. 29).

## THE STRUCTURAL GENE FOR IRBP MAPS TO CHROMOSOME 10

Using the probe H.4 IRBP we probed BglI-digested DNA from a panel of 29 rodent-human somatic cell hybrids (Fig 5) and carried out in situ hybridization to human chromosomes at metaphase, permitting assignment of the IRBP gene to chromosome 10 with a regional localization close to the centromere (p11.2→q11.2; ref. 27).

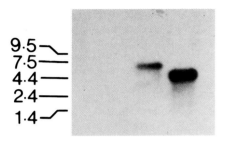

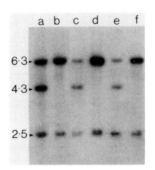

Fig 3 Northern blot
analysis of bovine and
human IRBP mRNAs. $^{32}$P-
labeled (nick-translated)
H.4 IRBP was hybridized
to polyadenylated RNA
from bovine (left) and
human (right) retinas.

Fig 4 Bgl II RFLP
recognized by H.4
IRBP. Southern blot
analysis of Bgl II
digests of DNA from
a 6-member family.
Father, lane a;
mother, lane b;
offspring, lanes
c,d,e,f.

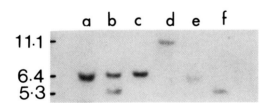

Fig 5 Chromosomal localization of human IRBP.
Southern blot analysis of Chinese hamster x human
hybrid cell DNAs using H.4 IRBP as a probe and
restriction digestion with Bgl I. Lanes d, e
and f contain mouse, Chinese hamster and human
DNA, respectively. A variety of chromosomes are
present in the hybrids in lanes a, b and c.
Chromosome 10 is present in the hybrid in lane b.

## H.4 IRBP IS A LINKED GENETIC MARKER FOR MULTIPLE ENDOCRINE NEOPLASIA TYPE 2A ON CHROMOSOME 10

Multiple endocrine neoplasia type 2A is an autosomal dominantly inherited cancer syndrome characterized by medullary carcinoma of the thyroid, phaeochromocytoma and hyperparathyroidism. Using H.4 IRBP, we have established linkage between the locus defined by IRBP and the MEN2A locus with a maximum lod score of 3.88 at a recombination fraction of 0.04 (30). Simpson et al. simultaneously reported linkage with MEN2A with the same probe (31).

## CONCLUSION

The availability of full-length cDNA for human IRBP and of genomic DNA clones containing sequences upstream from the transcription initiation site now permits studies on the IRBP gene and its regulation. Additionally, the IRBP probes that are currently being used worldwide in linkage studies for diseases that map to chromosome 10 are also proving valuable in determining whether IRBP is a candidate gene in certain types of retinitis pigmentosa.

## REFERENCES

1.    Adler, A.J., Evans C.D., and Stafford III, W.F. (1985) J. Biol. Chem. 260, 4850-4855.
2.    Adler, A.J., Stafford III, W.F., and Slayter, H.S. (1987) J. Biol. Chem. 262, 13198-13203.
3.    Taniguchi, T., Adler, A.J., Mizuochi, T., Kochibe, N., and Kobata, A. (1986) J. Biol. Chem. 261, 1730-1736.
4.    Fong, S.-L., Liou, G.I., Landers, R.A., Alvarez, R.A., and Bridges, C.D.B. (1984) J. Biol. Chem. 259, 6534-6542.
5.    Fong, S.-L., Liou, G.I., Landers, R.A., Alvarez, R.A., Gonzalez-Fernandez, F., Glazebrook, P.A., Lam, D.M.K., and Bridges, C.D.B. (1984) J. Neurochem. 42, 1667-1676.
6.    Gonzalez-Fernandez, F., Landers, R.A., Glazebrook, P.A., Fong, S-L., Liou, G.I.,

Lam, D.M.K. and Bridges, C.D.B. (1984) J. Cell Biol. 99, 2092-2098.

7. Redmond, T.M., Wiggert, B., Robey, F.A., Nguyen, N.Y., Lewis, M.S., Lee, L., and Chader, G.J. (1985) Biochem. 24, 787-793.

8. Saari, J.C., Teller, D.C., Crabb, J.W., and Bredberg, L. (1985) J. Biol. Chem. 260, 195-201.

9. Bridges, C.D.B., Liou, G.I., Alvarez, R.A., Landers, R.A., Landry Jr., A.M., and Fong, S-L. (1986) J. Exp. Zool. 239, 335-346.

10. Carter-Dawson, L., Alvarez, R.A., Fong, S-L., Liou, G.I., Sperling, H.G., and Bridges, C.D.B. (1986) Dev. Biol. 116, 431-438.

11. Fong, S.-L., Irimura, T., Landers, R.A., and Bridges, C.D.B. (1985) In The Interphotoreceptor Matrix in Health and Disease. Progress in Clinical and Biological Research, Vol. 190, Bridges, C.D.B., and Adler, A.J., Eds., Alan R. Liss, New York, 111-128.

12. Fong, S.-L., Lee, P.G., Ozaki, K., Hara, R., Hara, T., and Bridges, C.D.B. (1988) Vision Research, 28, 563-574.

13. van Veen, T., Katial, A., Shinohara, T., Barrett, D.J., Wiggert, B., Chader, G.J., and Nickerson, J.M. (1986) FEBS Letters 208, 133-137.

14. Johnson, A.T., Kretzer, F.L., Hittner, H.M., Glazebrook, P.A., Bridges, C.D.B., and Lam, D.M.K. (1985) J. Comp. Neurol., 233, 497-505.

15. Fong, S.-L., Balakier, H., Canton, M., Bridges, C.D.B., and Gallie, B. (1988). Cancer Res., 48, 1124-1128.

16. Bridges, C.D.B., Fong, S.-L., Landers, R.A., Liou, G.I., and Font, R.L. (1985). Neurochem. Int., 7, 875-881.

17. Kyritsis, A.P., Wiggert, B., Lee, L., and Chader, G.J. (1985) J. Cell Physiol., 124, 233-239.

18. Bridges, C.D.B., Landers, R.A., Fong, S.-L., and Liou, G.I. (1986) In Pineal and Retinal Relationships, O'Brien, P.J., and Klein, D.C., Eds., Academic Press, New York, 383-400.

19. Chader, G.J., Wiggert, B., Gery, I., Lee, L., Redmond, T.M., Kuwabara, T., and Rodrigues, M.M. (1986) In Pineal and Retinal Relationships, O'Brien, P.J., and Klein, D.C., Eds., Academic Press, New York, 363-382.

20. Bridges, C.D.B., Foster, R.G., Landers, R.A., and Fong, S.-L. (1987) Vision Res., 27, 2049-2060.

21. Bazan, N.G., Reddy, T.S., Redmond, T.M., Wiggert, B., and Chader, G.J. (1985) J. Biol. Chem., 260, 13677-13680.

22. Timmers, A.M.M. (1987) Ph.D. Thesis, Univ. of Nijmegen.

23. Bernstein, P.S., Law, W.C., and Rando, R.R. (1987) Proc. Natl. Acad. Sci. USA 84, 1849-1853.

24. Bridges, C.D.B., and Alvarez, R.A. (1987) Science 236, 1678-1680.

25. Lin, Z.S., Alvarez, R.A., and Bridges, C.D.B. (1987) Invest. Ophthal. & Vis.Sci., 28 (Abstr.), 252.

26. Liou, G.I., Fong, S-L., Beattie, W.G., Cook, R.G., Leone, J., Landers, R.A., Alvarez, R.A., Wang, C., Li, Y., and Bridges, C.D.B. (1986) Vision Res. 26, 1645-1654.

27. Liou, G.I., Fong, S.-L., Gosden, J., van Tuinen, P., Ledbetter, D.H., Christie, S., Rout, D., Bhattacharya, S., Cook, R.G., Li, Y., Wang, C., and Bridges, C.D.B. (1987) Somatic Cell. & Mol. Genet. 13, 315-323.

28. Liou, G.I., Li, Y., Wang, C., Fong, S.-L., Bhattacharya, S., and Bridges, C.D.B. (1987) Nucleic Acids Res., 15, 3196, 1987.

29. Chin, K.S., Mathew, C.G.P., Fong, S.L., Bridges, C.D.B. and B.A.J. Ponder (1988) Nucleic Acids Res. 16, 1645.

30. Mathew, C.G.P., Chin, K.S., Easton, D.F., Thorpe, K., Carter, C., Liou, G.I., Fong, S.-L., Bridges, C.D.B., Haak, H., Nieuwenhuijzen Kruseman, A.C., Schifter, S., Hansen, H., Telenius, H., Telenius-Berg, M., and Ponder, B.A.J. (1987) Nature, (London), 328, 527-528.

31. Simpson, N.E. et al. (1987). Nature 328, 528-530.

Molecular Biology of the Eye: Genes, Vision,
and Ocular Disease, pages 169–178
© 1988 Alan R. Liss, Inc.

## THE COLLAGEN GENE FAMILY AND ITS EVOLUTION

Gabriel Vogeli, Paul S. Kaytes and Linda Wood

Molecular Biology Research, The Upjohn Company
Kalamazoo, Michigan 49001

**ABSTRACT** A landmark in the evolution of higher
eukaryotes was the appearance of collagenous proteins in
the extracellular matrix. Characteristic for all the
collagen proteins is the triple helix formed by Gly-X-Y
repeats; many other repetitive elements are found within
the protein and the gene and are essential for the
function and thus for the evolution of collagens. We
propose here that repetitive clusters of hydrophobic/
hydrophilic amino acids found along type IV collagens
are responsible for the assembly of these collagens into
the sheets of the basement membrane.
  We show here that introns stabilize genes with
repetitive coding sequences against deletion mutations
and conclude that introns thus can control the "speed of
evolution". To demonstrate this, we present DNA
sequence data for the murine type I collagen and compare
it with the sequences from different vertebrate species.
The higher homology in the triple helical domains
reflects a lower mutation rate throughout evolution. We
explain this lower mutation rate by finding that introns
reduce the probability of deletion mutations 10 fold.

## 1) INTRODUCTION

The dictum of molecular biology that a mouse or an
elephant are the same in a test-tube, stems from the finding
that: 1) many of the biochemical reactions occurring in these
organisms are very similar and 2) the variations found
between the biochemical reactions usually do not account for
the striking differences between a mouse and an elephant.
Our contention is that the major divergence between a mouse
and an elephant arise from changes in the amount and the

arrangement of extracellular matrix molecules.  Consequently,
we argue that the forces of evolutionary selection have as
their prime targets the extracellular matrix.  An intense
evolutionary history has thus left its mark on these genes
and their regulatory elements.  The study of genes
synthesizing the extracellular matrix is aimed at answering
the following questions (For reviews see Ref. 1): 1) How is
the growth of tissues and organs controlled during normal
development, during regeneration and malignancies?  2) How
can collagen over production (2,3) be controlled during
fibrosis and diabetes?  3) Can we change the course of human
genetic diseases (4) or are we restricted to genetic
counseling?

The collagens (for a review see Ref. 1), composed of
three subunits with a typical Gly-X-Y amino acid repeat, are
one of the key elements in extracellular matrix proteins and
make up 30 % of all animal proteins.  Their highest concentration is in the vertebrate skeleton, the skin, and the
eye. To create, for example, the physical shape of the
vertebrate eye as an optical apparatus, the activity of the
collagen genes must be controlled very precisely in many
tissues during embryonal development.  Some understanding of
the evolution and the control of collagen synthesis has come
from the analysis of the collagen genes (5,6,7,8,9).

One of the salient features of the collagens is the
repetitive structure of the proteins, of the DNAs and of the
genes (5,6).  Here we examine in detail two repetitive
patterns:  First, we analyze hydrophilic/hydrophobic amino
acid clusters along the molecules type IV collagen.  From
this analysis we propose a model of basement membrane
assembly that explains the sheet-like structure of the
basement membranes and some of its functions.  Second, by
analyzing the repetitive DNA sequences coding for type I
collagen that are interrupted in the gene by introns (6), we
uncover an evolutionary explanation to the enigma of why the
collagen genes have maintained 50 introns (5) during their
evolution.

## 2) BASEMENT MEMBRANES AND TYPE IV COLLAGEN.

A landmark in the evolution of multicellular animals was
the assembly of collagenous proteins into basement membranes,
structures that separate compartments of cells with different
functions (11).  Since the advent of the coelenterates (12),
cells in contact with a basement membrane have been able to

From published data, we find that there are 14 introns
per 1000 bp of coding sequences in the helical region (7), but
only 6 introns per 1000 bp of coding sequences for the
terminal peptide domains (7,28). Hence we argue that the
number of introns may have an effect on the evolutionary
stability of the domains of collagen.

**The Function of Introns: Conservation of the Gly-X-Y repeat.**

As we have shown above, the amino acid sequences and the
DNA sequences within the helical portion of the type I
collagen genes are more conserved than in the terminal
propeptides. In contrast, one would expect that helical
regions with nucleotide repeats that reflect the Gly-X-Y
repeat are subject to a high rate of deletion mutation. High
rates of deletions occur between repeated sequences during DNA
replication in E.coli (22) and in humans (23).

To search for repetitive DNA sequences within the Gly-X-Y
repeats, we used published DNA sequences for exons from the
chick alpha 2 type I collagen gene (6, 7, 8) and compared them
with repeats found in the human gamma globin gene (25). The
analysis was done in two ways. First, the DNA sequence from
the exons was spliced together into one sequence and the total
number of repeats (10 ntd long with a similarity of 80 %) was
determined by the program of Queen and Korn (26). Second, the
analysis was done for each exon separately and then the
numbers from each individual exon were added.

### TABLE 1
**POSSIBLE DELETION SITES PER 100 BASE PAIRS OF CODING SEQUENCE
IN GENES WITH OR WITHOUT INTRONS:**

| | Without Introns | | With Introns | |
|---|---|---|---|---|
| | COLLAGEN | GLOBIN | COLLAGEN | GLOBIN |
| Repeats | 60 [677] | 4 [20] | 4 [44] | 1 [6] |

The total number of possible deletion sites (23) found by the
computer program (26) is in brackets. **COLLAGEN:** 17 exons
(6,7,8) out of 51 with a total of 1134 ntd were analyzed.
**GLOBIN:** 3 exons (25) out of 3 exons with a total of 441 ntd
were analyzed.

Table 1 shows that collagen genes "without introns" have a 10 fold higher number of possible deletion sites (60 sites) compared to the same collagen genes with introns (4 sites). In contrast gammaglobin genes with or "without introns" both have a low deletion site density (4 versus 1 site).

From this analysis we conclude that introns reduce by 10 fold the density of possible deletion sites and that introns stabilize genes with repetitive coding sequences. Hence, we argue that intron number can control the "speed of evolution" and that the introns have been maintained by the evolutionary pressure to keep the collagen gene intact.

## 4) CONCLUSIONS

The evolution of animals is driven by the members of the collagen gene family. Short Gly-X-Y repeats have been assembled into the collagen genes, genes that have been duplicated to provide the tissue and organ structure of the vertebrate body. To allow for the independent control of these different collagens, we postulate that the control and regulatory elements also underwent gene duplication and are thus also related to each other.

## REFERENCES

1.  Piez KA and Reddi AH (Edts.) (1984). Extracellular matrix biochemistry. Elsevier Science Publishing Co.,Inc., New York.
2.  Pierce RA, Glaug MR, Greco RS, Mackenzie JW, Boyd CD, Deak SB (1987). Increased procollagen mRNA levels in carbon tetrachloride-induced liver fibrosis in rats. J Biol Chem 262:1652.
3.  Martinez-Hernandez A, and Amenta PS (1984). The basement membrane in Pathology. Lab Invest 48:656.
4.  Tsipouras P, Ramirez F (1987). Genetic disorders of collagen. J Med Genet 24:2.
5.  Vogeli G, Ohkubo H, Avvedimento VE, Sullivan M, Yamada Y, Mudryj M, Pastan I, deCrombrugghe B (1981). A repetitive structure in the chick alpha 2 collagen gene. Cold Spring Harbour Symposium XLV:777. .

6.  Yamada Y, Avvedimento VE, Mudryj M, Ohkubo H. Vogeli G, Irani M, Pastan I, de Crombrugghe B (1980) The collagen gene: evidence for its evolutionary assembly by amplification of a DNA segment containing an exon of 54 bp. Cell 22:887.
7.  Wozney J, Hanahan D, Tate V, Boedtker H, Doty P (1981). Structure of the pro alpha 2 (I) collagen gene. Nature 294:129.
8.  Tate VE, Iner HM, Boedtker H and Doty P (1983). Chick pro alpha 2 (I) collagen gene: exon location and coding potential for the prepropeptide. Nucl Acids Res 11: 91.
9.  Yamada Y, Mudryj M, and de Crombrugghe B (1983). A uniquely conserved regulatory signal is found around the translation initiation site in three different collagen genes. J Biol Chem 258:14914.
10. Vogeli G, Horn E, Carter J, and Kaytes PS (1986) Proposed alignment of helical interruptions in the two subunits of the basement membrane (type IV) collagen. FEBS Lett 206:29.
11. Laurie GW, and Leblond CP (1983) What is known of the production of basement membrane components. J Histochem Cytochem 31:159.
12. Day RM, Lenhoff HM (1981) Hydra mesoglea: a model for investigating epithelial cell basement membrane interactions. Science 211:291.
13. Timpl R, Wiedemann H, Van Delden V, Furthmayr H, and Kuhn K (1981). A network model for the organization of type IV collagen molecules in basement membranes. Eur J Biochem 120:203.
14. Yurchenco PD, and Furthmayr H (1984). Self-assembly of basement membrane collagen. Biochem. 23:1839.
15. Wood L, Theriault N and Vogeli G (1988). cDNA clones completing the nucleotide and derived amino acid sequence of the alpha 1 chain of basement membrane (type IV) collagen from mouse. FEBS Lett 227:5.
16. Kaytes PS, Theriault NY, Vogeli G (1987). Homologies between the non-collagenous C-terminal (NC1) globular domains of the alpha 1 and alpha 2 subunits of type-IV collagen. Gene 54:141.
17. Kyte J, and Doolittle RF (1982). A simple method for displaying the hydropathic character of a protein. J Mol Biol 157:105. Program from Lipman DJ, Mathematical Research Branch, NIADDK, NIH.

18. Nath P, Laurent M, Horn E, Sobel ME, Zon G, Vogeli G (1986) Isolation of an alpha 1 type-IV collagen cDNA clone using a synthetic oligodeoxynucleotide. Gene 43:301.

19. Harbers K, Kuehn M, Delius H, and Jaenisch R (1984). Insertion of retrovirus into the first intron of alpha 1 (I) collagen gene leads to embryonic lethal mutation in mice. Proc Nat Acad Sci USA 81:1504.

20. Chu M, DeWet W, Bernard M, Ding J, Morabito M, Myers J, Willimas C, Ramirez F (1984) Human pro alpha 1 (I) collagen gene structure reveals evolutionary conservation of a pattern of introns and exons. Nature 310:337.

21. Bernard MP, Chu M, Meyers JC, Ramirez F, Eikenberry EF and Prockop DJ (1983). Nucleotide sequences of complementary deoxyribonucleic acids for the pro alpha 1 chain of human type I procollagen. Statistical evaluation of structures that are conserved during evolution. Biochem 22:5213.

22. Dixit AN, Seyer JM, and Kang AH (1977). Covalent structure of Collagen: Amino acid sequence of chymotryptic peptides from the carboxyl-terminal region of alpha 2-CB3 of chick-skin collagen. J Biochem 81:599.

23. Farabough PJ, Schmeissner U, Hofer M and Miller JH (1978). Genetic studies of the lac repressor. VII On the molecular nature of spontaneous hotspots in the lacI gene of Escherichia coli. J Mol Biol 126:847

24. Efstratiadis A, Posakony JW, Maniatis T, Lawn RM, O'Connell C, Spritz RA, DeRiel JK, Forget BG, Weissman SM, Slightom JL, Blechl AE, Smithies O, Baralle FE, Shoulders CC, Proudfoot NJ (1980). The structure and evolution of the human beta-globin gene family. Cell 21:653.

25. Slightom JL, Blechl AE and Smithies O (1980). Human fetal G gamma- and A gamma-globin genes: complete nucleotide sequences suggest that DNA can be exchanged between these duplicated genes. Cell 21:627.

26. Queen CL, and Korn LJ (1980) Computer analysis of nucleic acids and proteins. Methods of Enzym, Academic press, Edts Grossman L and Moldave K. 65:595.

27. Finer MH, Boedtker H and Doty P (1987) Construction and characterization of cDNA clones encoding the 5' end of the chick pro alpha 1(I) collagen mRNA. Gene 56:71.

28. Vogeli G, Avvedimento EV, Sullivan M, Maizel JV Jr, Lozano G, Adams SL, Pastan I, de Crombrugghe B (1980). Isolation and characterization of genomic DNA coding for alpha 2 type I collagen. Nucl Acids Res 8:1823.

**Molecular Biology of the Eye: Genes, Vision, and Ocular Disease, pages 179-187**
© **1988 Alan R. Liss, Inc.**

AN INTRODUCTION TO CRYSTALLIN GENE EXPRESSION

Joram Piatigorsky, John F. Klement, Robert A. Dubin,
H. John Roth, Eric F. Wawrousek, Charlotte A. Peterson,
Teresa Borras, George Thomas and Ana B. Chepelinsky.

Laboratory of Molecular and Developmental Biology,
National Eye Institute, Bethesda, MD 20892

ABSTRACT  Now that many of the crystallin genes have
been cloned and sequenced attention is being directed
to explaining their tissue-specific, temporal and
spatial regulation in the lens.  The 5' flanking
sequence of many crystallin genes contain regulatory
elements controlling their expression.  Gel retardation
and DNAse I protection experiments provide evidence
that numerous factors interact with these regulatory
elements to promote transcription.

INTRODUCTION

The crystallins are an attractive system for the study
of differential gene expression since they constitute 80-90%
of the soluble protein of the eye lens and are thus easily
identified markers for lens differentiation (1).  The
crystallins are composed of several families of soluble
proteins, the most common of which are the $\alpha$-, $\beta$-, $\gamma$- and $\delta$-
crystallins (2).  Each crystallin family contains several
related polypeptides.  The crystallins are found principally
in the lens, however low level expression of some
crystallins does occur elsewhere.  For example, $\delta$-crystallin
is the most abundant protein in the embryonic lenses of
birds and reptiles (3), but low amounts are also found in
other tissues (2,4).  The reason for the non-lenticular
expression of $\delta$-crystallin is probably the fact that it is
homologous to argininosuccinate lyase (5) and indeed appears
to share the gene for this metabolic enzyme (6).
Understanding crystallin gene expression, then, involves
explaining the preferential, high-level activity in the lens
and, at least in some cases, the low level activity in other
tissues.

In addition to their preferential expression in the
lens, the different crystallin polypeptides are also
temporally regulated during development (1,7).
Interestingly, the order of appearance of the different
crystallins is species-dependent, with α-crystallin
appearing first in the mouse, β-crystallin first in the frog
and δ-crystallin first in the chicken (see 7). Not only is
there a difference in the temporal regulation of the various
classes of the crystallins, there also are differences in
the order of appearance of the individual crystallin
polypeptides within the classes (8).   We may anticipate in
view of this complexity that multiple cis- and trans-acting
regulatory elements are used to control the expression of
these highly specialized genes encoding
structural/enzymatic proteins.


RESULTS AND DISCUSSION

5' Regulatory Sequences

The use of reporter genes has revealed the presence of
DNA sequences flanking the 5' end of crystallin genes which
play a central role in their regulation.   We have used the
bacterial chloramphenicol acetyltransferase (CAT) gene in
the pSVO-CAT vector (9) to test for crystallin gene
regulatory sequences.   This vector includes polyadenylation
and splicing signals of the SV40 early region.   Initially we
showed that 366 base pairs (bp) of 5' flanking and 46 bp of
exon 1 of the murine αA-crystallin gene are able to drive
the CAT gene in explanted epithelia from embryonic chicken
lenses but not in primary cultures of muscle fibroblasts
from the embryos (10).   By contrast, 88 bp of 5' flanking
sequence did not promote CAT gene expression in the lens
explants.   In collaborative experiments, we showed that 171
bp of 5' flanking sequence of the murine γ2-crystallin gene
are also able to promote CAT gene expression in the
embryonic chicken lens epithelial explants in a tissue-
specific manner (11).   Subsequent experiments with
transgenic mice established the presence of a lens-specific
regulatory sequence at the 5' end of the murine αA-(12) and
γ2-(13) crystallin genes.
Ongoing experiments in our laboratory (J. F. Klement)
on the chicken αA-crystallin gene have defined a different
regulatory sequence than the one in the mouse.   In the case
of the chicken gene, the sequence between position number

-162 and -121 contains one or more key control elements for gene expression; in the mouse gene there are two interacting control elements located between positions -111 and -60 (14). It is interesting that the chicken 5' flanking sequence is quite different from that found in the mouse gene. Perhaps the difference in the regulatory sequences between the chicken and mouse αA-crystallin genes is related to the difference in their temporal regulation.

We have also obtained evidence for negative regulatory elements in the 5' region of crystallin genes. Transfection of lens explants with a pSVO-CAT vector containing 603 bp of 5' flanking sequence of the chicken δ1-crystallin gene gave approximately 20 times less CAT activity than a similar construct containing only 120 bp of 5' flanking sequence (15). In addition, current experiments with the chicken βB1-crystallin gene, which is expressed exclusively in elongating lens cells (8), have also suggested that 5' flanking sequences contain elements that down-regulate gene expression (H. J. Roth). An intriguing feature of these experiments is that the down-regulation appears stronger in fibroblasts than in cultured lens cells. These initial tests raise the possibility that negative control contributes to the lens-specific regulation of this crystallin gene, however it is premature to draw any conclusions at this time.

3' Flanking Sequences

Numerous experiments have established that the 5' flanking region of crystallin genes contain their regulatory elements. It is entirely possible however that there are other regions which also contain control elements. Indeed, a tissue-specific enhancer has been found recently in the third intron of the δ1-crystallin gene of chickens (16). In the chicken (17,18) and human (19) β-globin and chicken histone H5 (20) genes an enhancer exists in the 3' flanking region. Consequently, we have examined the 3' flanking region of the murine αB-crystallin gene for regulatory sequences. These experiments were performed by constructing a minigene for the murine αB-crystallin gene (R. A. Dubin). This minigene consisted of 656 bp of 5' flanking sequence, 74 bp of the 5' portion of exon 1 linked to 308 bp of the 3' portion of exon 3 followed by 2.2 kb of 3' flanking sequence; thus exon 2 and both introns were deleted from the gene, allowing us to detect its shortened transcript in transfected lens cells. Deletion of the

entire 3' flanking sequence did not reduce the expression of
this minigene until the putative polyadenylation signal was
removed.  We presume that loss of the polyadenylation signal
resulted in lowered gene expression by reducing the
stability of the RNA.   We are presently exploring the
possibility that introns contain additional regulatory
elements for this gene.  One feature of the murine αB-
crystallin gene which makes it interesting to seek
additional regulatory signals is that antibody (S.P. Bhat,
personal communication) and Northern blot (R.A. Dubin)
experiments have indicated its expression in non-lens
tissues.  Our Northern blot experiments showed relatively
high expression in the heart, with a trace in the kidney and
lung of the 1 to 2 week-old mouse (R. A. Dubin).

Gene Expression Within the δ-Crystallin locus

The chicken δ-crystallin locus contains two, tandemly
arranged, extremely similar genes which are spaced 3.8 kb
apart (21).   Both genes are composed of 17 exons which
encode proteins having 91% identity in amino acid sequence
(22).  Despite this similarity, almost all (we estimate at
least 99%) of the δ-crystallin mRNA in the embryonic chicken
lens is derived from the δ1 gene (23), which is situated 5'
to the δ2 gene (21).   In addition to this marked difference
in absolute amount of mRNA production, initial primer
extension experiments suggest that the ratio of δ1 to δ2
mRNA may also be regulated during lens development (23).
The biological meaning for the difference in the amounts of
the two δ mRNAs is not known for certain.  We have proposed
that δ2 is the active argininosuccinate lyase gene (6).
This would make its lowered expression consistent with it
encoding a metabolic enzyme.  These data suggest that there
is a major difference in transcription between the two δ-
crystallin genes, but this has not been proved.  If
transcription is the cause for the difference in the
expression of the two δ-crystallin genes, relatively small
differences in sequence have an enormous effect on
regulatory activity, an extremely interesting situation.
Experiments in a HeLa whole cell extract (24) and in
transfected explants of embryonic chicken lens epithelia
(25) have suggested that the promoter for the δ2 gene may be
several-fold less efficient than that for the δ1 gene,
however this would not account for the large difference in
the amount of mRNA.  It is likely that the δ1 enhancer in
the third intron (15) is important for the high expression

of the $\delta 1$ gene, but it is not yet known whether there is a similar enhancer in the $\delta 2$ gene. It is possible that chromatin configuration also contributes to the difference in expression of the two $\delta$-crystallin genes. Alternative possibilities are that the amount of $\delta 2$ mRNA is limited by splicing efficiency, transport to the cytoplasm or stability. Clearly further experiments are necessary to understand gene regulation within the $\delta$-crystallin locus. This system illustrates that it is important to consider numerous regulatory mechanisms when studying crystallin gene expression.

## TRANS-ACTING FACTORS

Regulatory DNA sequences may exert their influence via interaction with nuclear proteins; such regulatory proteins (trans-acting factors) may be general (distributed in many tissues) or specific (found only in the tissues expressing the gene). DNA-binding proteins may be identified by incubating nuclear extracts with restriction fragments or synthetic oligonucleotides containing sequences known to be important for gene regulation. The presence of DNA-protein interactions can be inferred from gel retardation experiments (26). We have incubated the SV40 promoter in nuclear extracts from 14 day-old embryonic chicken lenses or HeLa cells (J. F. Klement). The latter contains a transcription factor, Sp1, which binds to the double-stranded sequence GGGCGG (27). DNAse I protection experiments showed that the lens nuclear extract, like the HeLa nuclear extract, contains either Sp1 or a protein which had extremely similar binding characteristics. Previous competition experiments in a HeLa whole cell extract (28) and microinjected murine lens cells (29) have also provided evidence for the requirement of Sp1 or an Sp1-like protein for transcription of the $\delta 1$-crystallin gene, which has one Sp1 binding site in its promoter. The chicken $\beta$B1-crystallin promoter has two sp1 binding sites (H. J. Roth). Not all crystallin promoters have this binding site however.

We are also performing gel retardation experiments with different crystallin promoters. Initial tests have indicated that different proteins bind selectively to the $\delta 1$- and the $\beta$A3/A1-crystallin promoters of the chicken (C. A. Peterson and T. Borras). The proteins responsible for

the retarded bands have not been purified or identified
beyond these experiments at the present time.

There are a number of other interesting sequences
which may bind regulatory proteins found in regions
suspected to have regulatory significance in crystallin
genes.  We have identified a 15 bp consensus sequence in
the 5' region of many crystallin genes (30), but no
functional studies have been performed on this sequence.  A
CCAAT sequence occurs in the chicken δ1- (31,32) and
βA3/A1- (C. A. Peterson) crystallin promoters, but this
sequence does not appear in all crystallin genes.  The CCAAT
sequence is known to bind several transcription factors in
different genes (33,34).  The chicken βA3/A1-crystallin 5'
flanking sequence has an unusual stretch of T nucleotides
which is intriguing and may play an interesting role in
regulating this gene (C. A. Peterson).


## FUTURE DIRECTIONS

The study of crystallin gene expression is clearly
launched and in an exciting phase of growth and development,
as the reports in this section show.  More detailed mapping
and identification of new regulatory sequences are
necessary.  No studies have revealed yet the existence of
crystallin gene regulatory elements of any significant
distance from its gene, but we may anticipate such reports
in the future.  It seems clear that numerous DNA-binding
proteins will be required for crystallin gene expression.
One important question concerns the relative role of
ubiquitous factors, such as Sp1, and lens-specific factors
in order to obtain proper expression of these specialized
genes.  It is possible that different use of common factors
or modifications of their structure in the lens could lead
to selective expression and regulation of crystallin genes.
The differences in the sequences and genomic organization of
the numerous crystallin genes make it likely that many
mechanisms are used to obtain their regulated, tissue-
specific expression.  The fact that some of the crystallin
genes are expressed in non-lens tissues adds another
dimension of interest and complexity to their expression.
Finally, we must keep in mind that tissue-specificity and
tissue-preference are not the only problems in crystallin
gene expression.  It is also necessary to understand the
quantitative aspects of their expression as well as their
precise spatial regulation within the lens.  The solutions

to these problems will require functional mutagenesis and protein-binding experiments. The foundation has been laid; we now have the privilege and opportunity to unravel the mysteries of how these genes encoding lens structural proteins and, in some cases metabolic enzymes, function.

## ACKNOWLEDGMENT

We thank Dr. Hans Bloemendal for a gift of a calf αB-crystallin cDNA which was used to isolate the corresponding gene in the mouse, Mrs. Barbara L. Norman for excellent technical assistance and Mrs. Dawn Chicchirichi for expert typing of the manuscript.

## REFERENCES

1. Piatigorsky J (1987). Gene expression and genetic engineering in the lens. Invest Ophthal & Vis Sci 28:9.
2. Wistow GJ, Piatigorsky J (1988). Lens crystallins: The evolution and expression of proteins for a highly specialized tissue. Ann Rev Biochem 57:479.
3. Piatigorsky J (1984). Delta crystallins and their nucleic acids. Mol Cell Biochem 59:33.
4. Clayton RM, Jeanny J-C, Bower DJ, Errington LH (1986). The presence of extralenticular crystallin and its relationship with transdifferentiation to lens. Curr Top Dev Biol 20:137.
5. Wistow G, Piatigorsky J (1987). Recruitment of enzymes as lens structural proteins. Science 236:1554.
6. Piatigorsky J, O'Brien WE, Norman BL, Kalumuck K, Wistow GJ, Borras T, Nickerson JM, Wawrousek EF (1988). Proc Natl Acad Sci USA (in press).
7. Piatigorsky J (1981). Lens differentiation in vertebrates. A review of cellular and molecular features. Differentiation 19:134.
8. Hejtmancik JF, Beebe DC, Ostrer H, Piatigorsky J (1985). $\delta$- and $\beta$-Crystallin mRNA levels in the embryonic and posthatched chicken lens: Temporal and spatial changes during development. Dev Biol 109:72
9. Gorman CM, Moffat LF, Howard BH (1982). Recombinant genomes which express chloramphenicol acetyltransferase in mammalian cells. Mol Cell Biol 2:1044.

10.  Chepelinsky AB, King CR, Zelenka PS, Piatigorsky J
     (1985). Lens-specific expression of the chloramphenicol
     acetyltransferase gene promoted by 5′ flanking
     sequences of the murine αA-crystallin gene in explanted
     chicken lens epithelia. Proc Natl Acad Sci USA 82:2334.
11.  Lok S, Breitman ML, Chepelinsky AB, Piatigorsky J, Gold
     RJM, Tsui L-C (1985). Lens-specific promoter activity
     of a mouse γ-crystallin gene. Mol Cell Biol 5:2221.
12.  Overbeek PA, Chepelinsky AB, Khillan JS, Piatigorsky J,
     Westphal H (1985). Lens-specific expression and
     developmental regulation of the bacterial
     chloramphenicol acetyltransferase gene driven by the
     murine αA-crystallin promoter in transgenic mice. Proc
     Natl Acad Sci USA 82:7815.
13.  Goring DR, Rossant J, Clapoff S, Breitman ML, Tsui L-C
     (1987). In situ detection of β-galactosidase in lenses
     of transgenic mice with a γ-crystallin/lacZ gene.
     Science 235:456.
14.  Chelelinsky AB, Sommer B, Piatigorsky J (1987).
     Interaction between two different regulatory elements
     activates the murine αA-crystallin gene promoter in
     explanted lens epithelia. Mol Cell Biol 7:1807.
15.  Borras T, Peterson CA, Piatigorsky J (1988). Evidence
     for positive and negative regulation in the promoter of
     the chicken δ1-crystallin gene. Dev Biol (in press).
16.  Hayashi S, Goto K, Okada TS, Kondoh H (1987). Lens-
     specific enhancer in the third intron regulates
     expression of the chicken δ1-crystallin gene. Genes &
     Development 1:818.
17.  Choi O-R, Engel JD (1986). A 3′ enhancer is required
     for temporal and tissue-specific transcriptional
     activation of the chicken adult β-globin gene. Nature
     323:731.
18.  Hesse JE, Nickol JM, Lieber MR, Felsenfeld G (1986).
     Regulated gene expression in transfected primary
     chicken erythrocytes. Proc Natl Acad Sci USA 83:4312.
19.  Trudel M, Costantini F (1987). A 3′ enhancer
     contributes to the stage-specific expression of the
     human β-globin gene. Genes and Development 1:954.
20.  Trainor CD, Stamler SJ, Engel JD (1987). Erythroid-
     specific transcription of the chicken histone H5 gene
     is directed by a 3′ enhancer. Nature 328:827.
21.  Hawkins JW, Nickerson JM, Sullivan MA, Piatigorsky J
     (1984). The δ-crystallin gene family: two genes of
     similar structure in close chromosomal approximation. J
     Biol Chem 259:9821.

22. Nickerson JM, Wawrousek EF, Borras T, Hawkins JW, Norman BL, Filpula DR, Nagle JW, Ally AH, Piatigorsky J (1986). Sequence of the chicken $\delta 2$ crystallin gene and its intergenic spacer: Extreme homology with the $\delta 1$ crystallin gene. J Biol Chem 261:552.

23. Parker DS, Wawrousek EF, Piatigorsky J (1988). Expression of the $\delta$-crystallin genes in the embryonic chicken lens. Dev Biol 126 (in press).

24. Das GC, Piatigorsky J (1987). Transcription of the two $\delta$-crystallin genes in a Hela cell extract. In Granner D, Rosenfeld MG, Chang S (eds): "Transcriptional Control Mechanisms: Cetus-UCLA Symposia on Molecular and Cellular Biology, New Series Vol 52," New York: Alan R. Liss, Inc., p 405.

25. Borras T, Nickerson JM, Chepelinsky AB, Piatigorsky J (1985). Structural and functional evidence for differential promoter activity of the two linked $\delta$-crystallin genes in the chicken. EMBO Journal 4:445.

26. Crothers DM (1987). Gel electrophoresis of protein-DNA complexes. Nature 325:464.

27. Gidoni D, Kadonaga JT, Barrera-Saldana H, Takahashi K, Chambon P, Tjian R (1985). Bidirectional SV40 transcription mediated by tandem Sp1 binding interactions. Science 230:511.

28. Das DC, Piatigorsky J (1986). The chicken $\delta 1$-crystallin gene promoter: Binding of transcription factor(s) to the upstream G+C-rich region is necessary for promoter function in vitro. Proc Natl Acad Sci USA 83:3135.

29. Hayashi S, Kondoh H (1986). In vivo competition of $\delta$-crystallin gene expression by DNA fragments containing a GC box. Mol Cell Biol 6:4130.

30. Thompson MA, Hawkins JW, Piatigorsky J (1987). Complete nucleotide sequence of the chicken $\alpha$A-crystallin gene and its 5' flanking region. Gene 56:173.

31. Ohno M, Sakamoto H, Yasuda K, Okada TS, Shimura Y (1985). Nucleotide sequence of a chicken $\delta$-crystallin gene. Nucleic Acids Res 13:1593.

32. Nickerson JM, Wawrousek EF, Hawkins JW, Wakil AS, Wistow GJ, Thomas G, Norman BL, Piatigorsky J (1985). The complete sequence of the chicken $\delta 1$ crystallin gene and its 5' flanking region. J Biol Chem 260:9100.

33. McKnight S, Tjian R (1986). Transcriptional selectivity of viral genes in mammalian cells. Cell 46:795.

34. Dorn A, Bollekens J, Staub A, Benoist C, Mathis D (1987). A multiplicity of CCAAT box-binding proteins. Cell 50:863.

Molecular Biology of the Eye: Genes, Vision, and Ocular Disease, pages 189–196
© 1988 Alan R. Liss, Inc.

# REGULATORY ELEMENTS OF THE CHICKEN δ1-CRYSTALLIN GENE[1]

H. Kondoh, Y. Ueda[2], I. Araki, S. Hayashi[3] and K. Goto

Department of Biophysics, Faculty of Science
Kyoto University, Kyoto 606, Japan

ABSTRACT  With the knowledge that the chicken δ1-crystallin gene is well regulated in mouse tissues and mice after gene transfer, we investigated regulatory elements associated with the gene by attaching various segments to genes coding for bacterial enzymes and transfecting chicken embryo primary cultures.  We found that promoter or upstream regions do not contain significant tissue-specific elements, but the third intron bears a lens-specific enhancer.  From various criteria, we conclude that the intragenic enhancer is the major determinant of the tissue specificity of the chicken δ1-crystallin gene.

## INTRODUCTION

It is widely accepted that gene transfer techniques provide straightforward experimental approaches to the mechanisms of tisssue-specific gene regulation.  One of the earliest examples is the observation that the cloned δ1-crystallin gene of the chicken is expressed in a lens-specific manner when it is introduced into mouse cells in primary culture (1).  We extended the study to transgenic and gene-transferred chimeric mice, and found that the

[1]This work was supported by grants from the Ministry of Education, Science and Culture of Japan.
[2]Present address:  Department of Applied Biological Science, Science University of Tokyo, Noda 278, Japan.
[3]Present address:  Department of Molecular, Cellular and Developmental Biology, University of Colorado, Colorado 80309-0347, U.S.A.

regulation of the chicken δ-crystallin gene in the mouse very finely mimics that in the chicken (2,3).   These results clearly indicated that virtually every genetic element for regulation of the gene is associated with the DNA sequence introduced into the mouse tissues, which included upstream (up to 6 kb) and downstream (up to 1 kb) regions in addition to the 9 kb long gene itself.   We investigated the regulatory elements by examining various segments for their effect on expression of genes coding for bacterial enzymes after transfection of primary-cultured chicken embryonic tissues.

## PROMOTER AND THE UPSTREAM REGION

We constructed fusion genes, δCAT (4) and δZtk (5) in which the δ1-crystallin promoter and the upstream region are linked to the bacterial chloramphencol acetyl-transferase (CAT) and β-galactosidase (β-gal) genes, respectively.  We introduced various deletions and substitutions in the δ-crystallin regions and examined their effects by measuring the activities of the encoded enzymes expressed in the chicken tissues.

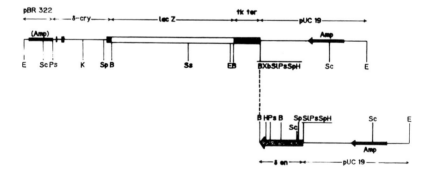

Figure 1.   Structure of plasmid pδZtk (upper, a deletion mutant form with 93 bp 5' flanking sequence is shown) and its derivative carrying the δ1-crystallin enhancer (lower).   Restriction sites: B, BamHI; E, EcoRI; H, HindIII; K, KpnI; Ps, PstI; Sc, ScaI; Sl, SalI; Sp, SphI; Ss, SstI; Xb, XbaI.

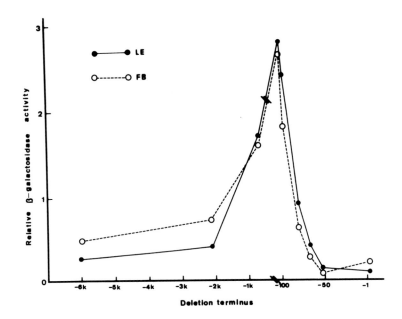

Figure 2.   Effect of deletions in the 5' flanking
sequence on δZtk expression.   Relative β-galactosidase
activity in δZtk-transfected cultures was plotted against
the breakpoints of the deletion.

The results of the deletion mutants of δZtk having
various lengths of the 5' flanking sequence are summarized
in Fig. 2.   Results of δCAT were essentially the same.
Both in lens epithelium (LE) and fibroblasts (FB), the
deletion to remove the region upstream of -93 resulted in
the highest level of expression.   The deletion to -69
reduced expression to one-fourth of the former and the
deletion to the points closer to the transcriptional
initiation site totally abolished the expression.   Thus,
the position around -90 is the 5' border of the promoter
region essential for its activity.   This result is in
generally good agreement with our previous observation
using mouse cells (6).

The region between -93 and -69 contains putative binding sequences for different kinds of transcription factors, i.e. GC-box sequence and CCAAT-box-like sequence. In vivo competition experiments indicated that factor binding to the GC-box is essential for the expression of the δ1-crystallin gene (7), but requirement of the latter sequence has not been established. We introduced linker-scanning mutations in this region and found that disruption of the GC-box totally abolished the expression, but that of CCAAT did not have an appreciable effect, ruling out the functional significance of the latter sequence.

A remarkable difference from the results of mouse cells injected with the whole δ1-crystallin gene was that the regions upstream of -300 exerted a repressing effect. Inclusion of the longer 5' flanking sequence resulted in lower activity. To examine if the upstream region bears any defined element(s) to reduce the transcriptional level, we deleted the region between -1285 to -322 from the δCAT gene having a 5' flanking sequence of 2200 bp. The level of CAT expression did not increase by this manipulation. Placement of the region -1285 to -322 in the upstream of CAT genes having viral promoters did not decrease the expression. Therefore, there appears no defined region to down-regulate gene expression, but rather the regions upstream of -300 may generally have a repressing effect on the δ-crystallin promoter in the transfection assay.

Expression of δCAT or δZtk was always roughly three times higher in LE than in FB. This difference is ascribed to difference in the transfection efficiency between the tissues, since the same range of difference was consistently observed with other enhancer-less genes (4). In addition, effect of varying length of the up-stream sequence and of the linker insertions/substitutions in the promoter region were always parallel between LE and FB. In a previous study, we suggested that the promoter region of the δ-crystallin gene is involved in generating tissue specificity (6). This proposition was based on the observation that replacement of the region with retroviral LTRs resulted in an apparent loss specificity of expression. We have evidence that the LTR elements we employed had lower activity in the lens cells than other tissues, and this down-effect of the LTRs was compensated

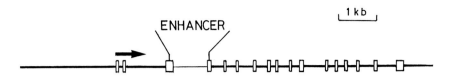

Figure 3.   Enhancer region of the δ1-crystallin gene.
Exons are indicated by boxes, and the direction of
transcription by the arrow.

by a lens-specific activating element described below.
From the present analysis of the promoter and upstream
regions, we concluded that these regions contain no major
determinant of tissue specificity.

### LENS-SPECIFIC ENHANCER IN THE THIRD INTRON

From the above results, lens-specificity determinants
were expected to be present within the gene or downstream
of it.   We examined various segments of the δ-crystallin
gene for a tissue-specific enhancer activity by placing
each of them in the downstream of δCAT or δZtk.   We found
that a segment which span the third intron bears a strong
lens-specific enhancer activity (Fig. 3)(4).  The effect
of the enhancer on δZtk expression is shown in Fig. 4.
This enhancer activates transcription from δ-crystallin
promoter by 20 to 40 folds in LE but not in other cell

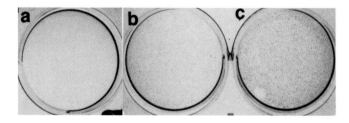

Figure 4.   Effect of δ1-crystallin enhancer on δZtk
expression.   a, b and c, LE cultures transfected with no
DNA, pδZtk and pδZtk-δen, respectively, and stained for β-
galactosidase activity with X-gal (5).

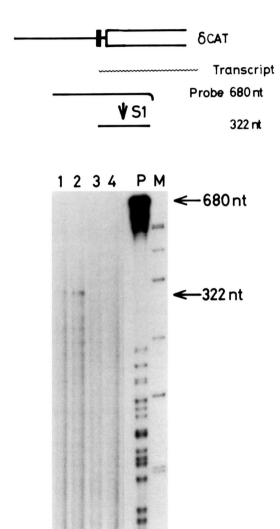

Figure 5.  S1 nuclease mapping of δCAT transcript.
Total cytoplasmic RNA (30 μg, except for 1, 10 μg) from LE
cells transfected with pδCAT or pδCAT-δen (with the δ1-
crystallin enhancer) was analyzed.  1 and 2, transfected
with pδCAT-δen; 3, transfected with pδCAT; 4, mock-
transfected; P, probe; M, molecular size marker.

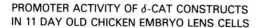

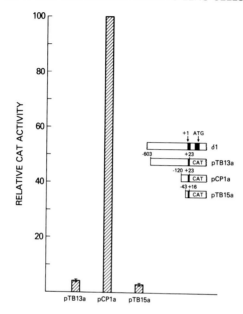

FIGURE 1. A total of 11 μg of DNA (10 μg of pTB13a, pCP1a or pTB15a) were introduced into 11 day-old chicken embryo PLE cells. Relative CAT activity was determined by standardizing nmoles of acetylated chloramphenicol against units of β-galactosidase activity.

δ-Crystallin synthesis is one of gradual turning off during development; indeed, δ-crystallin mRNA disappears from the lens between 3 and 5 months after hatching (10). Although we do not know the  molecular mechanism for the arrest of δ-crystallin gene expression, our experiments raise the possibility that negative control involving the sequence between positions -603 to -120 may have some role in this process.

One possibility concerning the mechanism by which negative control could modulate the expression of the δ1-crystallin gene is that there is an interaction with repressor molecules. To test this idea we performed in vivo competition experiments in order to titrate out repressors which bind to the sequence -603 to -120. Co-transfection experiments of δ-CAT constructs with plasmids carrying the sequence -603/-120 (at a molar ratio of 1:5) resulted in a small increase in CAT activity (Fig. 2). This is consistent with the possibility that the lens cells contain one or more trans-acting factors. The failure to obtain a greater effect in these competition experiments may be due to a concentration of factors greatly exceeding that of the competitor DNA.

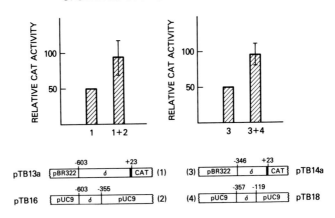

COMPETITION OF δ-CAT CONSTRUCTS WITH
UPSTREAM δ1 PROMOTER SEQUENCES

FIGURE 2. 2 μg of test plasmid (1 and 3) were mixed with either 8 μg (1 + 2) or 10 μg (3 + 4) of competitor plasmid. In each case 1 μg of pTB1 was included for normalization. CAT reactions were carried out for 2 hours and normalizations were done as in Fig. 1. In dishes 1 and 3, calf thymus DNA or pUC9 DNA, respectively, was used as carriers to equalize the total DNA correlation in every sample.

The δ1 promoter sequence -603/-120 did not reduce the activity of the SV40 early promoter (with or without the enhancer) or the thymidine kinase promoter of the Herpes simplex virus when inserted at their 5' end. It may be that negative factors cannot bind, or bind but cannot function, without being able to interact with other factors specifically bound to the δ1-crystallin promoter (Fig. 3).

Ehrlich et al. (11) described a similar interaction for
positive and negative factors of the PD1 gene.

## MODEL FOR THE INTERACTION
## OF THE POSITIVE AND NEGATIVE
## ELEMENTS OF δ1

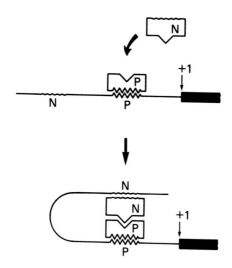

FIGURE 3.  A theoretical model for promoter function in
the δ1-crystallin gene.  N: putative negative trans-acting
factor.  P: putative positive trans-acting factor.  +1 is the
transcription initiation site of the δ1-crystallin gene.

A computer assisted comparison of sequences which
appear to down-regulate other eukaryotic and viral genes
(9) revealed two consensus sequences called box 1
(ANCCTCTCT) (Fig. 4) and box 2 (ANTCTCCTCC).  These
consensus sequences are present in the putative negative
regulatory domain of the δ1 gene.  The similarity to box 1
is found three times in the 5' flanking sequence of the δ1-
crystallin gene at positions -191, -224 and -294; the
similarity to box 2 is found once at position -356 in the δ1

gene.   No similarities to these boxes were found between positions -120 and -43 of the δ1-crystallin gene.

## SEQUENCE COMPARISONS OF NEGATIVE ELEMENTS
(data by Baniahmad et al., 1987)

### HOMOLOGY BOX 1

| Sequence | Position | Gene |
|---|---|---|
| ACC CTCTC T | -1.09kb | Chicken lysozyme |
| AAC CTCTC T | -1.11kb | Chicken lysozyme |
| ACC CTCTC T | -270bp | Rat insulin |
| CCC CTCTC C | -111bp | Rat insulin |
| GTC CTCTC T | -45bp | β-interferon |
| ACC CTCTC A | +141 | Mouse immunoglobulin heavy chain |
| GAC CTCTC T | +4 | Mouse immunoglobulin heavy chain |
| AGC CTCTC C | -367bp | Rat growth hormone |
| AGC CTCTC A | +5524 | Polyoma virus |
| ACA CTCTC C | -294 | Chicken δ1 crystallin |
| CAG CTCTC T | -227 | Chicken δ1 crystallin |
| AAC CTCTC A | -191 | Chicken δ1 crystallin |

ANCCTCTC$_C^T$    Consensus

FIGURE 4.   A compilation  of sequences which have been postulated by Baniahmad et al. (9) to have the ability to down-regulate promoter activity.  We have added δ1-crystallin to the list.   The boxed region contains the common element.   The vertical bars in the negative domain of the δ1-crystallin (below) mark the regions where the putative negative sequence is located.

In conclusion, we have provided evidence for both negative and positive regions in the 5′ flanking region of the δ-crystallin gene during transient expression in cultured lens epithelial cells.   The in vivo function of these regulatory elements are unknown.   Further experiments

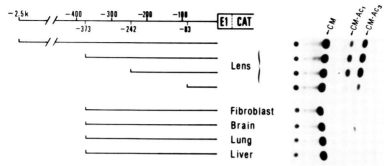

Figure 1. Expression of fusion genes introduced into a variety of primary cultures prepared from day-old chicken tissues. The 5' sequences of the fused α-crystallin-CAT gene are indicated by lines. Autoradiograms show CAT activities in cultures of tissues transfected with the fusion genes shown in the left.

To examine whether or not the fusion gene is expressed, it was introduced into a variety of primary culture cells prepared from day-old chick tissues (lens, fibroblast, brain, lung and liver cells) and the cells were harvested after 2 days of transfection. Figure 1 shows that the level of CAT activity was much higher in lens cells than in any other tissues, indicating tissue-specific expression of the fusion gene in primary culture cells. This also suggests that the 5' sequences -373 to +10bp are essential for expressing the α-crystallin gene in vitro in a tissue-specific manner.

DNA Sequences Required for Tissue-specific Expression

To narrow down the exact location of the DNA sequences responsible for tissue-specific expression of the crystallin gene, we constructed mutant genes with a series of 5' deletions using restriction endonuclease cleavage sites. Mutant genes were transfected to chick lens culture and CAT activity was determined. Mutant genes with DNA sequences -242 to +10 and -162 to +10 were still active as the original fusion gene. Mutant gene containing the sequences between -83 and +10, however, completely lost the CAT activity, indicating that DNA sequences between -162 and -83 are responsible for tissue-specific expression of the chicken α-crystallin gene.

Inhibition of Gene Expression with Regulatory DNA Sequences

The previous results suggest the presence of a positive regulatory factor which binds specifically to the regulatory DNA sequences between -162 and -83bp and then stimulates transcription of the α-crystallin gene in lens cells. If this hypothesis is correct, the level of the CAT activity should be reduced when a large amount of the regulatory DNA sequences are introduced into nuclei of lens cells. Regulatory DNA sequences will compete with those of the fusion genes for the binding factors in lens cells. Since most of these binding factors will bind to the regulatory DNA sequences, and few to the fusion genes, the result will be an inhibition of their promoter function.

As the amount of the regulatory DNA sequences increased with respect that of the gene, the level of expression decreased proportionally. The expression was reduced to 50% when the regulatory sequences were co-transfected in 150-fold molar excess over the reporter gene. In contrast, expression was not affected at all even when 300-fold molar excess of sequences -373 to -242bp, which do not contain the regulatory sequences, was co-transfected. These results support the hypothesis that a factor binding specifically to the regulatory sequences activates the transcription of the crystallin gene.

Identification of a Nuclear Factor which Binds to the Regulatory DNA Sequences

In order to detect a sequence-specific DNA binding factor, whose presence was suggested by the previous results, we carried out the gel mobility shift assay (gel retardation assay; 15,16). We localized a DNA binding region by interacting nuclear proteins prepared from day-old chick with specific DNA fragments digested with restriction endonucleases. The results showed that no protein-DNA complex was detected using DNA fragments containing the sequences -242 to -162. Similarly, no protein-DNA complex was observed using fragments containing the sequences -90 to +10. In contrast, DNA fragments containing the sequences -162 to -83 were able to form a nuclear protein-DNA complex, indicating that one or more protein binding sites lie within this region. These rsults showed a good correlation between the sequences involved in tissue-specific expression and the DNA binding activity.

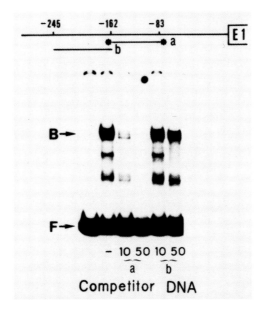

Figure 2.    DNA competition for the nuclear protein
binding to the regulatory DNA sequences.  Two unlabelled
competitors, the specific sequences (a; -162 to -83) and
the non-specific sequences (b; -245 to -162), were added in
either 10- or 50-fold molar excess over the regulatory DNA
sequences.


To determine if the protein-DNA complex was specific
for the regulatory DNA sequences, we added unlabelled
regulatory DNA sequences as well as other unlabelled DNA
fragments in the gel mobility shift assay (Figure 2).  Even
when 50-fold molar excess of the sequences -245 to -162
were used as competitor DNA, protein-DNA complex formation
was not affected at all (Figure 2).  In contrast, when the
sequences -162 to -83 were used as a specific competitor
DNA in 10- or 50-fold molar excess, protein-DNA complex was
not formed at all (Figure 2), indicating that this complex
was formed only with the specific DNA sequences containing
the regulatory DNA sequences.
        If the protein involved in protein-DNA complex
formation is a positive regulatory factor, such a factor
must be present only in lens cells because the α-crystallin
gene is expressed only in those cells.  We reacted the DNA

probe (sequences −162 to −83) with nuclear proteins prepared from different chick tissues and from HeLa cells to test whether the DNA binding protein activity correlated with tissue-specificity of the crystallin gene transcription. The mobility retardation assay showed that two rapidly migrating complexes with the same mobilities were detected both in lens and in HeLa extracts and the slowest of these was only in lens extract.  Competition experiments in the gel retardation assay showed that two protein-DNA complexes with fast electrophoretic mobilities were formed even in the presence of unlabeled regulatory sequences, indicating these two complexes were not specific for the regulatory sequences (data not shown).  In contrast, the slowest complex was not detected in the presence of a 10-fold excess of specific competitor DNA.  Thus far, this protein-DNA complex was obtained only with lens nuclear extracts, demonstrating that the regulatory DNA sequence-specific DNA binding activity is present only in lens cells.  Therefore, these results showed a good correlation between sequence-specific DNA-protein complex formation and the tissue-specificity of the crystallin gene.

  We reacted nuclear protein gel blots with the α-crystallin DNA probes (South-western blot analysis; 17,18) to determine if we could detect the protein responsible for the specific DNA binding activity in Figure 2.  The regulatory DNA sequences probe interacted with two proteins (61kDa and 110kDa proteins) in lens nuclear extracts in the presence of carrier DNA.  The large one was also detected in HeLa cell nuclear extract with the same probe, suggesting this protein is not tissue-specific.  Other DNA probes gave no signals in the presence of carrier DNA. Thus, the 61kDa protein present only in lens cells might be a candidate protein for the protein involved in the complex formation and the positive regulatory factor activating the α-crystallin gene.


## DISCUSSION

  We have shown the presence of a factor binding specifically to the cis-acting element of the chicken α-crystallin gene.  The gel retardation assay showed that the specific DNA binding activity is detected only in lens nuclear extracts, demonstrating a good correlation between the binding activity and the tissue-specificity of the crystallin genes.  Therefore, the factor involved in protein-DNA complex formation might be a transcriptional activator acting in a tissue-specific manner. Sequence-specific DNA binding activity was also detected in nuclear proteins prepared from brain cells of young chick embryos, suggesting the presence of a factor very similar to or the same as the one detected in lens cells. This might explain why crystallin mRNAs are expressed at a low level in brain cells of early embryos and why the presence of the positive regulatory factor might trigger the change from the differentiation state when they are cultured in vitro.

Competition experiments between DNA fragments containing the regulatory sequences and the crystallin gene fused to the CAT gene showed a remarkable reduction in CAT activity, indicating that the sequence-specific DNA binding proteins are positive regulators of crystallin gene transcription, a transcriptional activator acting in a tissue-specific manner. To reduce CAT activity by half, a 150-fold molar excess of the fragments over the gene was needed. A similar observation was reported in a competition experiment on δ-crystallin gene expression. A preliminary experiment showed that a 3000-fold molar excess of the fragments completely inhibited the gene expression. δ-crystallin gene enhancer did not inhibit α-crystallin gene transcription, demonstrating the presence of different types of activators in lens cells (Kondoh H and Gotoh K, personal communication). Altogether, these results suggest that more than a few positive regulators are present in lens nuclei.

We have also determined the molecular nature of the DNA binding protein by the South-western blot analysis, whereby nuclear protein bolts separated on SDS/polyacrylamide gel electrophoresis were probed with labeled specific double-stranded DNA. This method is very useful for determining the molecular weight of DNA binding proteins after the presence of sequence-specific DNA binding proteins was confirmed. Using this method a 60kDa nuclear protein has been identified as a trans-acting factor which interacts with cis-regulatory sequences required for soybeen seed protein gene expression (19). We have shown here that a 61kDa protein binds to the regulatory sequences and is detected only in lens cells. Therefore, it seems likely that this protein has features of tissue- and sequence-specific activators.

To obtain cDNA clones encoding sequence-specific DNA binding protein, we screened a λgt11 cDNA library by probing with specific double-stranded DNA. Several clones

were found. Northern blot analysis with this cDNA probe
showed that transcripts were detected only in lens cells,
suggesting that this cDNA clone might encode a candidate
for a sequence-specific DNA binding protein and a positive
regulator of the α-crystallin gene. This novel technique
is sure to pave the way for isolating DNA binding proteins
and for dissecting the molecular mechanisms involved in
tissue-specific expression.

## REFERENCES

1. Clayton RM (1971).    Comparative aspects of lens
   protein. In Davson H, Graham LT (eds): "The Eye" New
   York, London: Academic Press, p 399.
2. Bloemendal H (1981).    The lens protein. In Bloemendal H
   (ed): "Molecular and Cellular Biology of the Eye Lens"
   New York: John Wiley and Sons, p 221.
3. de Jong WW (1981). Evolution of lens and crystallins.
   In Bloemendal H (ed): "Molecular and Cellular Biology
   of the Eye Lens" New York: John Wiley and Sons, p 221.
4. Piatigorsky J (1981).    Lens differentiation in
   vertebrates. A review of cellular and molecular
   features. Differentiation 19:134.
5. Piatigorsky J (1984). Delta crystallins and their
   nucleic acids. Mol. Cell. Biochem. 59:33.
6. Yasuda K, Okada TS (1986).    Structure and expression of
   chick crystallin genes.  Oxford Surveys on Eukaryotic
   Genes 3:189.
7. Thomson I, Yasuda K, de Pomerai DI, Clayton RM, Okada
   TS (1981).    The accumulation of lens-specific protein
   and mRNA in cultures of neural retina from 3.5-day old
   chick embryos. Exp. Cell Res. 135:445.
8. Agata K, Yasuda K, Okada TS (1983).    Gene coding for a
   lens-specific protein, δ-crystallin, is transcribed in
   nonlens tissues of chicken embryos.  Develop. Biol.
   100: 222.
9. Okada TS (1984). Review: Recent progress in studies of
   the transdifferentiation of eye tissues in vitro.  Cell
   Differ. 13:177.
10. Yasuda K, Okuyama K, Okada TS (1983).  The accumulation
    of δ-crystallin mRNA in transdetermination and
    transdifferentiation of neural retina cells into lens.
    Cell Differ. 12:177.
11. Okazaki K, Yasuda K, Kondoh H, Okada TS (1985).  DNA

sequences responsible for tissue-specific expression of a chicken α-crystallin gene in mouse lens cells.  EMBO J. 4:2589.

12. Hayashi S, Kondoh H, Yasuda K, Soma G, Ikawa Y, Okada TS (1985). Tissue-specific regulation of a chicken δ-crystallin gene in mouse cells: involvement of the 5' end region.  EMBO J. 4:2201.

13. Chepelinsky AB, King CR, Zelenka PS, Piatigorsky J (1985).  Lens-specific expression of the chloramphenicol acetyltransferase gene promoted by 5' flanking sequences of the murine αA-crystallin gene in explanted chicken lens epithelia. Proc. Natl. Acad. Sci. USA. 82:2334.

14. Chepelinsky AB, Sommer B, Piatigorsky J (1987). Interaction between two different regulatory elements activates the murine αA-crystallin gene promoter in explanted lens epithelia. Mol. Cell. Biol. 7:1807.

15. Fried M, Crothers DM (1981).  Equilibria and  kinetics of lac repressor-operator interactions by polyacrylamide electrophoresis.  Nucleic Acids Res. 9:6505.

16. Singh H, Sen R, Baltimore D, Sharpe PA (1986).  A nuclear factor that binds to a conserved sequence motif in transcriptional control elements of immunoglobulin genes. Nature 319:154.

17. Bowen B, Steinberg J, Laemmli UK, Weintraub H (1980). The detection of DNA-binding proteins by protein blotting.  Nucleic Acids Res. 8:1.

18. Miskimins WK, Roberts MP, McClelland A, Ruddle FH (1983).  Use of a protein-blotting procedure and a specific DNA probe to identify nuclear proteins that recognize the promoter region of the transferrin receptor gene.  Proc. Natl. Acad. Sci. USA.  82:6741.

19. Jofuku KD, Okamura JK, Goldberg RB (1987). Interaction of an embryo DNA binding protein with a soybeen lectin gene upstream region.   Nature 328:734.

Molecular Biology of the Eye: Genes, Vision,
and Ocular Disease, pages 215–227
© 1988 Alan R. Liss, Inc.

ACTIVATION OF THE MURINE ALPHA A-CRYSTALLIN GENE
PROMOTER IN THE LENS

Ana B. Chepelinsky, Bernd Sommer[1], Eric F. Wawrousek
and Joram Piatigorsky.

Laboratory of Molecular and Developmental Biology, National
Eye Institute, National Institutes of Health, Bethesda, MD
20892.

ABSTRACT  We have investigated the cis-regulatory
elements of the murine αA-crystallin promoter
responsible for the lens-specific expression of this
gene.  Hybrid genes containing murine αA 5' flanking
sequences and the gene coding for the bacterial enzyme
chloramphenicol acetyltransferase (CAT) were
constructed and their expression studied in explanted
chicken lens epithelia and in transgenic mice.  Our
results indicated the presence of a proximal (-88/+46)
and a distal (-111/-88) domain which must interact for
promoter function in the explanted chicken lens
epithelia.  The sequence -88/-60 is essential for
promoter function.  The distal domain activates the
proximal domain when placed at the 5' end but not when
inserted at the 3' end of the CAT gene.  The distal
domain does not activate the enhancerless SV40
promoter.  Point mutations indicated that bases at
positions -108 and -109 are essential for the
activating properties of the distal domain.
Experiments with transgenic mice showed that the
sequence -111/+46 directs CAT gene expression
specifically to the lens.  Gel retardation and
methylation interference experiments provided evidence
for selective binding of different embryonic chicken
lens nuclear proteins to sequences -111/-84 and
-83/-55.

[1] Present address: Institut für Säugetiergenetik, GSF,
                Ingolstädter Landstr.  1
                8042 Neuherberg. Fed. Rep. Germany

## INTRODUCTION

α-Crystallin, the first crystallin to appear during lens differentiation in the mouse, is expressed specifically in lens epithelia and fibers (1).  The α-crystallin gene family consists of the αA and αB-crystallin genes.  In rodents, the αA-crystallin gene codes for two polypeptides ($\alpha A_2$ and $\alpha A^{ins}$) which are products of alternative RNA splicing (2-5) (see Fig. 1).  In the mouse, the αA-crystallin gene is located in chromosome 17 (6,7).

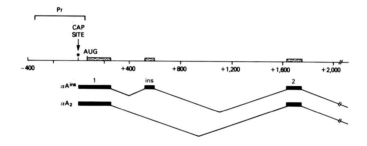

FIGURE 1.   Diagram of the murine αA-crystallin gene (2).   Solid bars: Exons. Exon "ins" is present in $\alpha A^{ins}$ mRNA and absent from $\alpha A_2$ mRNA.   Exon 3, present in both mRNAs, is not indicated.   Dotted bars: Coding sequences. Pr: DNA fragment containing 5' flanking sequence, initiation site of transcription and no coding sequences, inserted in expression vectors.

A DNA fragment containing 366 base pairs (bp) upstream from the initiation site of transcription and 46 bp of exon 1 was fused to the bacterial gene coding for chloramphenicol acetyl transferase (CAT) (8).   This αA-crystallin-CAT fusion gene was expressed specifically in lens cells when tested in transient experiments in explanted chicken lens epithelia (9) and in transgenic mice (10).   Furthermore, the developmental appearance of CAT activity closely followed the appearance of the endogenous αA-crystallin polypeptide in transgenic mice (10).   When the same αA-crystallin 5' flanking sequence (-366/+46) was inserted upstream of the SV40 large T antigen coding sequence, the expression of the transgene abolished lens fiber formation in transgenic mice (11).

Further dissection of the 5'flanking sequence allowed us to determine several <u>cis</u> regulatory elements of this promoter.

<u>cis</u> REGULATORY ELEMENTS OF THE MURINE αA-CRYSTALLIN PROMOTER

Distal Domain

We introduced different lengths of the 5' flanking sequences of the murine αA-crystallin gene containing 46 bp of exon one into the pSVO-CAT expression vector (8) (Fig. 2). To determine the location of the regulatory elements

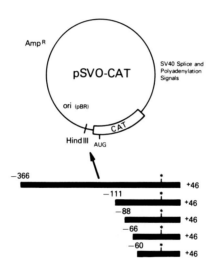

FIGURE 2.   5' flanking sequences of the murine αA-crystallin gene introduced into the pSVO-CAT expression vector (8).   Solid bars: αA-crystallin sequence. *: initiation site of transcription.

that activate this promoter, we studied CAT gene expression in transient assays in explanted chicken lens epithelia (9, 12).   When 5' flanking sequences between positions -366 and -112 were deleted, the promoter was still active.   By contrast, when an additional 23 bp were deleted the promoter activity was reduced 10-fold (Fig. 3).   We conclude that the

sequence between positions -111 and -88 is essential for the
activity of this promoter.

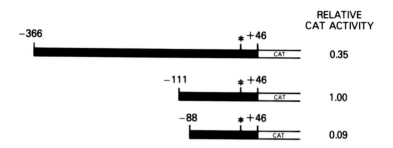

FIGURE 3.    CAT gene expression promoted by murine αA-
crystallin 5' flanking sequences in explanted chicken lens
epithelia (12).    Solid bars: murine αA-crystallin sequence.
Open bar: CAT gene.

A double-stranded synthetic oligonucleotide
corresponding to the sequence between positions -111 to -84
inserted in either orientation upstream of sequence -88 to
+46 restored promoter activity (12).    We thought that an
imperfect dyad of symmetry present in this sequence might be
responsible for its orientation-independence.    Some
regulatory proteins interact with DNA as dimers through α-
helix domains contacting dyads of symmetry (see ref. 13,14).
To test this hypothesis, we synthesized oligonucleotides
containing single or double point mutations in each half of
the dyad; the mutated oligonucleotides were inserted
upstream of -88 in the -88/+46 CAT vector.    While a double
point mutation in the 3' side of the dyad (positions -96 and
-97) did not affect promoter activity, the same double point
mutation in the 5' side of the dyad (positions -108 and
-109) abolished the activating property of this DNA
fragment.    In the first case, the activator element still
functioned in both orientations, while mutations in the
second case abolished activity in either orientation.

Proximal Domain

Since the activating element present in the distal
domain was able to function in both orientations, we were
interested in knowing whether it also shared other

23. Dignam JD, Lebovitz RM, Roeder RG (1983). Accurate transcription initiation by RNA polymerase II in a soluble extract from isolated mammalian nuclei. Nucl Acids Res 11:1475.

24. Garner MM, Revkin A (1986). The use of gel electrophoresis to detect and study nucleic acid-protein interactions. Trends Biochem Sci 11:395.

25. Crothers DM (1987). Gel electrophoresis of protein-DNA complexes. Nature 325:464.

26. Sen R, Baltimore D (1986). Multiple nuclear factors interact with the immunoglobulin enhancer sequences. Cell 46:705.

27. Staudt LM, Singh H, Sen R, Wirth T, Sharp PA, Baltimore D (1986). A lymphoid-specific protein binding to the octamer motif of immunoglobulin genes. Nature 323:640.

28. Maxam AM, Gilbert W (1977). A new method for sequencing DNA. Proc Natl Acad Sci USA 74:560.

29. Hendrickson W (1985). Protein-DNA interactions studied by the gel electrophoresis-DNA binding assay. Biotechniques 3:198.

30. Manley JL, Fire A, Cano A, Sharp PA, Gefter ML (1980). DNA-dependent transcription of adenovirus genes in a soluble whole-cell extract. Proc Natl Acad Sci 77:3855.

Molecular Biology of the Eye: Genes, Vision, and Ocular Disease, pages 229–237
© 1988 Alan R. Liss, Inc.

THE EXPRESSION OF RAT CRYSTALLIN GENES
IN VIVO AND IN VITRO

H.J.M. Aarts, R. Peek, P. van der Logt, N.H. Lubsen,
and J.G.G. Schoenmakers

Dept. of Molecular Biology, University of Nijmegen,
6525 ED  Nijmegen, The Netherlands

ABSTRACT  The changes in RNA levels during development of the rat lens show  that differential gene expression is found in the $\alpha$-, the $\beta$-, as well as in the $\gamma$-crystallin gene family of the rat. All $\beta$- and $\gamma$-crystallin genes are active during early lens development, but differential shut-down of transcription occurs during post-natal development. Within the $\alpha$-crystallin gene family differential activation may occur as transcripts of the $\alpha$A-crystallin gene could be detected earlier than transcripts of the $\alpha$B-crystallin gene. A comparison of the amount of crystallin RNA with the amount of the corresponding protein suggests that the translation efficiency of the crystallin mRNAs may vary widely. The suitability of two primary tissue-culture systems, namely transdifferentiating embryonic chicken neural retina cells and mouse lens epithelial cells, for the analysis of sequence elements involved in the differential expression of the rat crystallin genes was tested by assaying the efficiency of the promoters of the six rat $\gamma$-crystallin genes. These promoters were active in both systems, but only in the mouse system was a correlation between the $\gamma$-crystallin promoter activity and lens differentiation found.

INTRODUCTION

One of the attractive features of the lens as a model system for the study of gene regulation in terminally differentiated cells is the synthesis within the lens of a group of abundant lens-specific proteins, the crystallins. In the rat the crystallins comprise three major protein families, the α-, β- and γ-crystallins (for recent review see 1, 2). From studies at the protein level it has long been known that the crystallins are not uniformly distributed throughout the lens but that, for example, the lens nucleus and cortex differ in both crystallin concentration and composition (3, 4). Thus these studies suggested that the synthesis of the various crystallins is developmentally regulated. However, a detailed picture of the developmental expression pattern of the each of the various crystallin genes was still lacking. We have now determined these expression patterns at the RNA level in the rat lens (5, 6).

## THE DEVELOPMENTAL PATTERN OF EXPRESSION OF THE CRYSTALLIN GENES IN THE RAT LENS

We have striven to establish as complete a picture as possible of the developmental changes in expression of the crystallin genes in the rat lens and have therefore measured, at different developmental stages, the concentration of the RNA product of all the crystallin genes for which a clone is available, i.e. the αA-, the αB-, the βA3/A1-, the βB1-, the βB2-, the βB3-, the βs-, and the six γ-crystallin genes. We observed that differential gene expression occurs within all three crystallin gene families. Perhaps the simplest pattern is shown by the γ-crystallin gene family (5). Transcripts of all six members of this gene family can be detected at the earliest time that measurement of the RNA concentration is feasible, namely at 15 days of fetal development. A linear increase in the concentration of these transcripts is found up to birth. In the post-natal lens a differential shut-off of the transcription of the various γ-crystallin genes is observed: a decrease in the concentration of the RNA originating from the γA, γE and γF genes (for nomenclature, see 7) is seen at 1 month after birth, while at this time the same or even a slightly increased concentration of the transcripts of the γB, γC, and γD genes is found (see also table 1). The shut-off of the transcription from the γC and γD genes occurs around 3 months after birth. In the mature lens cortex (8 months after birth) only transcripts from the γB gene can be detected, albeit at a low level. Within the γ-crystallin gene family we thus find a simultaneous activation but a differential shut-down of the transcription of the individual members of the gene family. The distant relative

Molecular Biology of the Eye: Genes, Vision,
and Ocular Disease, pages 239–247
© 1988 Alan R. Liss, Inc.

β-CRYSTALLIN TRANSCRIPTION IN EMBRYONIC CHICK RETINA CELLS

R.M. Clayton, M.W. Head, S.K.A. Sedowofia and A. Peter

Department of Genetics, University of Edinburgh,
West Mains Road, Edinburgh EH9 3JN, U.K.

ABSTRACT  β-crystallin RNAs were found in a proportion
of cells of 6.5 and 8-day embryonic chick neural
retina. The number of cells which transcribe
δ-crystallin and β-crystallin RNAs imply that some
cells transcribe more than one crystallin RNA
species. There is some evidence that there is an
ontogenic change in distribution of such cells during
development and that some at least of the transcription may not be random with respect to cell type.

INTRODUCTION

Although crystallins had long been regarded as
quintessential organ-specific proteins, several authors,
using anticrystallin antibodies, reported finding
crystallins in certain non-lens tissues.  The earlier data
have been reviewed and discussed elsewhere (1).
More recently, immunohistology with mono-specific
antibodies to δ-crystallin, the major component of the
embryonic chick lens, have detected δ-crystallin antigenicity in 30% of the cells of the embryonic adeno-
hypophysis (2,3), in specific neuronal tracts of the
embryonic avian midbrain (4) and in a specifically located
sub-population of retinal glial cells (5).  cDNA probes
to coding sequences of δ-crystallin RNA detect its presence
in several non-lens tissues (6,7).
The potential for transdifferentiation of retina to
lens was found to be associated with the expression of
crystallin RNA at moderate or intermediate levels (8) but
in situ hybridisation showed that tissues which
transcribe δ-crystallin RNA are heterogeneous, with groups
of cells transcribing at relatively high levels amongst

histologically similar cells without such transcripts (9).

α-crystallin protein was reported in retina and iris by several investigators (1) and an antiserum to a fraction enriched with α-crystallin localised in retinal Muller-glia cells (10) while αA-crystallin RNA was detected in freshly isolated 8-day embryo neural retina (11).

β-crystallin antigenicity has been detected in retina. The simplest interpretation of the early data is that only some of the β-crystallin polypeptides are detectable (1). The 25kD β-crystallin RNA was not detected in freshly isolated 8-day embryo neural retina (12); however other β-crystallins remain to be investigated.

We report here on some data from a preliminary exploration of β-crystallin RNAs in the embryonic neural retina, and on a preliminary attempt to obtain a partial separation of cell types in order to examine the distribution among them of different crystallin RNAs.


## MATERIALS AND METHODS

We are currently using cDNA probes to the following crystallin RNAs: δ-crystallin RNA (pM56) (13), 25kD β-crystallin (026) (12) and three β-crystallin probes which were a generous gift from Dr. J. Piatigorsky (pCβ19/26 Cr42, pCβ23 Cr52, pCβ25 Cr61 (14). All probes were constructed by dG dC homopolymer tailing and were inserted into the Pst 1 site of the plasmid vector, pBR322. In situ hybridisation to sectioned whole eyes at 6.5 days of incubation, to squashes of neural retina at 8 days of incubation, and to cultured cells from 8-day neural retina was carried out as in Bower et al (15) and Jeanny et al (9) but under conditions of higher stringency as in Pardue (16). Cells or tissue fragments were cultured for 24 hours in medium containing sodium valproate or phenytoin, and neurotransmitter uptake and glial enzyme activities were measured according to Sedowofia and Clayton and Sedowofia et al (17,18). Cells were also grown in control medium, in valproate or·phenytoin from days 17 to 24, and harvested on day 24. Total cell RNA was prepared according to Chirgwin et al (19) and preparation of dot blots, hybridisation, highly stringent washing and hybrid detection were carried out according to Anderson and Young (20): SDS PAGE was as in Patek and Clayton (21).

RESULTS

We are currently examining sectioned eyes and tissue squashes of eyes from embryos of 3.5 to 16 days of incubation, but report here only on 6.5 and 8-day embryonic material, for which we have examined several eyes from two different chick strains.

6.5-day embryo eyes. δ-crystallin RNA was found located in both nuclei and cytoplasm of lens cells (Fig. 1A) while 19/26kD β, 23kD β and 25kD β RNAs were mainly nuclear in these cells Fig. 1 BCD). Fig. 1 EFGH represent sections through the central posterior neural retina and pigment epithelium of the corresponding eyes. All four RNA species were found in numerous cells scattered throughout the neural retina. Occasional pigment epithelium cells were also labelled by hybridisation to each of the four probes. The number of positive cells for each probe implies that at least some cells in neural retina transcribe more than one crystallin RNA.

8-day embryo neural retina. Some degree of cellular heterogeneity, both quantitative and qualitative is shown in squashes of all four RNAs, (Fig. 2 ABCD). This is especially marked for 25kD β-RNA, where small groups of heavily labelled cells are surrounded by cells of indistinguishable morphology which exhibit little or no hybridisation to the probe.

Cultured 8-day embryo neural retina cells. The 21-day cultured cells shown in Fig. 2 (FGHI) show that all four RNAs are partially processed to the cytoplasm.

Partial selection of retina cells. Phenytoin treatment for 24 hrs led to a 36% increase in the uptake of dopamine, a 177% increase in the uptake of noradrenaline and to a relative increase in 19/26kD RNA (Fig. 3A). Sodium valproate treatment for 7 days resulted in a 48% diminution in GABA uptake and a 170% increase in noradrenaline uptake in the neurons, and an increase of 27% and 29% respectively in the activity of glial carbonic anhydrase and cyclic nucleotide phosphorylase. There was a virtual absence of αA and αB crystallins, 22kD β-crystallin and 50kD δ-crystallin in 24 day old cultured cells. Further information will be presented elsewhere (Head and Clayton in prepn.).

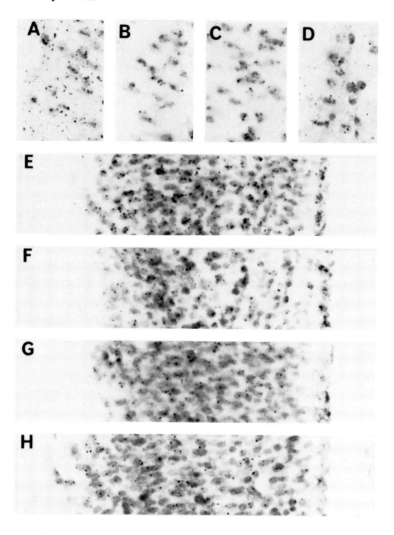

FIGURE 1. In situ hybridisation of δ- and β-crystallin
cDNA probes to sectioned 6.5 day embryo chick retina and
lens. A,B,C, and D, show lens fibre nuclei. E, F, G, and H,
posterior retina: vitreal border on the left; pigmented
epithelium on the right. Paired lens and retina fields
come from the same section. All fields x400. Specificity
of probes: (AE) δ-crystallin: (B,F) 19/26 β-crystallin (C,G)
23 β-crystallin: (D,H) 25 β-crystallin.

Clayton RM (1983b). The pattern of expression of chick δ-crystallin genes in lens differentiation and transdifferentiating cultured tissues. EMBO J 2:333.

16. Pardue ML (1985). In situ hybridisation. In Hames BD, Higgins SJ: "Nucleic Acid Hybridisation: a practical approach", Oxford, Washington DC: IRL Press p179.

17. Sedowofia SKA, Clayton RM (1985). Effects of anti-convulsant drugs on brain cultures from chick embryos: A comparison with cultures from embryos treated in ovo. Teratogen. Carcinogen. Mutagen. 5: 205.

18. Sedowofia SKA, Innes J, Peter A, Alleva E, Manning AWG, Clayton RM (1988). Submitted for publication.

19. Chirgwin JM, Przybyla AE, MacDonald RJ, Rutter WJ (1979). Isolation of biologically active ribonucleic acid from sources enriched in ribonuclease. Biochemistry 18:24, 5294.

20. Anderson MLN, Young BD (1985). Quantitative filter hybridisation. In Hames BD, Higgins SJ; "Nucleic Acid Hybridisation: a practical approach", Oxford, Washington DC: IRL Press, p73.

21. Patek CE, Clayton RM (1988). The influence of the genotype on the process of ageing of chick lens cells in vitro. Exp Cell Res 174:330.

22. Clayton RM, Errington LE, Jeanny J-C, Bower JD, Cuthbert J (1986a). Crystallins in non transparent structures in the embryo. In Duncan G (ed): "The Lens: Transparency and Cataract", Eurage Press, Netherlands: p201.

23. Osterer H, Beebe DC, Piatigorsky J (1981). β-crystallin mRNAs: Differential distribution in the developing chicken lens. Dev Biol 86:403.

24. Clayton RM (1982a). Cellular and molecular aspects of differentiation and transdifferentiation of ocular tissues in vitro. In Yeoman MM, Truman DES (eds): "Differentiation in vitro," Cambridge University Press, p83.

25. Wistow G and Piatigorsky J (1987). Recruitment of enzymes as lens structural proteins. Science 236: 1554.

26. Clayton RM, Head MW, Patek CE (1988). Non coordinate regulation of crystallin RNAs and proteins in lens and in transdifferentiating retina. in. J.H.Chen and G.C. Lavers, eds. "Cellular and Molecular Aspects of Eye Research" Post.Congr.Conf. 7th ICER. in press .

**Molecular Biology of the Eye: Genes, Vision, and Ocular Disease, pages 249–258**
© **1988 Alan R. Liss, Inc.**

PROTO-ONCOGENE EXPRESSION DURING IN VITRO DIFFERENTIATION
OF EMBRYONIC CHICKEN LENS EPITHELIAL EXPLANTS

Peggy S. Zelenka, Luke Pallansch, Malini Vatal,
and Pravendra Nath

Laboratory of Molecular and Developmental Biology
National Eye Institute, NIH, Bethesda, MD 20892

ABSTRACT  Explants of embryonic chicken lens epithelia
differentiate to form lens fiber cells when cultured in
the presence of IGF-I or related substances.  We have
investigated the expression of several proto-
oncogenes during this process using specific DNA
probes for proto-oncogene mRNA's and a sensitive
nuclear "run-on" transcription assay.  Of seven proto-
oncogenes investigated, three are very actively
transcribed in the lens epithelium: c-myc, c-fos, and
p53.  Cytoplasmic levels of c-myc mRNA are transiently
elevated during the first few hours of differentiation
in vitro, while cells are withdrawing from the cell
cycle.  A similar increase in c-myc mRNA levels is
produced by inhibitors of the lipoxygenase pathway of
arachidonic acid metabolism, suggesting that some
product of this pathway may exert a negative
regulatory effect on c-myc expression.

INTRODUCTION

Proto-oncogenes are normal, cellular homologs of the
transforming oncogenes carried by retroviruses.  Since
expression of viral oncogenes in infected cells disrupts the
regulation of cell division and cell differentiation, the
proto-oncogenes may be involved in the normal control of
these processes.  In support of this hypothesis, it has
been found that expression of c-myc and c-fos is transiently
elevated when quiescent cells are stimulated to re-enter the
cell cycle (1,2).  On the other hand, high levels of c-src
are found in differentiating neurons (3), and terminal
differentiation of human monocytic leukemia cells is

associated with elevated expression of c-fos (4). In addition, tissue-specific temporal patterns of proto-oncogene expression have been noted during embryogenesis (5,6). Thus, the proto-oncogenes promise to be key regulatory genes whose functions must be examined in order to understand cell differentiation during embryogenesis.

We have been investigating proto-oncogene expression associated with lens fiber cell differentiation in embryonic chickens. Differentiation of lens epithelial cells to form lens fibers cells occurs in vitro when explants of the central region of lens epithelia from early chicken embryos are cultured in the presence of IGF-I and related substances (7,8,9,10). Careful comparisons of fiber cell formation in vitro and in vivo have shown that in vitro changes in morphology and biochemistry closely parallel the changes that normally occur in vivo (11). Thus, we have used cultured explants of 6-day-old embryonic chicken lens epithelia for our initial studies of proto-oncogene expression during terminal differentiation of lens fiber cells.

RESULTS

To survey expression of a variety of proto-oncogenes in lens epithelial cells, we have used a nuclear run-on transcription assay (12). By modifying published procedures for this assay, we have been able to detect transcripts of specific genes in embryonic chick lens cells using as few as $10^6$ nuclei (Zelenka, Pallansch, and Vatal, unpublished). Using this technique we have found that three proto-oncogenes are very actively transcribed in lens epithelial cells of 6-day-embryos: c-myc, c-fos, and p53 (Fig. 1). Remarkably, transcription of these genes is comparable to transcription of the delta-crystallin gene, which codes for the principal protein product of embryonic chick lenses (13). We also observed a low level of transcription of c-src in these cells, but no significant transcription of c-myb, N-ras or c-raf (c-mil).

The cytoplasmic levels of mRNA for three of the actively transcribed proto-oncogenes (c-myc, c-fos, and c-src) were examined by "dot blot" filter hybridization assays (14). To determine whether levels of mRNA for any of these oncogenes changed significantly during lens fiber cell differentiation, we compared RNA extracted from lens epithelia with RNA extracted from lens fiber masses. The

results showed that specific changes in proto-oncogene
expression are associated with lens fiber cell
differentiation in vivo (Fig.2)(15).  In particular, c-myc
mRNA levels are higher in epithelial cells than in lens
fiber cells, c-fos levels are comparable in the two
populations, and c-src mRNA levels seem to increase
following lens fiber cell formation.

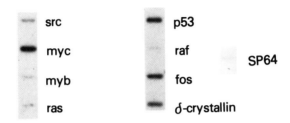

| | |
|---|---|
| src | p53 |
| myc | raf |
| myb | fos |
| ras | δ-crystallin |

SP64

FIGURE 1.   Transcription of proto-oncogenes in
embryonic chicken lens epithelial cells.  Nuclei from
explants of the central region of 6-day-old embryonic
chicken lens epithelia were used for "run-on" transcription.
The [$^{32}$P]-labeled RNA synthesized was applied to
nitrocellulose for hybridization to 10 ug each of linearized
plasmid DNA's containing specific sequences for the
indicated oncogenes and for delta-crystallin.  10 ug of DNA
from the vector plasmid SP64 were used a a control.

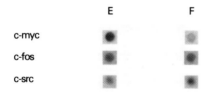

| | E | F |
|---|---|---|
| c-myc | | |
| c-fos | | |
| c-src | | |

FIGURE 2. Hybridization of $^{32}$P-labeled v-myc, v-fos,
and v-src DNA to RNA extracted from whole epithelia (E) or
fiber cells (F) of 6-day embryonic chick lenses.  Each dot
represents 20 ug of total RNA.

Since these results indicated that specific changes in
c-myc expression are associated with lens fiber cell
differentiation, we examined the time course of these

changes in more detail using cultured explants of the
central region of the lens epithelium during differentiation
in vitro (Fig. 3). Differentiation of the cultured explants
was initiated by supplementing the medium with chicken
vitreous humor, which contains an activity immunologically
related to IGF-I (10). mRNA was extracted from the explants
at different times following the addition of vitreous humor,
and analysed by agarose gel electrophoresis and
nitrocellulose filter hybridization. The results indicated
that cells in the central region of the lens epithelium
initially have very low levels of c-myc mRNA, much lower
than the levels observed in the whole epithelia used for the
experiments shown in Fig. 2. After only 0.5hr of
differentiation in vitro, however, c-myc mRNA levels
increased substantially. c-myc mRNA continued to accumulate
in the differentiating cells for at least 5hr, before
declining at 9hr. Thus, there seems to be a transient
increase in c-myc mRNA levels during the early stages of
differentiation. We attribute the high levels of c-myc mRNA
observed in the whole epithelia (Fig. 2) to cells in the
peripheral region of the epithelium, which are in the early
stages of differentiation in vivo.

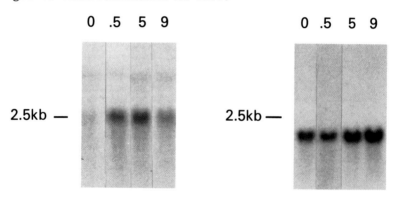

FIGURE 3. Time course of c-myc mRNA expression in
differentiating explants of 6-day embryonic chick lens
epithelia. RNA filter hybridization of total cytoplasmic
RNA to a $^{32}$P-labeled v-myc DNA probe at 0, 0.5, 5, and 9 h
after initiating differentiation with 20% vitreous humor
(left), and hybridization of the same blot to $^{32}$P-delta
crystallin cDNA (right).

Since previous work from this laboratory has demonstrated that turnover of the membrane phospholipid, phosphatidylinositol (PI), ceases when lens epithelial explants undergo differentiation in vitro (16) or in vivo (17), we considered the possibility that PI turnover might in some way regulate c-myc mRNA levels. One consequence of PI turnover in many cells is the release of arachidonic acid, which is then further metabolized to bioactive products. We, therefore, treated lens epithelial explants with inhibitors of arachidonic acid metabolism to test the possibility that some arachidonic acid metabolite might be responsible for the elevated levels of c-myc mRNA in the differentiating cells. The inhibitors used were indomethacin, which blocks the cyclo-oxygenase pathway (18), nordihydroguiaretic acid (NDGA), which blocks the lipoxygenase pathways (19), and eicosatetraynoic acid (ETYA), which blocks all known pathways of arachidonic acid metabolism, including metabolism by cytochrome P450 (20). The results showed that c-myc mRNA levels were significantly elevated by NDGA and ETYA, but were unaffected by indomethacin. This finding is consistent with the hypothesis that some lipoxygenase product of arachidonic acid metabolism may be a negative regulator of c-myc mRNA levels.

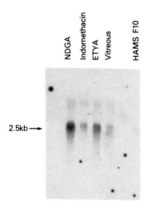

FIGURE 4.  Effect of inhibitors of arachidonic acid metabolism on c-myc mRNA analysed by RNA filter hybridization using a $^{32}$P-labeled chicken c-myc DNA probe. Explants were incubated 2 h in 20% vitreous humor containing either 20uM NDGA, 1uM indomethacin, or 50uM ETYA, in 20% vitreous humor alone, or in unsupplemented Ham's F-10 medium.

## DISCUSSION

Differentiation of embryonic chicken lens epithelial cells to form lens fibers is characterized by a number of morphological and biochemical changes, both in vivo and in the cultured explant in vitro system used in these studies (13).  The cells elongate to many times their original length, microtubules are assembled parallel to the long axis of the cells, the nuclei become pyknotic and are ultimately degraded.  mRNA for delta-crystallin, the principal protein of the embryonic chicken lens, accumulates in the cytoplasm, and the cells become highly speciallized for synthesis of this protein.  Phosphatidylinositol turnover ceases and the dividing cells withdraw from the cell cycle. By investigating the role of specific proto-oncogenes in this process, we hope to learn how these disparate events are regulated, and how they are expressed in a coordinated manner.

Our initial findings, using a nuclear run-on transcription assay, indicate that four proto-oncogenes are transcribed at significant levels in embryonic chicken lens epithelial nuclei.  They are c-myc, c-fos, p53, and c-src. C-myc and c-fos are both short-lived, nuclear DNA-binding proteins(21,2).  C-myc is associated with competence to traverse the cell cycle, and has been shown to play a role in DNA replication( 22,23).  It may also affect transcription of heat shock proteins(24). Increased expression of c-fos has been observed both in quiescent fibroblasts entering the cell cycle (1), and in differentiating monocytic leukemia cells, withdrawing from the cell cycle(4).  Its expression has also been shown to affect transcription of collagen genes(25).  The p53 gene product is overexpressed in certain tumors(26). It forms stable complexes with SV40 large T antigen(27) and with 68 and 70K heat shock proteins(28).  The gene product of c-src is a membrane-associated protein with tyrosine kinase activity(29).  Interestingly, one of the known substrates of the viral homolog, v-src, is calpactin I, a major component of the EDTA extractable protein from lens membranes (30,31).

The transient increase in c-myc mRNA in differentiating lens cells occurs at a time when entry of cells into S phase is blocked and cells are withdrawing from the cell cycle(15). This finding is surprizing in view of the known association between c-myc expression and DNA replication.

Nevertheless, similar transient increases in c-myc mRNA have also been observed in other cell types preceding cell cycle arrest(32-34). These observations suggest that the c-myc protein may play a role in these cells which is distinct from its role in DNA replication.

Specific changes in c-myc mRNA levels have been observed in response to the binding of polypeptide growth factors such as PDGF (1), EGF (35), NGF (35), and an IGF-related protein (15). However, little is known about the second messenger which transfers the signal from the recptor at the plasma membrane either to the nucleus, where transcriptional changes occur, or to the cytoplasm, where specific nucleases may post-transcriptionally regulate c-myc mRNA levels. Our observation that c-myc mRNA can be elevated by inhibitors of the lipoxygenase pathway of arachidonic acid metabolism raises the possibility that some lipoxygenase pathway metabolite may serve as a negative regulator of c-myc mRNA levels in these cells.

## REFERENCES

1.  Kelly K, Cochran BH, Stiles CD, Leder P (1983). Cell-specific regulation of the c-myc gene by lymphocyte mitogens and platelet-derived prowth factor. Cell 35:603

2.  Verma IM, Graham WR (1987). The fos oncogene. Adv Cancer Res 49:29.

3.  Sorge LK, Levy BT, Maness PF (1984). pp60c-src is developmentally regulated in the neural retina. Cell 36:249.

4.  Lee J, Mehta K, Blick MB, Gutterman JU, Lopez-Berestein G (1987). Expression of c-fos, c-myb, and c-myc in human monocytes: correlation with monocytic differentiation. Blood 69:1542.

5.  Muller R, Verma IM, Adamson ED (1983). Expression of c-onc genes: c-fos transcripts accumulate to high levels during development of mouse placenta, yolk sac and amnion. EMBO J 2:679-84.

6.  Van Beveren C, Mitchell RL, Henning-Chubb C, Huberman E, Verma IM (1987).Expression of the c-fos gene during differentiation. Adv Exp Med Biol 213:263.

7.  Philpott GW, Coulombre AJ (1968). Cytodifferentiation of precultured embryonic chick lens epithelial cells in vitro and in vivo. Exp Cell Res 52:140.

8.  Piatigorsky J (1973). Insulin initiation of lens fiber differentiation in culture: elongation of embryonic lens epithelial cells. Develop Biol 30:214.

9.  Beebe DC, Feagans DE, Jebens HA (1980). Lentropin: A factor in vitreous humor which promotes lens fiber cell differentiation. Proc Natl Acad Sci (USA) 77:490.

10. Beebe DC, Silver, MH, Belcher KS, Van Wyk JJ, Svoboda ME, Zelenka PS (1987). Lentropin, a protein that controls lens fiber formation, is related functionally and immunologically to the insulin-like growth factors. Proc Natl Acad Sci (USA)84:2327.

11. Piatigorsky J, Webster H deF, Craig SP (1972) Protein synthesis and ultrastructure during the formation of embryonic chick lens fibers in vivo and in vitro. Develop Biol 27:176.

12. Greenberg ME, Ziff EB (1984). Stimulation of 3T3 cells induces transcription of the c-fos proto-oncogene. Nature 311:433.

13. Piatigorsky J (1981). Lens differentiation in vertebrates. A review of cellular and molecular features. Differentiation 19:134.

14. Maniatis T, Jeffrey A, Kleid DG (1975). Nucleotide sequence of the rightward operator of phage lambda. Proc Natl Acad Sci USA 72:1184.

15. Nath P, Getzenberg R, Beebe D, Pallansch L, Zelenka P (1987). C-myc mRNA is elevated as differentiating lens cells withdraw from the cell cycle. Exp Cell Res 169:215.

16. Vu N-D, Chepko G, Zelenka P (1983). Decreased turnover of phosphatidylinositol accompanies in vitro differentiation of embryonic chicken lens epithelial cells into lens fibers. Biochim Biophys Acta 750:105.

17. Zelenka P (1980). Changes in phosphatidylinositol metabolism during differentiation of lens epithelial cells into lens fiber cells in the embryonic chick. J Biol Chem 255:1296.

18. Vane JR (1981). Inhibition of prostaglandin synthesis as a mechanism of action for aspirin-like drugs. Nature 231:232.

19. Tappel AL, Lundberg WO, Boyer PD (1953). Effect of temperature and antioxidants upon the lipoxygenase-catalyzed oxidation of sodium linoleate. Arch Biochem Biophys 42:293.

20. Tobias LD, Hamilton JG (1979). The effect of 5,8,11,14-eicosatetraynoic acid on lipid metabolism. Lipids 14:181.
21. Cole MD (1986). The myc oncogene: its role in transformation and differentiation. Ann Rev Genet 20:361.
22. Heikkila R, Schwab G, Wickstrom E, Like SL, Pluznik DH, Watt R, Neckers LM (1987). A c-myc antisense oligodeoxynucleotide inhibits entry into S phase but not progress from $G_0$ to $G_1$. Nature 328:445.
23. Studzinski GP, Brelvi ZS, Feldman SC, Watt RA (1986). Participation of c-myc protein in DNA synthesis of human cells. Science 234:467.
24. Kingston RE, Baldwin AS Jr, Sharp PA (1984). Regulation of heat shock protein 70 gene expression by c-myc. Nature 312:280.
25. Setoyama C, Frunzio R, Liau G, Mudryj M, de Crombrugghe B (1986). Transcriptional activation encoded by the v-fos gene. Proc Natl Acad Sci USA 83:3213-7.
26. Oren M (1985). The p53 cellular tumor antigen: gene structure, expression and protein properties. Biochim Biophys Acta 823:67.
27. McCormick F, Clark R, Harlow E (1980). Association of a murine 53,000-dalton phosphoprotein with simian virus 40 large T antigen in transformed cells. J Virol 34:213.
28. Pinhasi-Kimhi O, Michalovitz D, Ben-Zeev A, Oren M (1986). Specific interaction between the p53 cellular tumor antigen and major heat shock proteins. Nature 320:182.
29. Radke K, Gilmore T, Martin GS (1980). Transformation by Rous sarcoma virus: a cellular substrate for transformation-specific protein phosphorylation contains phosphotyrosine. Cell 21:821.
30. Erikson E, Erikson RL (1980). Identification of a cellular protein substrate phosphorylated by the avian sarcoma virus-transforming gene product. Cell 21:829.
31. Russell P, Zelenka P, Martensen T, Reid TW (1987). Identification of the EDTA-extractable protein in lens as calpactin I. Curr Eye Res 6:533.
32. Yen A, Guernsey DL (1986). Increased c-myc RNA levels associated with the precommitment state during HL-60 myeloid differentiation. Cancer Res 46:4156-4161.

33.  Levine RA, McCormack JE, Buckler A, Sonenshein GE
     (1986). Transcriptional and post-transcriptional
     control of c-myc gene expression in WEHI-231 cells.
     Mol Cell Biol 6:4112.
34.  Larsson L-G, Gray HE, Totterman T, Pettersson U,
     Nilsson K (1987). Drastically increased expression of
     myc and fos protooncogenes during in vitro
     differentiation of chronic lymphocytic leukemia cells.
     Proc Natl Acad Sci (USA)84:223.
35.  Greenberg ME, Green LA, Ziff EB (1985). Nerve growth
     factor and epidermal growth factor induce rapid
     transient changes in proto-oncogene transcription in
     PC12 cells.  J Biol Chem 260:14101.

**Molecular Biology of the Eye: Genes, Vision, and Ocular Disease, pages 259–268**
© **1988 Alan R. Liss, Inc.**

CELL CONTACTS AND GENE REGULATION
IN EMBRYONIC RETINA

A. A. Moscona and Lily Vardimon

Laboratory for Developmental Biology,
Department of Molecular Genetics and Cell Biology,
The University of Chicago, Chicago, Illinois 60637

INTRODUCTION

Cell interactions play a critical role in regulation of
gene expression during embryonic development. Cells
communicate and cooperate in making developmental decisions;
their interrelationships influence and determine their
differentiation, morphogenesis and stability of phenotypic
characteristics. These facts have long been known, but the
molecular basis for the regulation of gene expression by cell
interactions is only beginning to be examined in detail.

Developmental cell interactions include: 1. Long-range
cell communication by hormones and hormone-like factors
(systemic; localized) which induce, or modulate gene
expression in receptive target cells. 2. Short-range, cell-
contact communication; this requires cell adhesion,
interactions of cell membrane molecules, or cell junctions;
it is assumed that signals generated or mediated by cell
contacts are relayed into cells and influence regulation of
gene expression.

In the system described here, <u>embryonic neural retina</u>,
the induction of <u>glutamine synthetase</u> is synergetically
dependent on both kinds of cell communication: hormonal
effects and cell-contact (1).

RETINA, MULLER GLIA AND GS INDUCTION

In vertebrate retina, the enzyme glutamine synthetase
(GS), which catalyzes the conversion of glutamate to glutamine, is confined exclusively to <u>Muller glia cells</u>; it is
not found in the neurons. In chicken retina —used in the

studies discussed here- Muller cells are the only type of
glia; GS is a characteristic product of their differentiation
(2) and it plays a major role in their physiological
function: glutamate, a candidate-neurotransmitter released
from certain neurons (3), is taken up into Muller cells and
converted by GS to glutamine; neurons use glutamine to make
glutamate. This neuron-glia metabolic cooperation is
reflected in the involvement of cell contacts in regulation
of GS gene expression, as discussed below.

In adult retina, GS is a major constituent of Muller
glia cells; we have recently estimated that GS represents,
at least, 20% of their total protein content (4). The
reason for the surprisingly high level of this enzyme in
these cells is not known; perhaps, a very rapid turnover
of glutamate into glutamine is necessary for vision-related
activity of retinal neurons (3). Another possibility is
suggested by the discovery that certain enzymes serve also
as major structural proteins (5).

In embryonic retina, the level of GS enzyme is very low
during early developmental ages. In chick embryo retina, GS
level begins to rise steeply only on day 15-16 of development, increases multifold and reaches a high plateau soon
after hatching (1). Correspondingly, GS mRNA accumulation
increases very markedly and attains a high level in mature
retina, as was demonstrated by Northern blot analysis and
hybridization with a GS gene clone (6).

The special attractiveness of this system for analysis
of gene regulation is that GS in Muller cells can be induced
precociously, several days before its normal rise, by
prematurely supplying cortisol to the retina (1) (in birds,
corticosterone is the predominant adrenal cortex hormone,
but cortisol and dexamethasone are equally effective as GS
inducers). The hormone can be supplied by injection into
early embryos, or it can be presented directly to isolated
retina tissue in organ culture; for obvious reasons, most of
the work was done on in vitro cultures of retina tissue and
cells (7).

Treatment of early embryonic retina tissue with
cortisol elicits rapid accumulation of GS mRNA (6,8,9); it
is markedly elevated already by 2 hrs after cortisol
addition (8,9), rising more slowly thereafter (Fig. 1). The
rate of GS enzyme synthesis also inceases rapidly and its
level in Muller cells rises manyfold in 24 hrs.

Inhibition of RNA synthesis at the time of cortisol
addition prevents GS induction (7), i.e., neither GS mRNA
nor the enzyme increase. However, when only protein

synthesis is inhibited, cortisol elicits GS mRNA accumulation (8,10). Thus, in the presence of cyclohexamide (a translational inhibitor), cortisol elicits a similar increase in GS mRNA level as in the inhibitor's absence (Fig. 2; original results); following cycloheximide withdrawal, the stockpiled templates are translated, resulting in rapid increase of GS (10). These findings strongly suggest that the onset of GS mRNA accumulation is not dependent on preceding synthesis of an intermediary, or ancillary factor elicited by cortisol, but is due to direct stimulation by the hormone of GS gene transcription.

Direct evidence that the induction of GS is regulated at transcriptional level was obtained by means of the in vitro nuclear run-on transcription assay (9). Within 2 hrs after cortisol addition, the rate of GS gene transcription increased very markedly; this is consistent with the kinetics of GS mRNA accumulation described above.

The evidence that cortisol induces GS by stimulating GS gene transcription confirms earlier suggestions to this effect (7,8,10,11,12). Together with other findings (13), this result places the role of cortisol in GS induction within the framework of the generally accepted mechanism of corticosteroid hormone action (14): we have previously established (13) that, as in other target cells, also in the retina cortisol binds to specific intracellular receptors, and that the complexes translocate into nuclei and bind to DNA (15); the resulting GS mRNA accumulation is due to increase in GS gene transcription (Fig. 4).


## CELL INTERACTIONS AND GS REGULATION

The above description addresses, however, only one aspect of the mechanism of GS induction. The possibility that also cell-to-cell contacts are implicated arose unexpectedly, when we attempted to induce GS in separated retina cells. Embryonic retina tissue was dissociated into single cells; the cells were plated as a monolayer in culture dishes, or were maintained monodispersed as a cell suspension. The culture medium contained cortisol, yet GS was not induced; even after culturing the cells for several days in cortisol medium, the enzyme either did not increase at all above baseline, or rose minimally, whereas in undissociated retina tissue GS was consistently inducible (1,2,9).

Compared with intact tissue, in separated cells cortisol elicited, at best, only a small increase in GS mRNA level

(Fig. 3), i.e., it failed to optimally stimulate GS gene transcription (9). It is important to note that there was no general reduction of other mRNAs in these cells, as evidenced by the unchanged levels of two other transcripts used as reference markers: carbonic anhydrase II (CA II) mRNA (a Muller glia enzyme not inducible with cortisol), and replacement histone H3.3 mRNA (Fig. 3). This suggested that cell separation selectively precluded the stimulation by cortisol of GS gene activity. Another important point should be mentioned: the small increases of GS mRNA level that were noted in monolayer cultures always coincided with the presence of spontaneously forming cell clusters: in cultures with numerous clusters, cortisol elicited greater accumulation of GS mRNA than when the cells remained monodispersed (9).

We tried to bring about GS induction in the separated cells by using different culture media, "conditioned" media, hormone concentrations, glutamate, glutamine and other additives, but these attempts were unsuccessful. There remained the possibility that disconnection and separation of the cells caused them to become non-inducible; this, in turn, implied that cell contacts were required for GS induction, in addition to the hormone.

This assumption was directly tested by reaggregating the dissociated cells. The prediction was that, if cell contacts were required for the induction, restoration of cell contacts might reverse the loss of inducibility--assuming that this loss was reversible. The results supported the prediction (2).

Dissociated embryonic retina cells were reaggregated into multicellular aggregates by swirling the cell suspension in a small flask on a gyratory shaker-incubator (16). In this procedure, the cells gradually reassemble and reestablish tissue-like contacts and associations; neurons and glia reconstruct histological patterns resembling those of retina tissue (2,16). When cortisol was added to such cell aggregates, GS was induced and its level increased rapidly. Immunostaining of the induced aggregates with GS-specific antibodies showed intense immunofluorescence in Muller glia cells, especially in those juxtaposed with neurons (2). Hence, restitution of cell contacts restored competence for GS induction. Indeed, Northern blot-hybridization analysis (9) showed that, in the reaggregated cells cortisol stimulated GS mRNA accumulation (Fig. 3).

In the above experiments the cells were reaggregated soon after their dissociation from the tissue. Do they remain induction-competent also after longer separation? To test this, dissociated cells were cultured dispersed for 48 hrs, and only then were reaggregated. Cortisol induced GS also in these aggregates; GS mRNA accumulation increased and GS enzyme level rose markedly (9). Therefore, in this case as well, restitution of cell contacts restored GS incucibility. It is, of course, quite conceivable that prolonged cultivation of Muller cells in monolayer culture might modify their phenotype regulation (17) resulting in complete loss of GS inducibility, or in relaxation of its dependence on cell contacts.

Are specific cell contacts requried for the induction, or is random proximity of cells sufficient? Dissociated retina cells were dispersed in cortisol medium, and were agglutinated with lectins, or with cross-linking antiserum. In these randomly bunched cells there was no GS induction (18). In another approach, dissociated retina cells were plated in culture dishes at a density at which some of the flattened glia cells came into close proximity with small clusters of neurons. Cortisol was added; two days later the cultures were immunostained for GS and the cells were individually inspected. An induced increase of GS level was detected in some of the glia cells but, significantly, only in those that were in close contact with neurons; those that were separated from neurons even by a short distance did not immunostain for GS (19).

The following conclusions were indicated by these findings: induction by cortisol of GS in glia cells requires their interactions with neurons; these interactions involve direct cell-to-cell contacts, rather than some diffusable cell-released factor, since even small distances between cells precluded induction. The retina contains several types of neurons and it is not known which are involved in this cell contact effect. It is important to mention here that there are no detectable gap junctions in the retina used in this work.

Are cell contacts necessary only to initiate the induction, or are they continuously required also to maintain the induced expression of GS? Does cell separation cause de-induction? To answer this question, GS was induced with cortisol to a high level in retina tissue; then, the tissue was dissociated and the cells were plated in cortisol medium. The level of GS mRNA fell rapidly in the separated cells and declined by 90% within 20 hrs, despite exposure to cortisol. The level of GS enzyme also was markedly reduced (9). Therefore, cell separation aborted the pre-existing induction. Using the in vitro nuclear run-on transcription assay, we

determined that GS gene transcription declined rapidly in
the separated cells from its initially high rate (9), which
accounted for the drop in GS mRNA level and for the de-
induction. We conclude that cell contacts are necessary both
for initiating the induction of GS and for maintaining the
induced state of GS gene activity. In this context it is of
interest that, in brain astroglial cells GS induction is
mediated by cell contact with neurons, and is also elicited
by cortisol (20).

## HYPOTHESIS AND COMMENTS

On the basis of these and related findings we hypothe-
size that, the induction by cortisol of GS in retina glia
cells is dependent on their adhesion and contact-communication
with neurons (Fig. 4). The hypothesis proposes that molecular
interactions between the adherent cell surfaces confer on the
glia cell membrane conformational or chemical characteristics
that are signalled into the glia cell; these signals address
regulatory processes which capacitate the glia cell for
stimulation by cortisol of GS gene expression. Cell detachment and separation modify the cell membrane and abrogate
the signals, thereby causing loss of inducibility.

Identification of the postulated signals is, of course,
a major challenge in this system, as well as in other cases
where gene expression is regulated by cell contacts. One
approach is to determine which of the steps along the pathway of the induction mechanism is affected by the signals.
Among possible candidates are cortisol-binding receptors;
indeed, we found that their level (or binding activity)
partially declined in separated cells and increased again
when the cells were reaggregated (13). The fact that these
receptors are subject to control by cell contacts is, in
itself, of major importance. However, at present, there is
no clear evidence of a directly causal and exclusive relationship between changes in receptor level and GS inducibility in
the retina (13). Thus, although the possibility remains open
that GS induction is precluded in separated cells because of
the partial down-regulation of cortisol receptors, it is
equally conceivable that some other process critical for the
enhancement of GS gene activity also is influenced by cell
contact, and that its failure in separated cells is primarily
responsible for the absence of induction. In any case, the
importance of intercellular contact-communication in the
control of gene expression in this system should encourage

search for similar mechanisms in other systems (16,17).

We thank Lyle Fox and Linda Degenstein for their participation in these studies. This work was supported by research grants from the National Science Foundation, and the March of Dimes-Birth Defects Foundation.

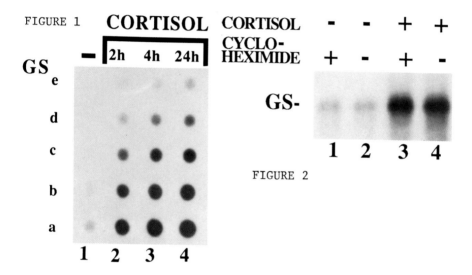

FIGURE 1. GS mRNA accumulation in cortisol-induced retina: dot blot analysis of total RNA from retina tissue of 13-day embryo. Non-induced tissue: lane 1; tissue treated with cortisol for 2, 4, 24 hrs: lanes 2, 3, 4. Undiluted (a) and serially diluted (b-e) RNA samples were hybridized to a clone of the GS gene (for detailed description, see reference 9).

FIGURE 2. Induction of GS mRNA accumulation in the absence of protein synthesis. Retina tissue from 13-day embryos was cultured for 4 hrs, in presence or absence of cortisol (lanes 1,2); control cultures were without cycloheximide (lanes 2,4). Analysis of total RNA by Northern blotting and hybridization to the GS gene clone.

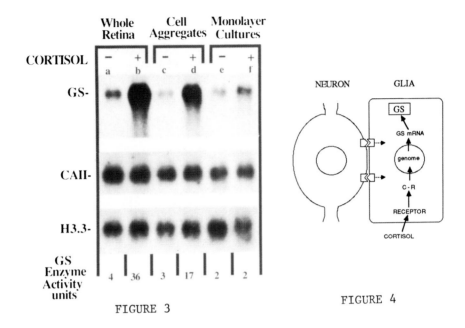

FIGURE 3                                    FIGURE 4

FIGURE 3.  Induction of GS mRNA accumulation requires cell
contacts:  Northern blot analysis.  Retina tissue from 10-day
embryos was cultured intact (lanes a,b), or was dissociated
into cells which were plated monodispersed in monolayer
culture (lanes e,f), or were immediately reaggregated
(lanes c,d).  All cultures were for 48 hrs.  Cortisol was added
for the last 24 hrs (lanes b,d,f).  Poly-A RNA was isolated and
was hybridized consecutively to the clones of the GS gene,
histone H.3 gene, and CA II cDNA (the latter as reference
markers).  Note low level of GS mRNA in monolayer cultures,
compared with cell aggregates and intact tissue.  No significant changes in the reference markers (details in reference 9).

FIGURE 4.  Proposed model of GS induction in retina glia
(Muller) cells.

REFERENCES

1. Moscona AA (1983). On glutamine synthetase, carbonic anhydrase and Muller glia in the retina. In Osborne N, Chader G (eds): "Progress in Retina Research," v.2, Oxford and New York: Pergamon Press, p 111.

2. Linser P, Moscona AA (1979). Induction of glutamine synthetase in embryonic neural retina: localization in Muller fibers and dependence on cell interactions. Proc. Natl. Acad. Sci. USA 76: 6476.

3. Brew H, Attwell D (1987). Electrogenic glutamate uptake is a major current carrier in the membrane of axolotl retinal glia cells. Nature 327: 707.

4. Fox L, Moscona AA (1988). Original results.

5. Wistow G, Piatigorsky J (1987). Recruitment of enzymes as lens structural proteins. Science 236:1554.

6. Vardimon L, Fox L, Degenstein L, Moscona AA (1986). Developmental regulation of glutamine synthetase and carbonic anhydrase II in neural retina. Proc. Natl. Acad. Sci. USA 83:9060.

7. Moscona AA, Moscona M, Saenz N (1968). Enzyme induction in embryonic retina: the role of transcription and translation. Proc. Natl. Acad. Sci. USA 61:160.

8. Petejunas G, Young AP (1987). Tissue-specific regulation of avian glutamine synthetase expression during development and in response to glucocorticoid hormones. Mol. Cellular Biol. 7:1070.

9. Vardimon L, Fox L, Degenstein L, Moscona AA (1988). Cell contacts are required for induction by cortisol of GS gene transcription in the retina. Proc. Natl. Acad. Sci. USA, in press.

10. Garfield S, Moscaon AA (1974). Glutamine synthetase in the embryonic chick neural retina: the effect of cycloheximide on conservation of labile templates for enzyme synthesis. Mech. Ageing Devel. 3:253.

11. Sarkar PK, Moscona AA (1973). Glutamine synthetase induction in embryonic neural retina: immunochemical identification of polysomes involved in enzyme synthesis. Proc. Natl. Acad. Sci. USA 70:1667.

12. Soh BM, Sarkar PK (1978). Control of glutamine synthetase messenger RNA by hydrocortisone in the embryonic chick retina. Dev. Biol. 64:316.

13. Saad AD, Moscona AA (1985). Cortisol receptors and inducibility of glutamine synthetase in embryonic retina. Cell Different. 16:241.

14. Ringold GM (1985). Steroid hormone regulation of gene expression. Ann. Rev. Pharmacol. Toxicol. 25:529.

15. Sarkar PK, Moscona AA (1975). Nuclear binding of hydrocortisone receptors in embryonic chick retina and its relationship to glutamine synthetase induction. Am. Zool. 15:241.

16. Moscona AA (1974). Surface specification of embryonic cells: lectin receptors, cell recognition and specific cell ligands. In Moscona AA (ed): "The Cell Surface in Development," New York: John Wiley & Sons, p. 67.

17. Moscona AA, Linser P (1983). Developmental and experimental changes in retinal glia cells: cell interactions and control of phenotype expression and stability. Curr. Topics Devel. Biol. 18: 155.

18. Linser P (1987). Neuronal-glial interactions in retina development. Am. Zool. 27:161.

19. Linser P, Moscona AA (1983). Hormonal induction of glutamine synthetase in cultures of embryonic retina cells: requirement for glia-neuron interactions. Devel. Biol. 96:529.

20. Wu DK, Scully S, deVelis J (1988). Induction of glutamine synthetase in rat astrocytes by co-cultivation with embryonic chick neurons. J. Neurochem. 50:929.

Molecular Biology of the Eye: Genes, Vision,
and Ocular Disease, pages 269–276
© 1988 Alan R. Liss, Inc.

# THE SELECTION OF RETINAL GANGLION CELLS THAT EXTEND THEIR AXONS FOR GENE EXPRESSION ANALYSIS

Lidia Matter-Sadzinski, Jean-Marc Matter,
and W. Maxwell Cowan

Department of Neurosurgery, Washington University School
of Medicine, St. Louis, MO 63110

ABSTRACT   We have developed an _in vitro_ assay system
that enables us to mark retinal ganglion cells which
extend their axons in a matrix of collagen, using
rhodamine-labeled microspheres.  Subsequent _in situ_
hybridization enables one to monitor the levels of
specific gene expression in this subpopulation of
ganglion cells.

## INTRODUCTION

During a relatively short period in the development of
the chick retina (from about the eighth to the fourteenth
days of incubation - E8 to E14), there is a transient phase
of enhanced expression of the $\beta$1-tubulin gene (1).  The
expression of this gene appears to be restricted to the
ganglion cell population and coincides with the major phase
of outgrowth of the optic nerve axons (1).  During the
development of the chick optic tectum, axonal outgrowth has
also been found to be associated with an increase in the
expression of the $\beta$1-tubulin gene (1,2).  Transient
expression of the $\beta$1-tubulin gene can be reproduced _in
vitro_, when retinal explants are embedded in a matrix of
collagen; these particular culture conditions are adequate
for the survival of ganglion cells and axonal outgrowth
(2).
It is critical in the analysis of the relationship
between axonal outgrowth and $\beta$1-tubulin gene expression to
restrict the gene expression analysis to those cells that
are actively extending axons.

In this report we describe an <u>in vitro</u> assay system that enables us to label retrogradely the ganglion cells that are extending their axons, and to determine, by <u>in situ</u> hybridization, the specific expression of the β1-tubulin gene in this subpopulation of cells.

## MATERIALS AND METHODS

1. <u>Embedding the retinal explants into a matrix of collagen</u>. Eyes were removed from 5 days-old chick embryos and the neural retina dissected away from the lens, vitreous, and pigment epithelium. Petri dishes (60 mm in diameter) were covered with 2.5 ml of Vitrogen 100 solution, prepared following the procedure recommended by the manufacturer (Collagen Corporation, Palo Alto). The dishes were preincubated for 30 minutes in a $CO_2$-incubator at 37°C. After polymerization of the collagen, the retinal explants (two per dish) were placed on the surface of the collagen and immediately covered with a drop ( ~ 150 μl) of the collagen solution. After 30 minutes in the $CO_2$-incubator, 4 ml of Dulbecco's modified Eagle medium (DMEM) supplemented with 10% heat-inactivated fetal calf serum (FCS; Gibco) was added and the explants were maintained in a $CO_2$-incubator at 37°C (2) (FIGURE 1).

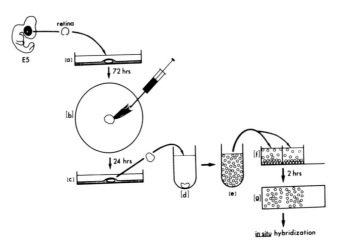

FIGURE 1.   Schematic representation of the experimental procedure used for labeling ganglion cells in the retinal explants.

2. <u>Labeling of ganglion cells</u>. On the 3rd day after explanting, by which time outgrowing axons had penetrated the collagen matrix, the culture medium was carefully removed and 200-400 nl of rhodamine-labeled microspheres (3) were injected into the collagen just ahead of the growing front of axons (within 100-150 $\mu$m of the leading axons). In some experiments, FITC-labeled microspheres (a gift from Dr. A. Burkhalter) were injected. The explants were then covered with 4 ml of culture medium and incubated for a further 24 hours at 37°C (FIGURE 1). The labeling of cells in the explants was monitored by fluorescence microscopy.

3. <u>Cell disaggregation and in situ hybridization</u>. At the end of the labeling period, the culture medium was removed and the retinal explants were transferred into 10 ml tubes (two retinas/tube), cut into 2-3 smaller pieces with forceps, and incubated for 15 minutes in 1.5 ml of a 2.5% trypsin solution (1:250, Gibco) at 37°C. To stop digestion, 2 ml of DMEM supplemented with 10% FCS were then added. After centrifugation for 5 minutes at 1200 rpm, the cells were suspended by gentle pipetting in 1 ml of DMEM and then incubated with DNaseI (130 $\mu$g/ml, Sigma) for 15 minutes. The suspension of disaggregated cells was then centrifuged for 5 minutes at 1200 rpm, after which the cells were resuspended in 2 ml of DMEM supplemented with 10% FCS, counted, and aliquots containing 5 x 10$^5$ cells were distributed into tissue culture chambers (4 chambers- 20 x 9 mm/slide, Lab-Tek) (FIGURE 1). After 2 hours incubation at 37°C in a CO$_2$-incubator, the culture medium was removed, the cells were washed twice with ice-cold D- PBS, fixed for 30 minutes with ice-cold 4% paraformaldehyde (prepared in D-PBS), dehydrated for 30 seconds in each of a graded series of ethanols (60%, 95%, 100%) and air dried. The slides were stored at 4°C in sealed boxes for up to six weeks.

Pretreatment of the slides for <u>in situ</u> hybridization was performed as described by Brigati <u>et al</u>. (4). After postfixation (4), the cells were dehydrated in a graded series of ethanols, air dried, and immediately overlaid with 10 $\mu$l of the hybridization mixture. This consisted of 50% v/v formamide, 2 x SSC, pH 7.0, 250 $\mu$g/ml of calf thymus DNA and 2 $\mu$g/ml of [$^{35}$S]-labeled DNA probe. The pAl cDNA probe contained the coding sequences of the $\beta$-actin gene (5). The cells were covered with a sterile glass coverslip (20 x 9 mm), incubated for 12 hours in a moist chamber at 37°C then washed twice, for 10 seconds each, in

2 x SSC at room temperature, followed by three washes (5 minutes each) at 50°C.  After drying, the slides were dipped in liquid Kodak NTB2 emulsion diluted with an equal volume of water, air-dried and exposed for 1-2 weeks at 4°C.  After development and fixation of the autoradiographs, a drop of Krystalon solution (Harleco) was placed on the slide, and the cells were covered with a glass coverslip.

## RESULTS

### 1. Retrograde Labeling of Retinal Ganglion Cells.

The first axons to emerge from the explants were recognizable within 24 hours of incubation and their outgrowth continued throughout the following 3 days.  On the 3rd day of culture, rhodamine-labeled microspheres (3) were injected into the collagen matrix just ahead of the growing axons.

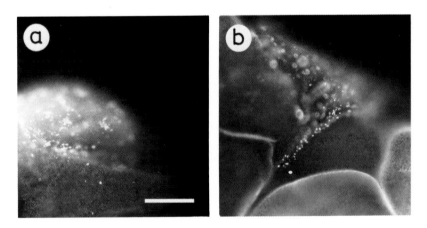

FIGURE 2. Retrograde labeling of ganglion cells with rhodamine-labeled microspheres in a typical retinal explant.  Bar: 500 μm.

Over a period of about 24 hours, the extending axons grow through the injection site and at this stage rhodamine-labeled cells can be observed in the retinal explants.  The labeled cells were usually clustered within

one region of the explant (FIGURE 2 a and b) corresponding
to the region from which the outgrowing axons arise.  This
suggests that the axons from neighboring ganglion cells
tend to remain closely grouped together.  When disaggregated retinal cells were seeded into tissue culture
chambers, about 95% of the inoculated cells attached to the
glass slide within 2 hours of incubation.  We found that
this step, which was crucial for the elimination of dead
cells and cellular fragments, did not alter the level of
$\beta$-actin gene expression (2).  After fixation, the
proportion of labeled cells (FIGURE 3a, 3b) was counted.
In most experiments between 0.5 and 2.0% of cells were
heavily labeled with the rhodamine-labeled microspheres
(TABLE 1).

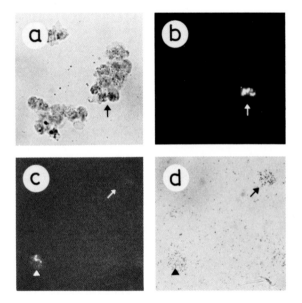

FIGURE 3.  $\beta$-actin gene expression in dissociated
retinal ganglion cells retrogradely labeled with microspheres.  (a) Thionin-labeled retinal cells; (b,c)
rhodamine-labeled cells seen with fluorescence optics; and
(d) <u>in situ</u> hybridization with the pA1 probe.

TABLE 1
RHODAMINE-LABELED CELLS

| Experiments | Labeled cells (%) | Relative Axon Abundance |
|:---:|:---:|:---:|
| 1 | 0.5 ± 0.1% | + |
| 2 | 0.9 ± 0.1% | ++ |
| 3 | 2.0 ± 0.1% | +++ |
| 4 | 0.01% | - |

In the developing chick retina, ganglion cells
represent about 7% of the total retinal cell population
(1); if we assume that the proportion is the same in our
retinal explants embedded in the matrix of collagen, these
results suggest that between 7% and 30% of the explanted
ganglion cells were labeled with rhodamine. Although the
number of axons growing into the collagen matrix was not
quantified, there seemed to be a fairly close correspon-
dence between the percentage of labeled cells  and the
relative abundance of axons (TABLE 1). The specificity of
the labeling procedure was evaluated in a series of
control experiments. When the rhodamine-labeled
microspheres were injected close to the explant, but in an
area in which there were no outgrowing neurites, only an
occasional labeled cell was detected (TABLE 1, experiment
4). In vivo, it has been found that microspheres labeled
with rhodamine are very efficiently transported along axons
(3), whereas FITC-labeled microspheres are relatively
poorly transported and not particularly useful as
retrograde markers (Dr. A. Burkhalter, personal communication). However, when FITC- or rhodamine-labeled
microspheres were added to the medium of primary neuronal
cell cultures, the percentages of FITC-and rhodamine-
labeled cells were similar (data not shown). In contrast,
no fluorescent cells could be detected in our retinal
explants when FITC-labeled microspheres were injected just
ahead of the growing axons. These control experiments
indicate that, under the conditions of our retinal explant
cultures, the rhodamine-labeled microspheres were
retrogradely transported from the site of the injection
back to the retinal ganglion cell bodies.

2. Analysis of Gene Expression in Rhodamine-Labeled
Ganglion Cells.

We have defined experimental conditions for the in
situ hybridization procedure that are compatible with the
presence of intracellular rhodamine-labeled microspheres.
To determine whether or not the presence of microspheres
interfered with the cellular program of gene expression, we
have compared the levels of $\beta$-actin mRNAs in the
rhodamine-labeled cells in retinal explants with those in
unlabeled explants. Since in vivo, the levels of these
mRNAs have been found to be similar in the ganglion cells
and in other retinal cell populations (unpublished
observations), these experiments are likely to be of
general relevance. As Figures 3c and 3d indicate, the
levels of $\beta$-actin mRNAs, revealed by in situ hybridization,
were similar in the rhodamine-labeled cells and in
unlabeled neurons (FIGURES 3c, 3d), indicating that the
expression of the $\beta$-actin gene was not affected by the
labeling procedure.


## DISCUSSION

As a first step towards defining the relationships
that may exist between the $\beta$1-tubulin gene expression and
axon formation, we have developed an in vitro assay system
that enables us to identify ganglion cells in retinal
explants and to analyze gene expression selectively in this
subpopulation of neurons.

The retinal ganglion cells could be uniquely identified by retrograde labeling, in vitro, with rhodamine-
labeled microspheres (3). The presence of the microspheres
did not seem to interfere with the cellular program of gene
expression; the patterns of $\beta$-actin gene expression were
similar in retinal explants subjected to the labeling
procedure and those in which no prelabeling had been
attempted. Preliminary results using this approach,
indicate that $\beta$1-tubulin gene expression in the rhodamine-
labeled cells similarly follows the pattern observed in
vivo.

We have previously shown, by in situ hybridization on
retinal tissue sections, that the expression of the $\beta$1-
tubulin gene in vivo is confined to the ganglion cell layer
(1) and that there is a transient increase in $\beta$1-tubulin
gene expression throughout the period when retinal ganglion

cells are sending their axons into the optic nerve (1). However, it had not been possible previously to establish that these two events were taking place simultaneously in the same cells. Preliminary results, obtained recently with the in vitro assay system described, indicate that the level of mRNA encoded by the β1-tubulin gene is significantly higher in rhodamine-labeled cells (i.e. cells with growing axons) than in unlabeled cells in the same explants.

The possibility of using β1-tubulin gene expression as a marker of axonal outgrowth, taken together with the potential for experimental manipulation of the in vitro system (e.g. by co-culturing tectal cells with the retinal explants) may make it possible, for the first time, to closely correlate the factors involved in axonal outgrowth and the cessation of such growth, with the regulation of specific gene expression in identified neuronal populations.

## ACKNOWLEDGEMENTS

We should like to thank Dr. Andreas Burkhalter for many helpful discussions.

## REFERENCES

1.  Matter J-M, Cowan WM (1988). Regulation of β-tubulin gene expression during the development of the chick retina and optic tectum. In preparation.
2.  Matter J-M, Matter-Sadzinski L, Cowan WM (1988). β1-tubulin gene expression is related to axonal outgrowth during the development of the chick retina and optic tectum. In preparation.
3.  Katz LC, Burkhalter A, Dreyer WJ (1984). Fluorescent latex microspheres as a retrograde neuronal marker for in vivo and in vitro studies of visual cortex. Nature 310:498.
4.  Brigati DJ, Myerson D, Leary JJ, Spalholz B, Travis SZ, Fong CKY, Hsiung GD, Ward DC (1983). Detection of viral genomes in cultured cells and paraffin-embedded tissue sections using biotin-labeled hybridization probes. Virology 126:32.
5.  Cleveland DW, Lopata MA, MacDonald RJ, Cowan NJ, Rutter WJ, Kirschner MW (1980). Number and evolutionary conservation of α- and β-tubulin and cytoplasmic β- and γ-actin genes using specific cloned cDNA probes. Cell 20:95.

Molecular Biology of the Eye: Genes, Vision,
and Ocular Disease, pages 277–291
© 1988 Alan R. Liss, Inc.

# IDENTIFICATION AND EXPRESSION OF DROSOPHILA PHOTOTRANSDUCTION GENES[1]

Craig Montell[2, 4], Drzislav Mismer[2, 5], Mark E. Fortini[2], Charles S. Zuker[3] and Gerald M. Rubin[2],

[2]Howard Hughes Medical Institute and
Department of Biochemistry, University of
California, Berkeley, CA 94720
[3]Department of Biology, University of California,
San Diego, CA 92093

ABSTRACT    The fruitfly, *Drosophila
melanogaster*, is an excellent organism in
which to study the roles of previously
identified photoreceptor cell proteins and to
isolate and characterize the roles of genes
and proteins important in phototransduction
that have not yet been identified in any
metazoan organism.  There are two important
advantages of studying phototransduction in
the fruitfly: 1) many of the relevant genes
have already been genetically identified  2)
DNA sequences can be stably and efficiently
introduced into the genome by P-element
mediated germline transformation.  Therefore,
it is possible to identify the DNA sequence
encoding a genetically defined locus by
complementing the mutant phenotype following
introduction of the wild-type gene into the
genome by germline transformation.  Using this

[1]This work was supported in part by a grant
from the National Institutes of Health to G. M. R.
and by and NIH postdoctoral felloship to C. M.

[4]Present address: Department of Biological
Chemistry, Johns Hopkins University, School of
Medicine, Baltimore, MD 21205.
[5]Present address: Synergen, Inc. 1885 33rd
St., Boulder, CO 80301.

approach, we have identified two genes, *trp* and *ninaC*. Both genes are expressed beginning late in development and encode proteins localized specifically to the photoreceptor cells. The *ninaC* proteins share significant homologies to two types of proteins which define two nonoverlapping domains. One domain shares amino acid homology to protein kinases and the other to all of the globular head region of the myosin heavy chain. The *trp* protein is not homologous to previously sequenced proteins but contains 8 putative transmembrane domains. Using a different approach, we have identified two opsin genes, Rh3 and Rh4, expressed specifically in the R7 ultraviolet sensitive subset of photoreceptor cells. Thus, a total of four related Drosophila opsin genes have now been isolated. Each of these opsin genes is expressed in a different subset of photoreceptor cells in the fly's compound eyes. Experiments directed at identifying the DNA sequences required for the proper spatial and quantitative expression of each of the opsin genes are described.


## INTRODUCTION

The goal of the work descibed here is to isolate and characterize the role of genes and proteins important for vision in the fruitfly, *Drosophila melanogaster*. The fruitfly is an excellent organism to study the molecular genetics of vision for several reasons. First, mutations have been isolated that affect the physiology of photoreceptor cells (reviewed in 1, 2). Many of these mutations were identified on the basis of eliciting abnormal electroretinogram (ERG) recordings. ERGs measure the change in potential due to extracellular current flow in the eye in response to light. The proteins affected by the *Drosophila* ERG mutations fall broadly into at least two categories. Some play a role in phototrans- duction and others are important for formation and/or function of specialized photoreceptor cell structures. The second advantage of using

Drosophila is that the techniques are available to
quickly and easily introduce cloned genes back into
the genome by P-element mediated germline
transformation (3, 4). The combination of these
two advantages enables the molecular identification
of new genes important in vision by complemention
of the mutant phenotype following introduction of
the wild-type gene by germline transformation.
Using genetics and germline transformation, we can
then characterize the roles of the isolated genes
by mutagenizing them *in vitro* and assessing the
effects of mutations following introduction of the
altered genes into the fly's chromosomes by
germline transformation.

In this paper, we summarize the isolation and
characterization of four genes important in
Drosophila vision. Two of these genes, *ninaC* and
*trp*, we identified on the basis of complementation
of mutants with ERG phenotypes (5, 6). The *trp*
gene encodes a protein which acts at an
intermediate step in the cascade subsequent to
photoreception but prior to the change in current
flow across the photoreceptor cell membrane (7).
The *ninaC* gene encodes two proteins required for
formation of the photoreceptor cell cytoskeleton
(8). We also describe the isolation and characterization of two genes encoding opsin which are
expressed in nonoverlapping subsets of the
ultraviolet-sensitive R7 photoreceptor cells (9,
10). Finally, we briefly describe analyses aimed
at defining the molecular basis controlling the
expression of the four Drosophila opsin genes in
different subsets of photoreceptor cells.


## RESULTS AND DISCUSSION

### The *ninaC* Proteins have Linked Kinase and Myosin Domains

The *ninaC* locus was originally identified on
the basis of an ERG phenotype resulting from a
reduced rhodopsin content (11). The decreased
rhodopsin content in *ninaC* has recently has been
shown to be due to a reduction of the diameter of
the rhabdomeres (8). Rhabdomeres are composed of

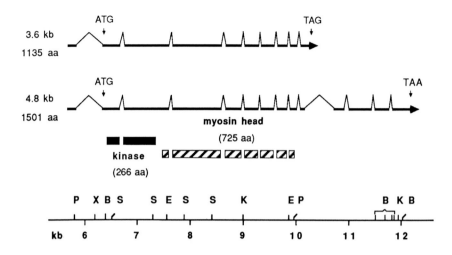

Figure 1.  Structure of *ninaC* mRNAs.  The
bottom line represents the genomic DNA demarcated
in kilobase pairs.  The location of the restriction
sites BamHI (B), EcoRI (E), KpnI (K), PstI (P),
SacI (S) and XbaI (X) are shown.  The bold
horizontal lines joined by the carot symbols
represent the exon and introns of the 3.6 and 4.8
kb mRNAs encoding the 1135 and 1501 aa proteins
respectively. The direction of transcription is
indicated by the arrowhead.  The black box
represents the region encoding the kinase domain
and the stripped box the myosin domain.  The sizes
of these domains is indicated in amino acids (aa).

---

closely packed arrays of microvilli which contain
rhodopsin and other components of the phototransduction cascade.  The microvilli contain a cytoskeletal infrastructure revealed in ultrastructural
studies as electron dense regions (12, 13).  In
*ninaC*, the microvilli are shorter than normal and
the cytoskeletal electron dense regions seen in
wild-type are markedly reduced (8).

We identified the *ninaC* gene by rescuing the
ERG phenotype by P-element mediated germline
transformation (6).  The *ninaC* gene is expressed as

two extensively overlapping mRNAs encoding proteins of 1135 and 1501 aa (figure 1). Both proteins contain two regions of homology with two types of proteins, a 266 amino acid putative kinase domain followed by a 725 amino acid domain similar to the head segment of the myosin heavy chain (MHC). The 1501 aa protein has in addition a third 448 amino acid C-terminal domain that is not similar to any previously sequenced protein. We showed by immunofluorescent localization that the two *ninaC* proteins are expressed predominantly in the rhabdomeres of the photoreceptor cells. Protein kinases play an important role in regulating a large variety of cellular functions including signal transduction and cell growth (reviewed in 14, 15). Myosins are proteins which convert the chemical energy in ATP into mechanical force used in a variety of cell processes (reviewed in 16-18). The globular head of the myosin heavy chain contains the actin binding region, the ATPase catalytic site and the light chain binding site (reviewed in 16-18). The *ninaC* proteins are the first examples of proteins which join putative protein kinase and myosin activities in the same molecule.

Overall, the *ninaC* kinase domain shares about 24-26% identity with other kinases. However, among the 16 amino acids invariant between 20 other protein kinases (14), 15 are identical in *ninaC* and the 16th is a conservative amino acid change. Further analysis of the homologies in the kinase domain indicates that *ninaC* is probably a serine/threonine kinase. The putative myosin domain of *ninaC* shares 24-27% identities with other myosins in separate pairwise alignments over about 725 amino acids. The MHC head is typically about 850 residues. The alignments with *ninaC* begin near amino acid 80 in other MHCs. This 80 amino acid N-terminal segment of the MHCs shows relatively little sequence conservation, even between pairs of MHCs that display very high levels of identity over the rest of the head (18). However, it is possible to make weak alignments expanding the *ninaC* myosin domain by 40 amino acids. Thus, the myosin domain may be 765 amino acids and begin just 8 residues from the end of the kinase domain. The percent

identity is not uniform over the entire head.  The
longest stretch of relatively high sequence
identity spans the putative ATP binding region.  In
this region the percent identity is greater than
50% over 51 amino acids residues in certain
pairwise comparisons

The myosin heavy chain (MHC) is a protein of
approximately 2000 amino acids consisting of two
major domains, the N-terminal S1 globular head
region of about 850 amino acids and an α-helical
rod in the C-terminal region.  In addition to the
large MHCs there are several examples of approximately 110 kd MHCs, first observed in *Acanthamoeba*
(19), which display the catalytic properties of
myosin but do not self-assemble into filaments (20,
21).  Two of these MHCs, referred to as myosin I
(M1HC), have been shown to consist of the head
region of the MHC fused not to the α-helical rod
but to a 35-50 kDa C-terminal tail of unknown
function (23, 24).  The structure of the *ninaC*
myosin domain is most analagous to the M1HCs which
consist of just the head of the MHC joined at the
C-terminus to a 36-51 kDa tail of unknown function
(22, 23).

The observations that *ninaC* mutants affect the
cytoskeletal structure of the photoreceptor cells
(8) and that the gene encodes novel proteins with
kinase and myosin domains which are expressed
predominantly in the photoreceptor cell rhabdomeres
allow us to suggest potential functions for the
*ninaC* proteins.  One possibility is that the *ninaC*
proteins are involved in organelle movement in the
photoreceptor cells.  Propulsion of organelles
along actin filaments may be an activity of myosin
I.  Adams and Pollard (24) found that movement of
organelles *in vitro* appears to be inhibited by
addition of antibodies specific to the myosin I but
not the myosin II of *Acanthamoeba*.  In insect
photoreceptor cells, pigment granules migrate close
to the rhabdomere border during periods of
illumination (reviewed in 25).  This response is
thought to attenuate the incoming light analogous
to the narrowing of the pupil in the vertebrate
eye.  The *ninaC* proteins might be involved in
mediating the movement of the pigment granules
which control this pupil mechanism.  Movement of

vesicles in the photoreceptor cells may also be a function of *ninaC*. The rhabdomeres of the photoreceptor cells appear to be maintained by removing old membrane through invagination. The membrane vesicles created by these invaginations merge to form multivesticular bodies which are presumably degraded after fusing with lysosomes (26). Other vesicles may be used to carry newly synthesized rhodopsin into the microvilli (Stark and Sapp, personal communication). The *ninaC* proteins may play a role in the intracellular migration of some of these vesicles in the photoreceptor cells. It is possible that one of the substrates for the kinase domain might be the *ninaC* proteins themselves. Organelle movement or any other activity mediated by the myosin domain might be controlled by autophosphorylation.

A number of *Drosophila* photoreceptor cell proteins, in addition to rhodopsin, have been shown to be modified by light dependent phosphorylation (27). An alternative possibility is that the *ninaC* proteins move along actin filaments in the rhabdomeral microvilli and regulate other proteins important in phototransduction by phosphorylation. Movement along the actin filaments in the very small, tightly packed microvilli might permit better access to proteins in the microvilli.

It has been shown that *ninaC* flies have smaller rhabdomeres and shorter rhabdomeral microvilli (8). No structural defect outside the photoreceptor cell rhabdomeres was observed. Consistent with these ultrastructural studies are the observations that *ninaC* encodes a putative myosin domain and that these kinase/myosin proteins appear to be expressed, as demonstrated by immunofluorescent localization, predominantly in the photoreceptor cell rhabdomeres. The shorter microvilli and rhadomeral diameter observed in *ninaC* flies may be a consequence of a requirement for the *ninaC* proteins to stretch the actin filaments to the normal extent. Thus, one or both of the *ninaC* proteins may be required for a late step in development of the photoreceptor cells, complete formation of the photoreceptor cell cytoskeleton.

The next experiments are to determine whether the *ninaC* proteins have the biochemical activities

suggested by the homologies to protein kinases and
to the head region of the MHC.  If so, then a
combined application of genetics, site-specific
mutagenesis and P-element transformation should
allow the roles of the individual proteins and
their kinase and myosin domains to be elucidated.


The *trp* Gene

     The *trp* mutation was also identified on the
basis of displaying an ERG phenotype (28).  The *trp*
mutant is characterized by a normal corneal
negative receptor potential.  However, the receptor
potential quickly returns to baseline during
continuous illumination.  The defect in *trp* does
not affect the rhodopsin and the Na$^+$ channels
appear normal.  Recently, Suss et al. performed a
series of experiments indicating that the defect in
*trp* is subsequent to the production of inositol
triphosphate (29).  These workers have suggested
that the defect in *trp* may be due impaired storage
or mobilization of Ca$^{2+}$.
     We have identified the *trp* gene by rescuing the
ERG phenotype following introduction of the
wild-type gene by P-element mediated germline
transformation (5).  We showed that *trp* is
expressed specifically in the eye of the adult fly
as a single 4 kb mRNA.  We have determined the
structure of the *trp* gene by obtaining the DNA
sequence of a full length cDNA and the corresponding genomic region (figure 2).  The *trp* gene does
not show significant homology to any previously
sequenced gene.  However, hydrophobicity
analyses of the deduced amino acid sequence,
according to the algorithm of Kyte and Doolittle
(30), indicates that *trp* is an integral membrane
protein with 8 transmembrane domains.  Since *trp*
appears to contain an even number of transmembrane
segments, the N and C terminal hydrophilic domains
would have to be on the same side of the membrane.
We have raised antisera to *trp*-β-galactosidase
fusion proteins and showed that the 140 kd *trp*
protein is expressed specifically in the
photoreceptor cells.
     Further investigations will be required to

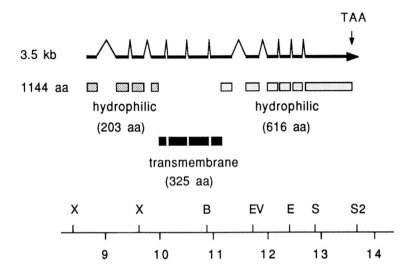

Figure 2.  Structure of *trp* mRNA.  The bottom line
represents the genomic DNA demarcated in kilobase
pairs.  The location of the restriction sites BclI
(B), EcoRI (E), EcoRV (EV), SacI (S), SacII (S2)
and Xho I (X) are shown.  The bold horizontal line
joined by the carot symbols represent the exon and
introns of the mRNA. The direction of transcription
is indicated by the arrowhead.  The black box
represents the region encoding the transmembrane
segments and the stripped box the N- and C-terminal
hydrophilic domains.  The sizes of these domains is
indicated in amino acids (aa).

determine whether *trp* is involved directly in $Ca^{2+}$
function.  The *trp* phenotype is not consistent with
the protein being a $Ca^{2+}$ channel. One attractive
possibilty is that *trp* is a $Ca^{2+}$ pump.  The $Ca^{2+}$-
ATPase also has an even number of multiple transmembrane domains (31); however, there is no primary
amino acid homology between *trp* and this protein.


Identification of Two Opsins Expressed in the
Ultraviolet Sensitive R7 Cells

     The compound eye of the fruitfly contains
approximately 800 repeat units called ommatidia.

Each ommatidium contains eight photoreceptor cells
which fall into three classes based on their
topological arrangement and spectral properties
(reviewed in 25). The major class consists of the
six outer photoreceptor cells, R1-6, which extend
the length of the retina and express a rhodopsin
that absorbs maximally at 480 nm. The two minor
classes of photoreceptor cells, R7 and R8, occupy
the distal and proximal central regions of the
ommatidia respectively. The R8 cells respond
maximally to blue light and the R7 photoreceptor
cells to ultraviolet light (32). In addition to
the compound eyes there are three small light
sensing organs, ocelli, arranged triangularly at
the vertex of the head.

The major visual pigment is encoded by the
genetically identified *ninaE* locus (33, 34). The
photopigments found in the R7 and R8 photoreceptor
cells are not affected by mutations in the *ninaE*
locus and thus must be encoded by other genes. A
distinct opsin might also be expressed in the
ocelli. Indeed, another opsin gene, Rh2, has been
identified (35) and shown to be expressed in the
ocelli (36-38). Microspectrophotometric studies
carried out mainly in the larger flies, Musca and
Calliphora, (reviewed in 25) have suggested the
existence of two distinct R7 photopigments. To
determine whether separate opsin genes are
expressed in photoreceptor cell seven of
Drosophila, we screened a Drosophila DNA library
for related opsin genes with oligonucleotide probes
corresponding to regions conserved between the
*ninaE* and Rh2 opsins. We isolated a DNA clone
which we found on the basis of a number of criteria
to encode a third Drosophila opsin, Rh3 (9).
Analysis of the deduced amino acid sequence of Rh3
indicates that it contains all the features typical
of opsins: eight potential transmembrane domains, a
putative retinal binding site, sites for N-linked
glycosylation near the N-terminus and serine and
threonine residues near the C-terminus which may
serve as site for light dependent phosphorylation.
On the basis of in situ hybridization to tissue
sections we found that Rh3 appears to be expressed
predominantly in the R7 cells. This was confirmed
by comparing the expression of Rh3 RNA in wild-type

and in a mutant, sevenless, which does not form the R7 cells.

To determine whether a second opsin gene is expressed in the R7 cells, we used an Rh3 DNA clone to screen a Drossophila library for related opsin genes. In this way, we identified another Drosophila opsin gene, Rh4, which is expressed specifically in the ultraviolet sensitive R7 photoreceptor cells (10). The two R7 opsins, Rh3 and Rh4, are expressed in nonoverlapping subsets of R7 cells. The Rh4 opsin shares 72% amino acid identity with Rh3 but is only about 35% homologous with the other two Drosophila opsins, *ninaE* and Rh2. Twenty eight amino acids are conserved among all four invertebrate and five vertebrate opsin genes thus far sequenced suggesting that these residues play an important role in rhodopsin function.


Analyses of Opsin Promoters

We would like to identify the factors responsible for regulating the expression of each of the four opsin genes in different subsets of photoreceptor cells. As a first step in this direction, the promoters of each of the four opsin genes are being analyzed to identify the DNA sequences required for normal levels and patterns of expression. DNA fragments containing the promoters of each gene were fused to either the *Escherichia coli* chloramphenicol acetyltransferase (CAT) or *lacZ* (β-galactosidase) genes and introduced into flies by P-element transformation. Expression of the *E. coli* genes was then used to assay the ability of various sequences to direct the normal pattern of expression.

To determine the minimum sequence requirements required for proper expression of these genes, a series of deletions were constructed and the patterns of expression assayed following germline transformation. For each of the four opsin genes, less than 0.3 kb of 5' flanking sequence was required and sufficient to direct normal expression. Further analyses of the *ninaE* promoter resulted in the identification of two small regions

which have the properties of enhancer elements
(39). Additionally, an 11 nucleotide sequence,
CTAATT(G/C)RRTT (R denotes a purine), has been
identified which is conserved among all Drosophila
photoreceptor specific genes including the opsins,
*ninaC* and *trp* (38). This sequence has been shown
by site-specific mutagenesis to be required for
proper quantitative expression of the opsin genes.


Concluding Remarks

    The next phase of the projects with *ninaC* and
*trp* will be to study their roles taking advantage
of the genetics and germline transformation. For
example, we will attempt to eliminate just the
*ninaC* kinase activity and not the myosin activity
and vice versa by site-specific mutagenesis. The
affects of these alterations on the morphology of
the photoreceptor cells and intracellular organelle
movement will then be assessed following
introduction of the altered genes back into flies
of the appropriate genetic background. The
continuing analyses of the opsin promoters will
include more detailed mutagenesis of the promoters
and a search for DNA binding proteins which may be
important for regulating the expression of these
genes.


REFERENCES

1.     Pak WL (1979). Study of photoreceptor function
    using *Drosophila* mutants. In Breakfield, X,
    (ed): "Neurogenetics, Genetic Approaches to the
    Nervous System," New York: Elsevier/North-
    Holland, p 67.
2.     Hall JC (1982). Genetics of the nervous system
    in Drosophila. Q. Rev. Biophys. 15: 223.
3.     Spradling AC, Rubin GM (1982). Transposition of
    cloned P elements into *Drosophila* germline
    chromosomes. Science 218: 341.
4.     Rubin GM, Spradling AC (1982). Genetic
    transformation of *Drosophila* with transposable
    element vectors. Science 218: 348.
5.     Montell C, Jones K, Hafen E, Rubin G. (1985).

Rescue of the *Drosophila* phototransduction mutation *trp* by germline transformation. Science 230: 1040.

6. Montell C, Rubin, GM (1988). The Drosophila *ninaC* locus encodes two photoreceptor cell specific proteins with domains homologous to protein kinases and the myosin heavy chain head. Cell 52: 757.

7. Minke B (1982). Light-induced reduction in excitation efficiency in the trp mutant of Drosophila. J. Gen. Physiol. 79: 361.

8. Matsumoto H, Isono K, Pye Q, and Pak WL (1987). Gene encoding cytoskeletal proteins in *Drosophila* rhabdomeres. Proc. Natl. Acad. Sci. 84: 985.

9. Zuker CS, Montell C, Jones K, Laverty T, Rubin GM (1987). A rhodopsin gene expressed in photoreceptor cell R7 of the *Drosophila* eye: homologies with other signal-transducing molecules. J. Neurosci. 7: 1537.

10. Montell C, Jones K, Zuker C, Rubin G (1987). A second opsin gene expressed in the ultraviolet-sensitive R7 photoreceptor cells of *Drosophila melanogaster*. J. Neurosci. 7: 1558.

11. Stephenson RS, O'Tousa J, Scavarda NJ, Randall LL, Pak WL (1983). *Drosophila* mutants with reduced rhodopsin content. In Cosens D, Vince-Prue D (ed): "Biology of Photoreceptors," Cambridge, England: Cambridge University Press, p 471.

12. Blest AD, Stowe S, Eddey W (1982). A labile, $Ca^+$-dependent cytoskeleton in rhabdomeric microvilli of blowflies. Cell Tissue Res. 223: 553.

13. Saibil H. (1982). An ordered membrane-cytoskeleton network in squid photoreceptor microvilli. J. Mol. Biol. 158: 435.

14. Hunter T, Cooper JA (1986). Viral oncogenes and tyrosine phosphorylation. In Boyer PD, Krebs EG (eds): "The Enzymes, Vol. XVII, Control by Phosphorylation, Part A,"Orlando, Florida: Academic Press, p 192.

15. Edelman AM (1987). Protein serine/threonine kinases. Ann. Rev. Biochem. 56: 567.

16. Harrington WF, Rodgers ME (1984). Myosin. Ann. Rev. Biochem. 53: 35.

17. Emerson CP, Bernstein SI (1987). Molecular genetics of myosin. Ann. Rev. Biochem. 56: 695.

18. Warrick HM, Spudich JA (1987). Myosin structure and function in cell motility. Ann. Rev. Cell Biol. 3: 379.

19. Pollard TD, Korn ED (1973). *Acanthamoeba* myosin I: isolation from *Acanthamoeba castellanii* of an enzyme similar to muscle myosin. J. Biol. Chem. 248: 4682.

20. Albanesi JP, Fujisaki H, Hammer JA III, Korn E. D, Jones R, Sheetz MP (1985). Monomeric *Acanthamoeba* myosins I support movement in vitro. J. Biol. Chem. 260: 8649.

21. Fujisaki H, Albanesi JP, Korn ED (1985). Experimental evidence for the contractile activities of *Acanthamoeba* myosins IA and IB. J. Biol. Chem. 260: 11183.

22. Jung G, Korn ED, Hammer JA III (1987). The heavy chain of *Acanthamoeba* myosin IB is a fusion of myosin-like and non-myosin like sequences. Proc. Natl. Acad. ScI. 84: 6720.

23. Hoshimaru M, Nakanishi S (1987). Identification of a new type of mammalian myosin heavy chain by molecular cloning. J. Biol. Chem. 262: 14625.

24. Adams RJ, Pollard TD (1986). Propulsion of organelles isolated from *Acanthamoeba* along actin filaments by myosin-I. Nature 322: 754.

25. Hardie RC (1983). Functional organization of the fly retina. In Autrum H, Ottoson D, Perl ER, Schmidt RF, Shimazu H, Willis WD (eds): "Progress in Sensory Physiology," New York: Springer-Verlag, p 1.

26. Stark WS, Sapp R (1987). Ultrastructure of the retina of *Drosophila melanogaster*: the mutant *ora* (*outer rhabdomeres absent*) and its inhibition of degeneration in *rdgB* (*retinal degeneration-B*). J. Neurogenetics 4: 227.

27. Matsumoto H, O'Tousa JE, Pak WL (1982). Light-induced modification of *Drosophila* retinal polypeptides in vivo. Science 217: 839.

28. Cosens DJ, Manning A (1969). Abnormal electroretinogram from a Drosophila mutant. Nature 224: 285.

29. Suss E, Barash S, Stavenga DG, Stieve H, Selinger Z, Minke B (1988). Interaction between

chemical excitation and the trp and nss phototransduction mutations in fly photoreceptors. (submitted).

30. Kyte J, Doolittle RF (1982). A simple model for displaying the hydropathic character of a protein. J. Mol. Biol. 157: 105.

31. MacLennan DH, Brandl CJ, Korczak B, Green NM (1985). Amino-acid sequence of a $Ca^{2+}+Mg^{2+}$-dependent ATPase from rabbit muscle sarcoplasmic reticulum, deduced from its complementary DNA sequence. Nature 316: 696.

32. Haris WA, Stark WS, Walker JA (1976). Genetic dissection of the photoreceptor system in the compound eye of Drosophila melanogaster. J. Physiol. 256: 415.

33. O'Tousa JE, Baehr W, Martin RL, Hirsh J, Pak, WL, Applebury ML (1985). The *Drosophila ninaE* gene encodes an opsin. Cell 40: 839.

34. Zuker CS, Cowman AF, Rubin GM (1985). Isolation and structure of a rhodopsin gene from *D. melanogaster*. Cell 40: 851.

35. Cowman AF, Zuker CS, Rubin GM (1986). An opsin gene expressed in only one photoreceptor cell type of the Drosophila eye. Cell 44: 705.

36. Pollock JA, Benzer S (1988). Of four Drosophila opsin genes, only Rh2 is transcribed in the ocellus. Nature (submitted).

37. Feiler R, Harris W, Kirschfeld K, Wehrhahn C, Zuker C (1988). Genetically-engineered cell-specific misexpression of an opsin gene in Drosophila leads to altered visual behaviour and physiology, and allows a detailed analysis of a novel photopigment. Nature (submitted).

38. Mismer D, Michael WM, Laverty T, Rubin GM (1988). Analysis of the Rh2 opsin gene in *Drosophila melanogaster*. Genetics (in press).

39. Mismer D, Rubin GM (1987). Analysis of the promoter of the *ninaE* opsin gene in *Drosophila melanogaster*. Genetics 116: 565.

Molecular Biology of the Eye: Genes, Vision,
and Ocular Disease, pages 293–303
© 1988 Alan R. Liss, Inc.

RECOMBINANT DNA MAPPING OF RETINITIS PIGMENTOSA GENES

A.F.Wright (1), S.S.Bhattacharya (1,2), I.W.Craig (3),
M.Jay (4), M.Dempster (1), N.Fraser (3) T.Meitinger(3),
   B.Jay (4), A.C.Bird (4) and  H.J.Evans (1).

   (1) M.R.C. Clinical and  Population Cytogenetics Unit,
       Western  General Hospital, Edinburgh  EH4 2XU.
   (2) Department of Human  Genetics, University  of
       Newcastle-upon-Tyne, Newcastle-upon-Tyne NE2 4AA.
   (3) Genetics Laboratory, Department of Biochemistry,
       University of Oxford, Oxford OX1 3QU.
   (4) Department of Clinical  Ophthalmology,
       University of London, Moorfields Eye Hospital,
       London EC1V 2PD.

   ABSTRACT   The results of genetic linkage studies
   on 34 families with X-linked Retinitis Pigmentosa
   are presented.  Three restriction fragment length
   polymorphisms   (RFLP)  located  in   band   Xp21
   (DXS206,  DXS84,  OTC)  were found to be  loosely
   linked to the disease locus.  Two loci located in
   the  region Xcen - Xp11.3 (DXS7,  DXS255)  showed
   closer linkage, particularly in families in which
   a   tapetal-like  reflex  was  not  evident   in
   heterozygous females.  The evidence in favour  of
   two  loci on the short arm of the X chromosome is
   discussed.

INTRODUCTION


     Retinitis  Pigmentosa  is a group  of  progressive
retinal  degenerations  associated  with  visual  field
loss, night blindness and migration of pigment into the
retina  (1,2).  Although  as  many as 40%  of  affected
subjects have no identifiable family history,  distinct
genetic  subtypes  can be identified  corresponding  to
autosomal  dominant,  autosomal recessive and  X-linked
varieties (3-5). On the basis of segregation analyses,

it has been estimated that most isolated (simplex)
cases are due to recessive inheritance but some are
likely to be autosomal dominant or X-linked, while
others may represent new mutations or phenocopies
(3,5). Despite some promising leads, the chromosomal
assignment of autosomal dominant and recessive genes
for Retinitis Pigmentosa remains elusive, but progress
has been made towards the localization of the X-linked
gene(s) (XLRP). The initial report of linkage to a
restriction fragment length polymorphism (RFLP)
identified by DNA segment L1.28 (DXS7) (6), close to
band Xp11.3, has been confirmed in some families (7-
10), while others have shown tighter linkage to RFLPs
located some 15-20 centiMorgans more distal on the X
chromosome short arm, including OTC and 754 (DXS84)
(11, 12).

The possibility of a gene causing XLRP located
within band Xp21 was first proposed by Francke et al.
(13) on the basis of a male patient with Duchenne
Muscular Dystrophy, Retinitis Pigmentosa, McLeod
Syndrome and Chronic Granulomatous Disease, bearing a
cytologically visible deletion in this band. This
localization was favoured by Nussbaum et al. (7) on the
basis of two triply informative meioses in a large XLRP
family in which female carriers showed a characteristic
tapetal-like reflex, previously reported to identify a
distinct subtype of XLRP (14). In contrast, the result
of a large multi-point analysis of 20 XLRP families
involving nine RFLP marker loci essentially excluded
the XLRP locus segregating in these families from the
Xp21 region and favoured a location proximal to L1.28
(DXS7) and distal to 58-1 (DXS14) (15).

The idea that there may in fact be two loci for
XLRP is not new (14) although the clinical evidence was
always subject to the alternative and more parsimonious
explanation of allelic rather than non-allelic
heterogeneity. Nevertheless, one of the criteria
reported to distinguish some XLRP families from others,
the presence of a tapetal-like reflex in carrier
females, was reported to be present in the families
showing close linkage to Xp21 markers (11, 12). This
clinical sign has been variously described as a golden
or white glistening appearance that is especially

prominent near the macula (2,16) and is found in some ,
but not necessarily all, carriers in some families, but
not at all in other families (2,14,16-20).

We report here the results of further linkage
studies in 34 XLRP families using Xp21 probes XJ-1.1
(DXS206), 754 (DXS84) and OTC as well as the more
proximal probes L1.28 (DXS7), M27B (DXS255) and 58-1
(DXS14) located in the region Xp11.3-Xcen (21-22).


## RESULTS


A preliminary survey of the XLRP families used in
our linkage analysis and ascertained through the
Genetic Clinic, Moorfields Eye Hospital, London showed
that there was no evidence of tapetal-like reflex in
carrier females in 18 out of 21 kindreds. In the
remaining three, at least one female identified as a
carrier either on the basis of genetic or other
clinical grounds showed a tapetal-like reflex. The
appearance of this reflex has been described by Bird
(2) in one of these families (P336). Only a minority of
carriers showed the reflex in each family.
Unfortunately, none of the latter families was
sufficiently informative to confirm or refute the
proposal that this locus is closely linked to Xp21
probes.

Linkage Analysis using Xp21 probes.

The results of probing the 34 XLRP families with
Xp21 probes XJ-1.1 (DXS206), 754 (DXS84) and OTC are
shown in Table 1. This includes data from new families
not published previously.

TABLE 1
Genetic  distances ( W ) (in centiMorgans)  and
corresponding lod scores ( Z ) between XLRP and
RFLP loci.
Values are maximum likelihood estimates and
the number of informative kindreds ( No. )
is shown for each locus.

| Locus | W | Z | No. |
|---|---|---|---|
| DXS206 | 26 | 0.37 | 4 |
| DXS84 | 25 | 3.17 | 22 |
| OTC | 20 | 3.52 | 15 |
| DXS7 | 10 | 9.12 | 15 |
| DXS14 | 21 | 3.73 | 13 |

Fifteen families were informative at the OTC locus    and
a maximum likelihood value of the genetic distance
( W  ) of 20 centiMorgans (cM) was obtained at   a   lod
score of 3.52. Twenty two families were informative for
RFLP locus DXS84 identified with probe 754,   giving a W
value  of 25 cM at a lod score of 3.17.   Four   families
were   informative  for DXS206 (XJ-1.1) which gave   a   W
value  of  26 cM at a lod score of  0.37.   The   results
clearly show loose linkage between XLRP and these   Xp21
probes.
     Figure   1 shows a family with XLRP in which DXS206
(XJ-1.1) is segregating,   in which either 3 or 4 out of
seven informative meioses are recombinant, depending on
the linkage phase in the carrier mother.

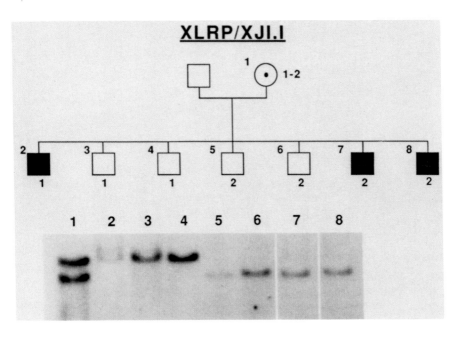

Figure 1. Segregation of DXS206 (XJ-1.1) RFLP in an XLRP kindred, showing a minimum of three recombinants out of 7 informative meioses.

Linkage Analysis using Xp11.3 - Xcen RFLPs

The results of linkage analysis using more proximally located probes L1.28 (DXS7), M27B (DXS255) and 58-1 (DXS14), assigned to Xp11.3 - Xcen, were as follows. Table 1 shows that 15 families were informative for L1.28 (DXS7), which gave a W value of 10 cM at a lod score of 9.12. Thirteen families were informative for probe 58-1 (DXS14), which showed a W value of 21 cM at a lod score of 3.73. These results are consistent with the previous multi-point analysis (15) supporting the gene order DXS7 - XLRP - DXS14 - Xcen and suggest that DXS14 may lie relatively close to the centromere.

Eight families were informative for the multi-allele RFLP identified with probe M27B (DXS255), located in the region Xp11.3 - Xcen (22). The results to date are shown in Table 2.

TABLE 2

Results of Linkage Analysis in XLRP using M27B (DXS255). Families were classified on the basis of the presence or absence of a tapetal-like reflex in carrier females. The number of definite recombinants and the total number of informative meioses is shown. NK, not known.

| Family | Tapetal Reflex | Recs. | Total Meioses |
|---|---|---|---|
| F15, F38 F51, F53 | − | 1 | 31 |
| F43 | + | 1 | 3 |
| F47, F54 F56 | NK | 4 | 14 |

In four families in which there was no evidence of a tapetal-like reflex in carrier females, only one definite recombinant was observed out of 31 informative meioses. In one small family, in which a tapetal-like reflex was observed in a carrier, there was one definite recombinant out of three informative meioses. Three families, in which it was not possible to classify them in this way, showed four definite recombinants out of 14 informative meioses.

It is known from ultrastructural studies that Müller cells in normal retinas contain a large number of intermediate filaments, some of which may be GFAP filaments (8,9). Hence, one might inquire as to the mechanism that leads to the appearance of GFAP-immunoreactivity in Müller cells in retinas with photoreceptor degeneration. Is the immunostaining due to depolymerization, proteolysis, or chemical modification of the existing filaments or is it due to decreased GFAP degradation? Alternatively, could it be due to de novo synthesis as a result of transcriptional activation of the GFAP gene, increased mRNA stability or translation of preexisting GFAP mRNA? In the present study, we show that photoreceptor degeneration resulting from mutations, or constant light exposure results in the synthesis and accumulation GFAP mRNA in Müller cells.

## RESULTS

Immunocytochemical localization of GFAP.

The immunocytochemical localization of GFAP in normal and *rd* retinas are presented in Fig.1. In BALB/c and B6 retinas, staining was found in cell bodies and processes located just underneath the ganglion cell layer (Fig. 1A). From the location of the stained cell bodies and their processes, we infer that these cells are the astrocytes. No immunostaining was seen in other parts of the retina except in the far periphery where a few radially-oriented processes were found to be immunoreactive. In the retinal dystrophic mutant, *rd*, however, there was intense staining of radially-oriented processes across the retina. The staining extended from inner limiting membrane all the way to the scleral edge of the inner nuclear layer (Fig.l B). Similar results were obtained with retinas from BALB/c mice that had been maintained under constant light. These studies suggest that in normal retina, astrocytes are GFAP-immunoreactive while Müller cells remain unstained; and that photoreceptor degeneration results in the appearance of GFAP-immunostaining in Müller cells.

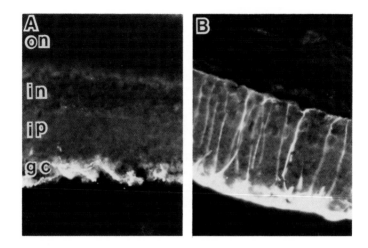

Figure 1. Immunocytochemical localization of GFAP in normal and photoreceptor-deficient mouse retina. Sections of aldehyde-fixed retina were reacted with anti-GFAP and the antigen was visualized by indirect immunofluorescence method. (A) Normal retina and (B) *rd/rd* retina. Outer nuclear layer (on); inner nuclear layer (in); inner plexiform layer (ip) and ganglion cell layer (gc).

GFAP levels.

The GFAP-immunoreactivity observed in the Müller cells could result from various causes such as depolymerization, proteolysis, or chemical modification of the existing filaments or decreased GFAP degradation. Alternatively, it could be due to de novo synthesis of GFAP as a result of induction of the GFAP mRNA, increased mRNA stability or translation of pre-existing mRNA. If the appearance of immunoreactivity is not due to new GFAP synthesis but is the result of other causes, we reasoned that the GFAP content of normal and dystrophic retinas should be similar. An immuno-blotting experiment was carried out to examine this possibility. Results of the experiment showed that there is a 5 to 10 -fold increase in GFAP content in retinas with photoreceptor degeneration (7). This increase is probably due to the synthesis of new GFAP molecules.

GFAP mRNA levels.

In order to determine whether the increased GFAP content is due to increase in GFAP mRNA content, we extracted RNA from normal and dystrophic retinas and determined the GFAP mRNA levels by northern blot analysis (10). Results of these experiments are shown in Fig. 2.

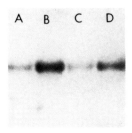

Figure 2. Northern blots of RNA extracted from mouse retinas. Total RNA, extracted from 10-12 eyes, was separated in formaldehyde-containing agarose gels and transferred to nitrocellulose. Blots were hybridized to $^{32}$P-labeled, GFAP DNA probe. (A), B6 ; (B), B6 rd/rd ; (C), BALB/c and (D) BALB/c kept in constant light for two weeks.

A small amount of GFAP mRNA (2.7 Kb) was found in the normal retina. In the *rd* retina there was a 8-10 fold increase in the GFAP mRNA levels while in retinas with light damage, there was a 15-20 fold increase. In control experiments, hybridization with bovine opsin probe showed that the levels of opsin mRNAs were drastically reduced (7). In contrast, the level of GAD mRNA was unchanged in these retinas (7). These data demonstrate that there is a 10-20 fold increase in the GFAP mRNA levels in retinas with photoreceptor degeneration.

GFAP mRNA Localization.

From the northern blot analysis one cannot infer that the increase in GFAP mRNA levels in dystrophic retinas is due to increase in GFAP mRNA content in Müller cells, since it could as well arise from enhanced transcription of the gene in astrocytes. In order to resolve this issue, we have carried out in situ hybridizations with retinas from normal and photoreceptor-deficient mice (7). Figure 3 presents results of the in situ hybridization experiments. In normal retinas, labeled cell bodies were found in the ganglion cell layer. These labeled cells are probably the astrocytes, a result in accordance with earlier immunocytochemical data. Control experiments with bovine opsin and L-glutamic acid decarboxylase probes established that there was no preferential loss of mRNA from the nuclear layers in the retina.

Since retinas with light damage showed a larger increase in GFAP mRNA content, we used these retinas for in situ localization. As shown in Fig. 3B, in retinas with light damage, there was a substantial increase in the density of silver grains in the INL, and patches of silver grains were prominent around cell bodies located in the middle of this layer. The labeling was specific since prior treatment of sections with RNAse before hybridization, abolished INL labeling.

Although a double labeling method using a Müller cell-specific marker could be used to determine whether the labelled somata were those of Müller cells, we decided to approach this problem using the more direct, single cell technique. It is possible to dissociate and morphologically identify the different cell types in the mammalian retina (11). In situ hybridization with morphologically identified cells should demonstrate whether there is an increase in GFAP mRNA content in Müller cells. Retinas isolated from mice with light damage were treated with papain and dissociated by gentle trituration. The cell suspension was fixed with paraformaldehyde and cells were allowed to attach to gelatin subbed slides. After hybridization and washing, the cells were processed for autoradiography, and examined (12). Results of the experiments given in Fig. 3 showed that cells which could be identified as Müller cells based on their morphological features,were strongly labeled.

## DISCUSSION

Although it is quite clear that photoreceptor loss leads to expression of the GFAP gene in Müller cells, the cellular mechanism behind this phenomenon is unknown. One possibility is that some aspect of photoreceptor-Müller cell contact interaction keeps the GFAP gene repressed in the normal retina and

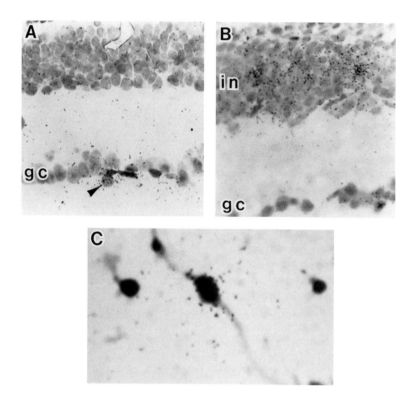

<u>Figure 3.</u> Cellular localization of GFAP mRNA in mouse retina and in dissociated cells by <u>in situ</u> hybridization. Eyes from BALB/c mice (A) and animals kept in constant light for two weeks (B), were fixed in paraformaldehyde and sectioned in a cryostat. Tissue sections were processed for <u>in situ</u> hybridization as described in elsewhere (7). (C), Dissociated cell from retina with two weeks of light damage.

that photoreceptor loss leads to derepression of the gene. This notion is supported by the finding that when embryonic retinal cells are dissociated and plated <u>in vitro</u>, the glial cells in these cultures express GFAP (13). It could also be argued that the photoreceptor membranes released, induce GFAP synthesis (Fig.4). Alternatively, lymphokine and monokine factors produced

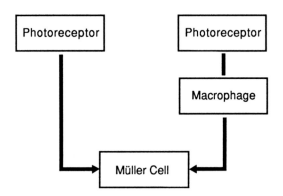

Figure 4. Two possible mechanisms for GFAP induction in Müller cells. In the mechanism shown on left, membranes or other cellular components derived from degenerating photoreceptors, act directly on Müller cells. In the mechanism shown on the right, macrophages that invade the retina as a result of photoreceptor degeneration, release factors that stimulate GFAP synthesis in Müller cells.

by macrophages that invade dystrophic retinas, may be involved in activation of the GFAP gene. For example, a glial cell-stimulating factor (GSF) released by ConA-stimulated mouse lymphocytes, has been shown to increase GFAP content in astrocyte cultures (14).

It might be mentioned here that induction of glutamine synthetase, a Müller cell-specific enzyme, appears to be under a different type of control as the enzyme cannot be induced maximally if Müller cells are maintained in the absence of neurons (15). It would be interesting to examine the influence of photoreceptor degeneration on the expression of other Müller cell-specific proteins such as glutamine synthetase and carbonic anhydrase in the mouse retina.

Since we know little about the function of intermediate filaments, it is difficult to understand the significance behind GFAP induction in Müller cells. It is possible that GFAP induction is adventitious and is actually the result of activation of an

position 55; ('), putative leader sequence; (><), putative
cleavage site of the leader; (---), amino acid sequence
identical with that of tryptic peptide; (=), polyadeny-
lylation signal. See text for discussion.

```
        *       *       *               **
     MF'SKLAHLQRFAVLSRGVHSSVASATSVATKK   OAT
     :   :   :   :   :       :
     MLFNLRILLNNAAFRNGHNFMVRNFRCGQPLQ   OTC
        *       *           *   *
```

Figure 4. Comparison of the leader sequences of the
human OAT and ornithine transcarbamylase (OTC). OAT,
putative leader sequence of the human ornithine aminotransferase; OTC, leader sequence of the human ornithine
transcarbamylase; *, basic amino acid residue; :, conserved residue. Single letter amino acid designations
are as follows: M, Met; F, Phe; S, Ser; K, Lys; L, Leu; A,
Ala; H, His; Q, Gln; R, Arg; V, Val; G, Gly; T, Thr; N,
Asn; I, Ile; C, Cys; P, Pro.

---

enzyme, revealed the presence of a putative 32 amino acid
leader sequence in OAT (Fig. 3). The leader sequence of
OAT is similar to that of OTC and other nuclear-encoded
mitochondrial proteins in its lack of acidic amino acid
residues and its normal content of basic amino acid
residues (Fig. 4) (19). An interesting conservation of
five specific non-polar residues in the leader sequences is
present which, along with the positively-charged nature of
this sequence, may play an important role in the directed
transport of the precursors to the mitochondria (Fig. 4).
Presumably, a processing of the OAT precursor takes place
in the mitochondria to yield the mature OAT without the
leader of 407 amino acid residues with a molecular mass of
45,136 daltons which matches approximately the size of the
purified OAT.

A comparison of the OAT sequence to other protein
sequences including those in the Protein Sequence Data Bank
revealed an interesting homology between OAT and chicken
aspartate aminotransferase (AAT). Aspartate aminotransferase has been studied extensively, including a
crystallographic analysis to delineate its tertiary
structure(20). This enzyme is very similar to OAT in that

it is also a nuclear-encoded, pyridoxal phosphate-requir-
ing, mitochondrial matrix transaminase(21). The homology
between OAT and AAT is not particularly high (27%) but is
significant in that a region of good homology between the
two sequences contains the active site of AAT including the
pyridoxine-binding lysine at position 261 (Fig. 5). The
OAT protein also contains a lysine at position 310 in close
analogy with AAT, and this may be the pyridoxine-binding
lysine. This homology indicates that OAT and AAT may be
linked in evolution, and that the active site of OAT may be
structurally similar to that of AAT.

Using the human OAT cDNA as a probe, we have begun to
examine the OAT gene. A genomic southern analysis indicated that the OAT gene is a very complicated gene family
consisting of multiple copies of OAT-related gene sequences. Preliminary results of hybridization experiments
using specific probes and varying temperatures indicated
the presence of at least four copies of OAT or OAT-related
gene sequence, one of which is the functional OAT gene
corresponding to the cDNA (data not shown). We have mapped
the OAT gene sequences to chromosomes 10 and X, and
determined that the functional OAT gene is on the former
(22). The chromosomal mapping result appeared to confirm
the presence of the OAT gene family and agrees with the
autosomal recessive inheritance of GA. Numerous genomic
clones representing most of the members of the OAT gene
family have been isolated, and their partial sequence

```
LOCALLY HOMOLOGOUS REGIONS BETWEEN ;OATAA    AND ;AATCHK

ALIGNMENT  1, DISTANCE   -65,  181- 317 ( 6),  128- 266 ( 4)
          190       200       210       220       230       240       250
IQKY K AKIVFAAGNFWGRTLSAISSSTDPTSYDGFGPFMPGFDIIPYNDLPALERALQDPNVAAFMVEPIQGEAGVVV
     :  :       ::     :                :           : :      ::
LQRFFKFSRDVYLPKPSWGNH TPIFRDAG LELQAYRYYDPKTCSLDFTG  AMEDISKIPEKSIILLHACAHNPTGVD
130       140       150       160       170       180       190       200
          270       280       290       300       310
PDPGYLMGVRELCTRHQVL FIADEIQTGLARTGR  WLAVDYENVRPDIVLLGK ALSGGLY
     :              :    :     :           : ::    :      :::
PREEQWKELASVVKKRNLLAYFDMAYQGEASDINRDAWALRHFIEQGIDVVLSQSYAKNMGLY
210       220       230       240       250       260
```

Figure 5. Locally homologous regions between the
human ornithine aminotransferase (OAT) and chicken aspartate aminotransferase (AAT) sequences. Amino acid
residues 181 to 317 for OAT and 128 to 266 for AAT are
shown.

analysis confirmed the chromosome 10 gene to be the functional gene and at least one of the X chromosome genes to be a pseudogene.

We have also begun to investigate the status of the OAT gene and its expression in tissues from GA patients. DNA and RNA analysis of the OAT gene in 20 GA patients demonstrated grossly normal OAT gene and mRNA in all of the cases except one patient who appears to have a partial heterozygous deletion of the OAT gene and no OAT mRNA(23). Western analysis also demonstrated that OAT protein is essentially undetectable in this patient (data not shown). Thus, this is the first real demonstration that an OAT gene defect indeed does exist in GA, and that this gene defect forms the molecular basis of pathology in this disease. In those GA patients that have detectable OAT mRNAs, a subtle defect must be present at the sequence level that results in non-translation of the mRNA or abnormality of the translated protein to explain the lack of OAT activity. It is hoped that continued investigation of the OAT gene and its expression in the tissues from GA patients will reveal the exact nature of the molecular genetic defect in OAT present in this disease, and that this knowledge will help us in considering the possibility of a gene therapy for this disease in the future.

## REFERENCES

1.  Valle D, Simell O (1983).  The hyperornithinemias: gyrate atrophy of the choroid and retina.  In Stanbury JB, Wyngaarden JB, Fredrickson DS, Goldstein JL, Brown MS (eds):  "The Metabolic Basis of Inherited Disease", New York:  McGraw Hill, pp. 389-396.
2.  Simell O, Takki K (1973).  Raised plasma ornithine and gyrate atrophy of the choroid and retina. Lancet 1:1030-1033.
3.  Valle D, Kaiser-Kupfer MI, DelValle LA (1977).  Gyrate atrophy of the choroid and retina:  Deficiency of ornithine aminotransferase in transformed lymphocytes. Proc Natl Acad Sci (USA) 74:5159-5161.
4.  Trijbels JMF, Sengers RCA, Bakkeren JAJM, DeKort AFM, Deutman AF (1977).  L-ornithine-ketoacid-transaminase deficiency in cultured fibroblasts of a patient with hyperornithinemia and gyrate atrophy of the choroid and retina.  Clinica Chimica Acta 79:371-377.

5. Ohura T, Kominami E, Tada K, Katunuma N (1984). Gyrate atrophy of the chroid and retina: decreased ornithine aminotransferase concentration in cultured skin fibroblasts from patients. Clin Chim Acta 136:29-37.
6. Peraino C, Pitot HC (1963). Ornithine-δ-transaminase in the rat: I. Assay and some general properties. Biochim Biophys Acta 73:222-231.
7. Shiotani T, Sanada Y, Katunuma N (1977). Studies on the structure of rat liver ornithine aminotransferase. J Biochem 81:1833-1838.
8. Sanada Y, Suemori I, Katunuma N (1970). Properties of ornithine aminotransferase from rat liver, kidney and small intestine. Biochim Biophys Acta 220:42-50.
9. Deshmukh DR, Srivastava SK (1984). Purification and properties of ornithine aminotransferase from rat brain. Experientia 40:357-359.
10. Ohura T, Kominami E, Tada K, Katunuma N (1982). Crystallization and properties of human liver ornithine aminotransferase. J Biochem 92:1785-1792.
11. Mueckler MM, Himeno M, Pitot HC (1982). In vitro synthesis and processing of a precursor to ornithine aminotransferase. J Biol Chem 257:7178-7180.
12. Inana G, Totsuka S, Redmond M, Dougherty T, Nagle J, Shiono T, Ohura T, Kominami E, Katunuma N (1986). Molecular cloning of human ornithine aminotransferase mRNA. Proc Natl Acad Sci (USA) 83:1203-1207.
13. Young RA, Davis RW (1983). Efficient isolation of genes by using antibody probes. Proc Natl Acad Sci (USA) 80:1194-1198.
14. Young RA, Davis RW (1983). Yeast RNA polymerase II genes: isolation with antibody probes. Science 222: 778-782.
15. Kozak M (1981). Possible role of flanking nucleotides in recognition of the AUG initiator codon by eukaryotic ribosomes. Nucleic Acids Res 9:5233-5252.
16. Law SW, Dugaiczyk A (1981). Homology between the primary structure of α-fetoprotein, deduced from a complete cDNA sequence, and serum albumin. Nature 291:201-205.
17. Mueckler MM, Pitot HC (1985). Sequence of the precursor to rat ornithine aminotransferase deduced from a cDNA clone. J Biol Chem 260:12993-12997.
18. Schatz G, Butow RA (1983). How are proteins imported into mitochondria? Cell 32:316-318.

19. Horwich AL, Fenton WA, Williams KR, Kalousek F, Kraus JP, Doolittle R, Konigsberg W, Rosenberg LE (1984). Structure and expression of a complementary DNA for the nuclear coded precursor of human mitochondrial ornithine transcarbamylase. Science 224:1068-1074.
20. Ford GC, Eichele G, Jansonius JN (1980). Three-dimensional structure of a pyridoxal-phosphate-dependent enzyme, mitochondrial aspartate aminotransferase. Proc Natl Acad Sci (USA) 77:2559-2563.
21. Graf-Hausner U, Wilson KJ, Christen P (1983). The covalent structure of mitochondrial aspartate aminotransferase from chicken. J Biol Chem 258:8813-8826.
22. Barrett DJ, Bateman JB, Sparkes RS, Mohandas T, Klisak I, Inana G (1987). Chromosomal localization of human ornithine aminotransferase gene sequences to 10q26 and Xp11.2. Invest Ophthalmol Vis Sci 28:1037.
23. Inana G, Hotta Y, Zintz C, Takki K, Weleber RG, Kennaway NG, Nakayasu K, Nakajima A, Shiono T (1988). Expression defect of ornithine aminotransferase gene in gyrate atrophy. Invest Ophthalmol Vis Sci, in press.

Molecular Biology of the Eye: Genes, Vision, and Ocular Disease, pages 329–338
© 1988 Alan R. Liss, Inc.

NORRIE DISEASE: LINKAGE ANALYSIS
USING THE L1.28 AND THE HUMAN
ORNITHINE-AMINOTRANSFERASE (OAT) cDNA PROBES.

Julielani T. Ngo,[1] J. Bronwyn Bateman,[1]
Victoria Cortessis,[2] Robert S. Sparkes,[3] T. Mohandas,[4]
George Inana,[5] and M. Anne Spence.[2]

Jules Stein Eye Institute and Department of
Ophthalmology
UCLA School of Medicine, Los Angeles, CA 90024

ABSTRACT   A  recombinational  event  between  the  Norrie
disease  locus  and  the DXS7 locus identified by the L1.28
probe  has been detected in a family affected with X-linked
recessive  Norrie  disease.   Inclusion  of  this  family
significantly  reduces  the  maximum lod score of 9.32 at a
recombination  frequency  of  0.00  to a score of 7.58 at a
recombination frequency of $0.038 \pm 0.036$.  This observation
indicates  that  the  L1.28  probe  is  useful for prenatal
diagnosis but the gene for Norrie disease is not within the
DNA  sequence  identified  by  the probe.  In light of this
recombinational event, the human ornithine aminotransferase
(OAT)  cDNA  which  recognizes OAT-related sequences in the
same region on the X chromosome as the L1.28 probe was used
to  study  this  family.   A Pvu II-associated restriction
fragment  length  polymorphism (RFLP) of 4.8 kb in size was
found.   In this family, the affected males do not express
this  4.8  kb  fragment while the obligate carriers and the
normal male do.  This finding suggests linkage between this
locus and the Norrie disease locus.

[1]This  work  is  partially  supported  by NIH grants EY-07026
(JTN) and EY-06772 (JBB), the Research to Prevent Blindness
Inc.  William  and  Mary Greve International Scholar Award,
and the George Gund Foundation.
[2]Present  address: Department of Psychiatry/Biomathematics,
UCLA School of Medicine, Los Angeles CA 90024.
[3]Present  address:  Department of Medicine/Pediatrics, UCLA
Schoole of Medicine, Los Angeles CA 90024.

[4]Present address: Division of Medical Genetics, Harbor/UCLA Medical Center, Torrance CA 90509.
[5]Present address: National Eye Institute, National Institutes of Health, Bethesda MD 20892.

## INTRODUCTION

Norrie disease displays an X-linked recessive mode of inheritance (McKusick No. 310600) (1). It is a rare disorder characterized by congenital or infantile blindness which is due to retinal detachment (2). Hearing loss is common and may be acquired (1). In addition, about thirty percent of the patients show signs of mental retardation and/or psychotic behavior (3). Unlike many X-linked recessive ocular diseases, carriers show no ocular signs. Classically, genetic counseling has been limited to Bayesian calculations until an affected son proves his mother to be a carrier. Recently, with the advance in molecular technology, human gene probes have been generated and mapped close to several disease loci. These probes are useful for diagnostic purposes if a restriction fragment length polymorphism (RFLP) is identifiable. A polymorphic X-chromosomal locus identified by the L1.28 probe in the DXS7 region, was initially found to be closely linked to Norrie disease locus with a lod score of 3.50 at 0.00 genetic distance (4,5). Accumulation of additional families with Norrie disease has brought the maximum lod score to 6.92 at 0.00 recombination frequency (6,7). Using the L1.28 probe which has been assigned to the region p11.2-p11.3 on the X chromosome (8,9), we studied a six-member, three generation family in which two males were affected and identified a recombinational event between the DXS7 and the Norrie disease loci. This finding suggests that the Norrie disease locus is not within the gene sequence identified by the L1.28 probe. A second probe, the human ornithine aminotransferase (OAT) cDNA (10), which recognizes OAT-related sequences on the X chromosome also has been used to study this family; the OAT and the OAT-related sequences have been mapped to two human chromosomes in regions 10q26 and Xp11.2 by our group (11) and in 10q23 and Xp11-Xp21 by another (12). Ornithine aminotransferase (L-ornithine:2-oxo-acid aminotransferase, EC 2.6.1.13) is present in many human tissues (13) including eye (14) and catalyzes the major catabolic pathway of ornithine. Severe deficiency in OAT activity has been found to be associated with gyrate atrophy, an autosomal recessive disorder (15-18) characterized by myopia, cataracts and severe progressive degeneration of the choroid and retina (15,19). Although there is no known correlation between the Norrie disease and deficiency of OAT activity (chromosome 10), the X chromosomal location of the OAT-related sequences makes it a good candidate marker for the disease.

## MATERIALS AND METHODS

Restriction enzymes and Klenow fragment of DNA polymerase I were obtained from New England Biolabs (Boston, MA); and labelled nucleotide ($^{32}$P-alpha dCTP) from Amersham Corp. (Illinois).

Human genomic DNA was isolated from lymphocytes following described methods(20). Ten micrograms of genomic DNA were digested with Pvu II and Taq I (10U/ug). Agarose gel electrophoresis was used to separate the fragments which were transferred to nylon membrane (S & S) by the method of Southern (21).

The L1.28 probe defining the DSX7 locus (8,9) was cloned into a pBR322 vector as an EcoR I insert and was a gift from Dr. Peter Pearson, Leiden. The OAT probe was a 2.1 kb cDNA insert representing a nearly full length copy of the human OAT mRNA (10).

The filter was hybridized with radioactively labelled OAT or L1.28 probe by random priming (22) in 1% bovine serum albumin (BSA), 0.5 M sodium phosphate pH 7.0, 1 mM EDTA, 7% SDS, and 25 ug/ml denatured salmon sperm DNA for 24 h at 60°C. The filter was then washed in 2X sodium chloride/sodium citrate (SSC), 0.1% SDS and then in 0.2X SSC, 0.1% SDS at 57°C. The filter was then dried briefly and exposed to Kodak XAR-5X-ray film for 2-5 days.

Using somatic cell hybrids and in situ hybridization, OAT and OAT-related sequences have been mapped to chromosomes 10 and X (11). In the Pvu II digestion, assignment of the OAT-related sequences to the X chromosome was carried out using hybrid clones 84-21 and 84-5. Clone 84-21 contains chromosome 10 but not the X chromosome. Clone 84-5 contains the X chromosome but not chromosome 10.

The lod scores for this pedigree were calculated by the LIPED program (23) for an X-linked disease. For the L1.28 probe, all lod scores were based on a frequency of 0.32 for the 9.5 kb allele and 0.68 for the 12.3 kb allele

(9), and 0.0001 for the Norrie disease allele. Analysis for the OAT probe was independent of allelic frequencies since genotypes were known for each key individual of the family. The frequency of 0.0001 for the disease locus was used for linkage analysis. The lod score is the log of the odds of linkage and is a function of the distance between two loci on a chromosome, expressed in centimorgans. The calculation of the lod score is based on pedigree analysis and reflects proximity of the gene in question with the marker gene. Generally, a lod score of 3 or greater is interpreted as confirmation of linkage, and a score of -2 excludes linkage.

## RESULTS

The pedigree of this family is shown in Figure 1. Alleles detected by the L1.28 probe are designated as L for the 12.3 kb RFLP and 1 for the 9.5 kb RFLP. Similarly, the allele identified by the OAT probe is assigned as A for the presence of the 4.8 kb RFLP and B for the absence of the 4.8 kb RFLP. For identification, individuals are assigned a number in the upper right hand corner of the circle or square.

FIGURE 1

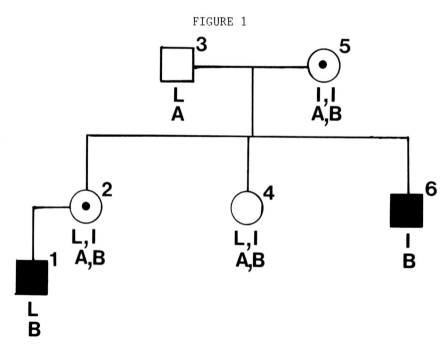

☐   = male

○   = female

■   = affected

⊙   = carrier

Figure 1. Pedigree of the six member family with two males affected with the Norrie disease. Individual #2 and #5 are obligate carriers.

L1.28 probe

    In this family, obligate carriers are either homozygous for the 9.5 kb allele (1) (individual #5) or heterozygous with the presence of the 9.5 (1) and 12.3 (L) kb alleles. The unaffected male in generation I (individual #4) is hemizygous for the 12.3 kb band. The affected male in generation II (individual #6) is hemizygous for the 9.5 kb allele (1) and the affected male in generation III (individual #1) is hemizygous for the 12.3 allele (L). A cross-over event has occurred in individual #2 and individual #1 is a recombinant offspring.

    Lod scores between the DSX7 and the Norrie disease loci are reported in Table 1.

TABLE 1

LOD SCORES

| Recombination fractions ($\theta_f$) | | | | | |
|---|---|---|---|---|---|
| Probes   0.00 | 0.05 | 0.10 | 0.20 | 0.30 | 0.40 |
| L1.28   $-\infty$ | $-1.00$ | $-0.70$ | $-0.40$ | $-0.22$ | $-0.10$ |

Table 1. Lod scores between the Norrie disease and the RFLP identified by the L1.28 probe.
L1.28: Assumed frequencies for the alleles were 0.32 for 1

and  0.68  for  L.  L and l are allelic fragments identified
by the L1.28 probe in TaqI digested genomic DNA.
The frequency of the Norrie disease is assumed to be 0.0001
in the analysis.OAT probe
    Using hybrid clones 84-21 and 84-5, bands of size 9.4,
8.9,  7.5, 7.3, 6.0, 5.8, 5.0, 4.8, 3.4, 2.8, 2.6, 1.0, and
0.95  kb  were  mapped  to  the X chromosome after a Pvu II
digestion.  The  4.8  kb  fragment  (A.B)  is  found  to be
polymorphic     between     the     affected    and   unaffected
individuals. Obligate carriers (individuals #1 and #5) both
express  this  fragment  as  well  as  the  unaffected male
(individual    #4)    (A);   affected   males   in   this   family
(individual #1 and #6) do not have this band (B).


                        DISCUSSION

        We   have   investigated   linkage   in  a family with two
males  affected  with  the  Norrie  disease using the L1.28
probe. Analysis of the segregation of the two alleles ( 9.5
and   11.2 kb) reveals a recombinational event in individual
#2,    an    obligate   carrier.  Similar   to   individual   #2,
individual  #4  is  also a heterozygote with respect to the
L1.28  probe; however, her carrier status is undeterminable
as  we  cannot  identify  which  maternal 9.5 kb allele she
received.
        Several    investigators    have    reported    close  linkage
between   the   Norrie   disease   locus   and   the   DXS7 locus
identified  by the L1.28 probe with a combined lod score of
6.92  at zero recombination (4-7,27,28). With the inclusion
of  our  family,  the  lod score becomes minus infinity at a
zero   recombination   fraction.  A   maximum  lod  score is now
7.58  at  a  recombination fraction of 0.038 $\pm$ 0.036. Since
this   recombination   frequency   is   low,   the   L1.28  will
continue to be useful but it may not be completely reliable
for diagnostic purposes.
        Due to this recombinational event and the ambiguity in
determining   the   carrier   status  in individual #4, we have
used  the  OAT  probe  to  further  study this family.  The
functional  OAT  gene  has  been  mapped  to chromosome 10
(11,12,24)  and  at  least  three  other  OAT-related gene
sequences   are   present   on   the   X  chromosome (11,25).
Hybridization  of  this  probe to Pvu II restricted genomic
DNAs   creates   a   complex   pattern   containing  both  OAT
(chromosome  10)  and OAT-related sequences (X chromosome).

Molecular Biology of the Eye: Genes, Vision,
and Ocular Disease, pages 339–348
© 1988 Alan R. Liss, Inc.

MOLECULAR STUDIES OF THE RETINAL DEGENERATION
IN THE rd MOUSE[1]

Debora B. Farber, Narendra Tuteja and Cathy Bowes

Jules Stein Eye Institute and Department of Ophthalmology
UCLA School of Medicine, Los Angeles, California 90024-1771

ABSTRACT.    Deficient    cGMP-phosphodiesterase    activity
resulting   in   elevated  cGMP levels has been associated with
the   retinal   degeneration   of   rd   mice.    The enzyme  is
synthesized  normally  and in the appropriate concentrations
in   rd   retina but its levels are always lower than those of
control   retina.    In addition, the activation/deactivation
processes   of   cGMP-PDE,   which involve the participation of
bleached rhodopsin, G-protein and 48 kDa-protein, occur to a
minimal   extent   in  rd retina.  To pinpoint any modification
in the  rd  cGMP-PDE composition that may have occurred at the
molecular level, we have obtained the cDNA for the γ subunit
of   cGMP-PDE   from   a   normal   mouse   retinal   library,   and
hybridized  it,  together with cDNAs for opsin, the α, β and γ
subunits   of   G-protein,   and   48   kDa-protein,   to   the
corresponding mRNAs from normal and rd retinas.  Our results
showed   that   none of these mRNAs are qualitatively abnormal
in   size or concentration, or delayed in their expression in
the  rd retina.

INTRODUCTION

The  rd  mouse  is affected with a genetic disease which
causes  the degeneration of the retinal photoreceptor cells.
The   autosomal   recessive   rd gene, located in linkage group
XVII   of   chromosome   5 (1) is expressed in the visual cells
when they differentiate during postnatal life.

[1]This  work  was  supported  by  NIH  grants EY02651 and
EY0331,  by  the  National  Retinitis Pigmentosa Foundation,
Fighting   Blindness,   Baltimore   and  by  The  George  Gund
Foundation.

At the light microscope level (2), the photoreceptors of
normal and rd retinas look alike up to 10 days of age.
Thereafter, there is rapid degeneration of the rd visual
cells--observed as progressive loss of outer segments and
reduction of the outer nuclear layer--and finally, the
pigment epithelial cells juxtapose the cells of the inner
retina which survive the disease. Most of the degeneration
process occurs during the first three weeks of life. At the
electron microscope level (3,4), the initial signs of
pathological changes are detected by the 8th postnatal day
as disorganization of the outer segments and swelling of the
mitochondria of the inner segments.

Several years ago, we found that elevated levels of cGMP
in the rd retina occur before any signs of degeneration can
be detected, and that they are restricted to the
photoreceptors (5). Accumulation of cGMP could result
either from an increase in its synthesis or a decrease in
its degradation. The activity of guanylate cyclase, the
enzyme which synthesizes cGMP, is comparable in both control
and rd retinas while the visual cells are viable, whereas
the activity of cGMP-phosphodi- esterase (cGMP-PDE), the
enzyme which hydrolyzes cGMP, is below normal (6). In fact,
in control mouse retina, cGMP-PDE activity increases
considerably during the period of maturation of the visual
cells, but the activity of the rd enzyme remains low
throughout life, at the level attained by 6–7 days of age,
which is only 5-6% of control (6). This abnormality in cGMP
hydrolysis is specific to retinal photoreceptors. Other
tissues of the rd mouse such as skin, brain, muscle, blood
(including plasma, serum, lymphocytes and erythrocytes),
show cGMP-PDE activities comparable to those of the control
mouse tissues (7).

cGMP-PDE from rod photoreceptors is a unique enzyme,
different from cGMP-PDEs from other tissues. It is composed
of three subunits, α and β with catalytic activity and γ
with inhibitory properties. The activation/deactivation of
the enzyme is a complex process regulated by light, GTP and
several proteins including rhodopsin, G-protein and a 48 kDa
protein. In the rd retina, many factors could contribute to
a lower activity of cGMP-PDE such as a reduced number of
molecules of the enzyme, an abnormal cGMP-PDE molecule, the
presence of an excess of cGMP-PDEγ or another inhibitor, a
lesion in any of the proteins involved in the process of
activation, etc.

We studied the biosynthesis of the rd cGMP-PDE and found
that it is comparable to that in normal retina in terms of
rate and amount of protein formed, and that it starts at the

expected time during postnatal development (8). In other words, cGMP-PDE synthesis is not defective prior to the degeneration of the photoreceptor cells. However, the levels of cGMP-PDE present in the rd retina are always lower than those of control retina, suggesting that the rd enzyme is more labile. This could be the result of a change in the cGMP-PDE composition or structure or of the presence of a more active proteolytic system in rd than in control retina (8). Preliminary studies seem to indicate that the latter is not the case. Thus, we have embarked on the cloning and sequencing of the cDNAs for the different subunits of cGMP-PDE from normal and rd mouse to compare their nucleotide and corresponding amino acid sequences. We hope that this will allow us to pinpoint any modifications at the DNA level and to determine whether there are post-translational changes responsible for the rd mutation. In this article, we report the characterization of the γ–subunit of cGMP-PDE from normal mouse retina.

On the other hand, we used different approaches to investigate the components of the rod photoreceptors that are involved in the activation/deactivation of cGMP-PDE. With regard to rhodopsin, we found that there is an abnormality in its phosphorylation/dephosphorylation (9). Rhodopsin does not incorporate $^{32}$P from ATP in vitro at any age in the rd retina, even at the time when its concentration is comparable in normal and rd photoreceptors. Responsible for this abnormality could be either rhodopsin kinase, rhodopsin itself or the phosphatase that dephosphorylates rhodopsin. Preliminary studies in collaboration with Paul Hargrave, (University of Florida at Gainsville), indicate that rhodopsin kinase and the rhodopsin molecules of rd retina function normally. We suggested earlier that rd rhodopsin may be stably phosphorylated in vivo and that phosphorhodopsin phosphatase activity could be deficient, in which case we would not be able to detect $^{32}$P incorporation in vitro (9). Furthermore, since phosphorylated rhodopsin does not support cGMP-PDE activation (10), this hypothesis would be consistent with our findings in the rd disease. We are currently investigating this possibility.

Using cDNA probes for the γ–subunit of cGMP-PDE, the α, β and γ subunits of G-protein, opsin and the 48 kDa–protein, we have investigated whether the mRNAs that code for the corresponding proteins are present and qualitatively comparable to normal in size and concentration in the rd retina, and whether the time of onset of expression of these mRNAs and the translated proteins is the same in both retinas. A delay in the appearance and action of any of these mRNAs and/or proteins could be associated with the etiology of the rd disease.    In this article, we also present the results of our studies addressing these issues.

## MATERIALS AND METHODS

C57BL/6N adult, normal mice (+/+), C57BL/6J rdle/rdle homozygous, retinal degeneration mice (rd/rd), and C57BL/6J rdle/+ heterozygous, morphologically normal mice (rd/+) were obtained either from Simonsen (Gilroy, CA) or from our colonies from stock originated at the Jackson Laboratory (Bar Harbor, ME), and breeding couples supplied the young animals.    All mice were reared under diurnal lighting conditions and were sacrificed at appropriate postnatal days by decapitation.    The eyes were enucleated and the retinas were dissected rapidly and frozen on dry ice.

Total RNA was isolated using the method of Chirgwin et al. (11), and was used to prepare mouse retinal cDNA libraries    in λgt10    or for Northern blots, after fractionation by electrophoresis under denaturing conditions on formaldehyde–agarose gels and transfer to nylon membranes.

About 50,000 recombinant clones were screened with a $[\gamma\text{-}^{32}P]$-5'end-labeled 30 mer probe that we had synthesized, corresponding to nucleotides 91-120 of the $\gamma$ subunit of bovine cGMP-PDE cDNA sequence (12). A positive clone was plaque-purified and its DNA was isolated and digested with EcoR I. The inserted DNA was purified by electrophoresis, subcloned into the EcoRI site of M13mp18, and sequenced by the standard dideoxy method.

Bovine cDNA clones used in these studies are shown in Fig. 1. They were radiolabeled by primer extension (11) and heat and alkali denatured before addition to the hybridization mix.    Hybridizations were carried out as previously described (14).    RNA slot blots were used for quantitative purposes, and the resulting autoradiograms were densitometrically scanned (15).

## RESULTS

The nucleotide sequence of the isolated cGMP-PDEγ cDNA insert containing 482 bp is shown in Fig. 2. This cDNA fragment has the complete coding moiety of the gene for cGMP-PDEγ (261 bp), and 121 bp of the 5'- and 100 bp of the 3'-untranslated regions, respectively. We did not find the polyadenylation signal in the 3'-untranslated sequence because the cDNA insert does not have the entire

3'-untranslated region.

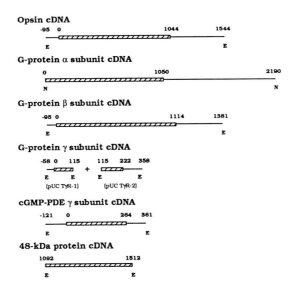

**FIGURE 1.** cDNA insert fragment sizes are numbered in base pairs 5' to 3' with 0 marking the first base pair in the coding region. Untranslated sequences are indicated by thin lines and coding regions by hatched lines. E, EcoR I; N, Nco I.

The deduced amino acid sequence of cGMP-PDEγ is also shown in Fig. 2. The 87 amino acids correspond to a molecular weight of 9.7 kDa and their composition determines the basic character of the protein.

When the $^{32}$P-labeled cGMP-PDEγ cDNA and the other specific probes that we had available were used to analyze the corresponding mRNAs in normal and <u>rd</u> mouse retinas, hybridizations such as those exemplified in Fig. 3 were obtained. The Northern blots contained RNA from 10-11 day old <u>rd</u> and <u>rd/+</u> littermate retinas, from adult <u>+/+</u> retinas, and also RNA from brain, spleen and liver, used as negative controls. In addition, a probe consisting of pCHO B cDNA, which hybridizes a specific mRNA constitutively expressed in all mammalian tissues, was used to confirm that the amount of RNA loaded on all the Northern blots was comparable.

The onset of expression of the same mRNAs studied above was determined by hybridizing the $^{32}$P-labeled cDNA probes to

```
       -121
       CCAGATCTCAGGAAGCCACAGCGCCGGTTATCTGTCCAGTGCTTGCCTGCATGAGGAC
                                                            -1
       ACCAGCCCAGCCTGACAGAGTCCAGAAGCTAAGGGTCACTGCAGTGTCTCTGCCAGCCTCACC
```

| | | | | | | | | | | | | | | | | |
|---|---|---|---|---|---|---|---|---|---|---|---|---|---|---|---|---|
| ATG | AAC | CTG | GAG | CCA | CCC | AAG | GGT | GAG | ATT | CGG | TCA | GCC | ACC | CGG | GTG | 1-48 |
| Met | Asn | Leu | Glu | Pro | Pro | Lys | Gly | Glu | Ile | Arg | Ser | Ala | Thr | Arg | Val | 1-16 |

| | | | | | | | | | | | | | | | | |
|---|---|---|---|---|---|---|---|---|---|---|---|---|---|---|---|---|
| ATA | GGA | GGA | CCA | GTC | ACC | CCC | AGG | AAA | GGA | CCA | CCT | AAG | TTT | AAG | CAG | 49-96 |
| Ile | Gly | Gly | Pro | Val | Thr | Pro | Arg | Lys | Gly | Pro | Pro | Lys | Phe | Lys | Gln | 17-32 |

| | | | | | | | | | | | | | | | | |
|---|---|---|---|---|---|---|---|---|---|---|---|---|---|---|---|---|
| CGG | CAA | ACC | AGG | CAG | TTC | AAG | AGC | AAG | CCC | CCC | AAG | AAA | GGC | GTG | CAA | 97-144 |
| Arg | Gln | Thr | Arg | Gln | Phe | Lys | Ser | Lys | Pro | Pro | Lys | Lys | Gly | Val | Gln | 33-48 |

| | | | | | | | | | | | | | | | | |
|---|---|---|---|---|---|---|---|---|---|---|---|---|---|---|---|---|
| GGG | TTT | GGG | GAT | GAC | ATC | CCT | GGA | ATG | GAA | GGC | CTG | GGG | ACA | GAT | ATC | 145-192 |
| Gly | Phe | Gly | Asp | Asp | Ile | Pro | Gly | Met | Glu | Gly | Leu | Gly | Thr | Asp | Ile | 49-64 |

| | | | | | | | | | | | | | | | | |
|---|---|---|---|---|---|---|---|---|---|---|---|---|---|---|---|---|
| ACC | GTC | ATC | TGC | CCT | TGG | GAG | GCC | TTC | AAT | CAC | CTA | GAG | CTG | CAC | GAG | 193-240 |
| Thr | Val | Ile | Cys | Pro | Trp | Glu | Ala | Phe | Asn | His | Leu | Glu | Leu | His | Glu | 65-80 |

| | | | | | | | | | | |
|---|---|---|---|---|---|---|---|---|---|---|
| CTG | GCC | CAG | TAT | GGC | ATC | ATT | TAG | TCAGATCCCTGCTATGTGAGCCCTGGGAAGA | | 241-295 |
| Leu | Ala | Gln | Tyr | Gly | Ile | Ile | TER | | | 81-87 |

```
       AACCTGCTGAAGACTCCCTCCCCCCTCTGCCAACCCGTGGAATTGTAATATGGTTAAGCTGTT     296-358

       CTT                                                              359-361
```

FIGURE 2. Nucleotide sequence of the γ subunit of cGMP-PDE for mouse retina and the corresponding amino acid sequence of the protein.

slot-blotted retinal RNA isolated at every postnatal day during development of rd and rd/+ mice, and analyzing the resulting autoradiograms by laser densitometry. Fig. 4 is an example of the quantitation of opsin mRNA levels as a function of age. Expression of opsin mRNA is first detectable, although minimally, during postnatal day 5 in both rd and control retina. The amount of hybridization increases significantly in both species until postnatal day 11-12. At this age, rd opsin mRNA begins to decrease, and by day 29, it is no longer detectable above background. In contrast, opsin mRNA in the control rd/+ retina increases steadily through adulthood.

Table I summarizes the results that we obtained for the developmental expression of mRNAs coding for opsin, the α, β and γ subunits of G-protein and the 48 kDa-protein. The mRNAs encoding the β subunit of G-protein and 48 kDa-protein are already expressed at low levels at birth (P0) in both rd and rd/+ retinas and only begin to increase by postnatal day 6. As with opsin, these mRNAs levels decrease from 11-12 days of age in the rd retina. A hybridization signal can be observed for the γ subunit of G-protein mRNA in both normal and rd retina by postnatal day 6 and for the α subunit of G-protein by postnatal day 7.

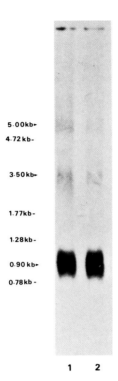

FIGURE 3. mRNA hybridization to the γ subunit of cGMP -PDE. Lane 1, normal retina mRNA; lane 2, <u>rd</u> retina mRNA.

## DISCUSSION

Degeneration of the visual cells of the <u>rd</u> retina starts during the most rapid period of photoreceptor development and coincides with the time at which the components of the cGMP-PDE system are initially detected. We have cloned and sequenced the γ subunit of cGMP-PDE and have used it as a probe, together with cDNA probes for the proteins involved in the activation/deactivation of the enzyme, to analyze the corresponding mRNAs.

Our results indicate that cGMP-PDEγ has been highly conserved during evolution. At the nucleotide level, there is 91.75% homology between mouse and cow coding sequences and at the amino acid level, the homology between the proteins of these species is 97.7%. Only two amino acids were found to be different (16).

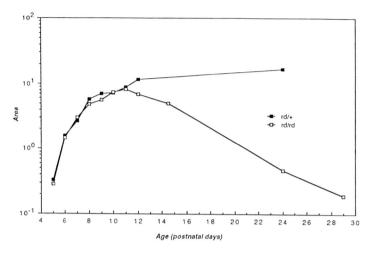

FIGURE 4. Developmental expression of opsin mRNA in r̲d̲ and r̲d̲/+ mouse retinas.

TABLE 1
DEVELOPMENTAL EXPRESSION OF RETINAL
mRNAs IN r̲d̲/r̲d̲ AND r̲d̲/+ MICE

| Age | | 0 | 1 | 2 | 3 | 4 | 5 | 6 | 7 | 8 | 9 | 10 | 11 | 12 | Adult |
|---|---|---|---|---|---|---|---|---|---|---|---|---|---|---|---|
| mRNA | sample | | | | | | | | | | | | | | |
| Gβ | rd/+ | ± | ± | ± | ± | ± | ± | + | + | + | + | + | + | + | ++ |
| | rd/rd | ± | ± | ± | ± | ± | ± | + | + | + | + | + | + | <+ | ± |
| 48K | rd/+ | ± | ± | ± | ± | ± | ± | + | + | + | + | + | + | + | ++ |
| | rd/rd | ± | ± | ± | ± | ± | ± | + | + | + | + | + | <+ | <+ | - |
| opsin | rd/+ | - | - | - | - | - | - | ± | + | + | + | + | + | + | + | ++ |
| | rd/rd | - | - | - | - | - | - | ± | + | + | + | + | + | <+ | - |
| Gγ | rd/+ | * | * | * | * | * | * | * | ± | + | + | + | + | + | + | + |
| | rd/rd | * | * | * | * | * | * | * | ± | + | + | + | + | <+ | - |
| Gα | rd/+ | - | - | - | - | - | - | - | - | - | + | + | + | + | + | ++ |
| | rd/rd | - | - | - | - | - | - | - | - | - | + | + | + | <+ | <+ | - |

Symbols: ±, just detectable; +, obvious hybridization; ++, most intense; <+, lower in r̲d̲ than in control; -, no hybridization; *, too low to be significant.

mRNAs coding for cGMP-PDEγ, opsin, the α, β and γ subunits of G-protein and 48 kDa-protein from age matched r̲d̲

photoreceptor synaptic function and in the disease process
and also the possibility of a transport abnormality in the
visual cells of the affected dogs.

Robert Sparkes summarized different strategies utilized
in gene mapping. Genetic linkage analysis has been greatly
revitalized through the use of DNA restriction fragment
length polymorphisms (RFLPs). The advantage of the RFLPs is
that the gene or DNA sequence does not need to be known to
be mapped. In addition, all genes or DNA sequences can be
"made" polymorphic with the use of different restriction
endonucleases, and what is investigated is the cosegregation
of an RFLP from a particular gene with the DNA probe that is
being used. Since the number of gene probes currently
available is quite large, the candidate gene approach may be
convenient for the selection of the best probes. Candidate
genes may be identified by considerations such as the
following: 1) phenotypic linkage information may help to
determine on what chromosome the linkage studies with RFLPs
should be focused (an example of this has been the linkage
of Retinitis Pigmentosa gene on chromosome 1 with the Rh
blood type); 2) a biochemical abnormality may be known which
would suggest the involvement of a given gene in the
disease; 3) information from mapping in the mouse may give
clues to the location of a gene in a human chromosome; 4)
chromosome abnormalities (as has been the case in the study
of retinoblastoma) may indicate what chromosome or part of a
chromosome would be important to study.

A second method commonly used for gene mapping is
somatic cell hybridization analysis. Hybrids formed by the
fusion of normal human cells and a rodent cell line
preferentially, and in a random fashion, lose human
chromosomes. Thus, different hybrid clones will have
different human chromosome content. By hybridizing a panel
of different clones to a given gene probe (human or other)
it is possible to assign a human gene or related sequences
to any human chromosome or to more than one chromosome (as
has been done with the ornithine aminotransferase gene,
which is present both in chromosomes 10 and X). In situ
hybridization is another technique which is being
increasingly used for gene mapping. In this method,
tritiated DNA probes are hybridized directly to human
metaphases. Although a large number of metaphases may need
to be analyzed, generally one or more peaks of activity can
be identified over one or more chromosomes. Finally, gene
mapping has been carried out in the mouse through the
analysis of recombinant inbred strains. In humans, it may

be possible to map any DNA probe to a particular gene by studying RFLPs for this probe in one or more large families which have been fully characterized by a linkage map.

Richard Weleber discussed the clinical grounds and linkage evidence for heterogeneity in X-linked recessive Retinitis Pigmentosa (RP). This is the least frequently seen inheritance type of RP, but one of the most severe, characterized by high myopia, astigmatism, foveal and macular lesions, and a visual acuity of 20/200 or less by 30-40 years of age. Manifestations in all affected males are the same, but the fundi of carrier women appear different, suggesting the existence of two forms of X-linked RP. In the classic form (McKusick 31260), carrier women may show scattered patches of pigmentary degeneration of the retina and choroid, whereas in the second form (McKusick 30320), the carriers have a brilliant, golden tapetal fundus reflex. The presence of the tapetal sheen has led some investigators to surmise that the disorder in carrier women is different from that in the hemizygous affected males. However, affected males occasionally show the tapetal sheen within the first to second decade of life, after which the sheen slowly fades and is replaced by diffuse retinal pigment epithelium atrophy. Dr. Weleber believes that the carrier state for X-linked RP is a slowly progressive retinal dystrophy in its own right, with regional involvement determined by the outcome of lyonization for cells of specific areas of the retina. The patchy distribution of pigmentary changes correlates well with the concept of the randomness of lyonization.

Linkage studies indicate that one locus for RP is close to or proximal to band 11.3 of the short arm of the X chromosome. Bhattacharya and colleagues first demonstrated relative close linkage of classic type RP to the RFLP probe called L1.28, which detects locus DXS7, located within band 11.3 of the short arm. Investigators have confirmed this linkage and the LOD score now is over 20 at a $\theta$ of approximately 0.09. Recently, a looser linkage with DXS14, which has also been localized within band 1 of the short arm and seems to lie proximal to DXS7, has been shown. The possibility of another gene for RP on the X chromosome has been suggested from studies of carrier women with tapetal sheen in large kindreds of X-linked RP. In these pedigrees, in addition to linkage to DXS7, linkage to an RFLP at the ornithine transcarbamylase (OTC) locus was also detected, supporting the presence of a gene distal to DXS7 on the short arm of the X chromosome. Recently, linkage associations were reported between RP and several markers in the region of band 21 of the short arm. Additional support for one RP locus in this region came from a patient with chromosomal deletion of band 21 in association with Duchenne muscular dystrophy (DMD), McLeod red cell phenotype, chronic granulomatous disease and RP. DNA from this patient was used to generate other new probes for the deleted region, allowing precise localization of the gene for DMD. Absence of RP in other patients with DMD who showed smaller deletions within the deletion zone of the original patient suggested that the second RP gene is most probably localized in the proximal portion of band 21.

Fielding Hejtmancik described his studies on the mapping of the gene responsible for blue cone monochromacy (BCM), an infrequent X-linked retinal disorder characterized by poor central visual acuity and color discrimination, early onset of nystagmus, variable degrees of myopia and astigmatism, and photodysphoria. The physiologic functions of both rods and blue cones are preserved. The frequency is estimated to be less than one in 650,000 persons.

Previous attempts to map BCM with serological markers suggested that BCM is not closely linked to either the Xg blood group or glucose-6 phosphate dehydrogenase. However, since protanopsia and deuteroanopsia had been mapped to Xq28, this region was studied using DNA probes and RFLPs. Three families provided more than 20 potentially informative meioses. Two loci, DXS15 and DXS52, showed significant linkage with LOD scores of 3.58 and 2.39 at $\theta$s of 0.05 and 0.07, respectively. Analysis with factor 8 suggested linkage with a LOD score of 1.31 at a $\theta$ of 0. Thus, BCM mapped to the tightly-linked cluster DXS25-DXS52-F8, all within Xq28.

The red and green pigment genes of BCM-affected males were examined in collaboration with Jeremy Nathans (Johns Hopkins University). Two families had similar deletions of the red pigment gene, as shown by a common junctional fragment, whereas other affected males showed absence of the red pigment gene or deletion of the green pigment gene. Thus, in these families, BCM results from deletion or rearrangement of the red and/or green pigment genes.

Dr. Hejtmancik indicated that both linkage analysis and direct identification of deletions must be performed to determine carrier condition in BCM families. In one case, absence of the junctional fragment described above indicated that a female at risk for being a carrier had not inherited the deletion associated with BCM in her family.

triphosphate (dTTP; NEN Research Products, Boston, MA). The hybridization reaction was initiated by replacing the prehybridization solution with 14-20 ng nick translated HSV-1 cloned DNA (specific activity >2 x $10^8$ CPM/μg) in 7 ml of a solution containing 57% formamide, 5X SSC, 1X Denhardt's solution, 50 mM sodium phosphate, pH 6.5, 10% dextran sulfate and 100 μg/ml denatured salmon sperm DNA. Hybridization was performed overnight @37C.

Hybridized filter papers were washed three times in 2X SSC containing 0.1% SDS at 55C. Autoradiography was performed with Kodak X-Omat AR film (Eastman Kodak Co., Rochester, NY) and DuPont Cronex Lightning Plus screens (DuPont NEN Research Products, Wilmington, DE) at -70C for 8 days. [14]

## RESULTS

Virological

Normal and VZV-infected rabbit corneal epithelial cell cultures are represented in Figure 1.

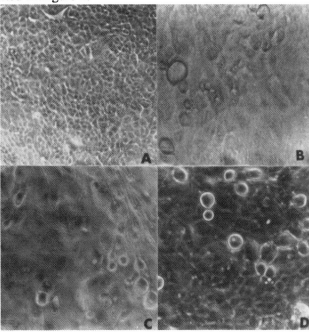

Figure 1: Legend on page following

Figure 1: Varicella Zoster Virus Cytopathology in Non-Infected and VZV-Infected ACV-Suppressed Rabbit Corneal Cell Monolayers. A) Control, Sham-Infected corneal Epithelial cell monolayer (day 5; X850). B) Early VZV CPE in ACV-Suppressed epithelial cell culture (day 4 post suppression; X800). C) Characteristic linear VZV CPE in reactivated corneal cell culture. (day 14 post inoculation, day 5 post reactivation; X800). D) VZV CPE in a reactivated corneal cell culture (day 15 post inoculation, day 6 post reactivation; X825).

No drug toxicity was evident in any non-VZV infected cell culture containing ACV (50 µg/ml). VZV-infected, non ACV-suppressed cell cultures demonstrated CPE from days 4-7 PI. These non-ACV-suppressed monolayers were completely destroyed by progressive cytopathology by day 9 PI. Seventeen percent of VZV-infected, ACV-suppressed cultures demonstrated a transient VZV CPE on days 3-4 PS. VZV CPE was not evident in the ACV-suppressed cultures after day 4 PI. Cell-free VZV was recovered from only 9% of VZV-infected ACV-suppressed cultures on days 4-9 PS indicating active VZV suppression in >90% of the cultures. After removal of ACV suppression on day 9 PI, VZV was recovered from 38% of the reactivated cultures.

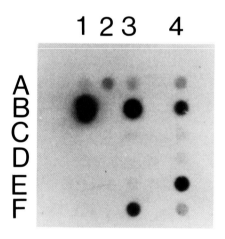

Figure 2: Dot blot hybridization with [32P]-labeled VZV DNA of extracted DNA from control (non-VZV-infected) and ACV-suppressed corneal epithelial cell cultures.

Row 1: A= 5 µg total DNA spots from sham inoculated control corneal cell monolayers;  B= 5 µg spot from VZV-infected non-suppressed culture on day 5 PI; Row 2: A= VZV-infected ACV-suppressed culture, day 2 PS; Rows 3 and 4: 5 µg spots from VZV-infected ACV-suppressed cultures: Row 3- A, day 2 PS; B, day 3 PS; E, day 5 PS; F, day 5 PS; Row 4- A, day 6 PS; B, day 6 PS; E, day 8 PS and F day 9 PS.

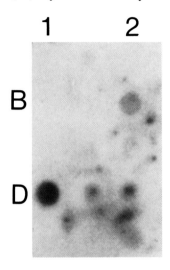

Figure 3: Dot blot hybridization with [32P]-labeled VZV DNA of extracted DNA from reactivated corneal epithelial cell cultures.
Rows 1 and 2: 5 µg spots from reactivated VZV-infected cultures, Row 1- D, day 10 post inoculation (day 2 post reactivation); Row 2- B, day 12 post inoculation (day 4 post reactivation).

Dot Blot Hybridization

The VZV probe did not hybridize to non-infected corneal epithelial DNA extracts.  In VZV-infected non-ACV-suppressed cultures VZV DNA was detected at concentrations of 10 pg/5 µg nucleic acid spot on days 3-4 PI.  VZV DNA concentrations increased in these non-ACV-suppressed cultures to 100 pg/5 µg nucleic acid spot on days 5-7 PI.  In VZV-infected ACV-suppressed cultures, VZV DNA was detected at approximately 7-10 pg/5 µg nucleic acid spot on days 1-4 PS and at <1-3 pg/5 µg spot during active ACV suppression (days 5-9 PS).  After removal of ACV suppression on day 9 PS, VZV DNA concentrations in the reactivated cultures increased to 50-100 pg/5 µg nucleic acid spot by days 12 -16 PI (Figures 2 and 3).

## DISCUSSION

Knowledge concerning VZV ocular pathogenicity and systemic infection disease processes has lagged behind other diseases of viral etiology, especially other herpes group virus infections. Because of this problem, characterization of VZV-host cell interactions and critical evaluation of the VZV latent state remain unclear.

Several in vivo models of VZV infection have been developed; however, most of these systems do not approximate the human disease state [15-18]. In situ hybridization studies in a guinea pig model of VZV infection that mimics human ocular disease (microdendrite development and systemic dissemination of the VZV infection) [8] and in human trigeminal ganglia at autopsy [19] have directly demonstrated the presence of the VZV genome in neurons as well as glial elements in the ganglion. This result may in part be due to VZV characteristics of cell-to-cell spread and may be an important difference between VZV and HSV latency states. Whether or not the VZV genome during periods of latency is retained in a static or dynamic state, and the contribution of VZV RNA (sense and/or anti-sense) awaits clarification in experimental models and in human tissue samples.

The present study used ACV to inhibit (restrict) the expression of the VZV genome, either by terminating DNA synthesis or selectively inhibiting viral thymidine kinase (TK) activity [20]. Limiting expression of the VZV genome with concurrent induction of a high ratio of corneal epithelial cells that contain the VZV genome is the ultimate goal of in vitro viral latency/suppression models. Since VZV is a herpes group virus, the criteria used to analyze and evaluate the in vitro drug-suppression model were identical to parameters used for HSV in vitro models [21,22]. They were: survival of VZV-infected corneal epithelial cells, absence of VZV particles in the ACV-suppressed cultures, persistence of the VZV genome in the surviving cells and, most importantly, the ability to reactivate the VZV infection after removal of ACV inhibition.

In our model, a transient VZV CPE was evident in ACV-suppressed cultures on days 3-4 PS. After day 5 PS, in the presence of continued ACV-suppression, no VZV CPE was evident, epithelial cell monolayers remained healthy and virus was not recovered from supernate culture. When ACV suppression was removed on day 9 PS, 38% of the cultures reactivated VZV as determined by virus recovery from supernatant cultures and development of VZV CPE. These virological data suggest that a suppressed VZV infection in rabbit corneal cell monolayers could be maintained and reactivated.

Detection of VZV DNA retained in this culture system by dot blot hybridization demonstrated that the VZV genome was consistently detected at approximately 1-3 pg levels during active ACV-suppression. The state (activity) of the VZV genome and the location of the VZV DNA retained in

cultures in DMEM supplemented with 10% fetal calf serum,
penicillin (100 U/ml), streptomycin (100ug/ml) and L-
glutamine (540ug/ml) at 37°C with 5% CO2.  Stocks of HCMV
(AD169) were prepared by low multiplicity passage (0.01
plaque forming units/cell) in HLF cells.  MCMV (Smith) was
passaged in MEF cells.


### Recombinant Plasmids

HIV$_{SF-2}$ molecular clone was cleaved with HindIII to
generate a 1475bp fragment comprising sequences upstream of
the 3' LTR, U3 and 77 bp into the 'R' region of the LTR.
This fragment was inserted upstream of the chloramphenicol
acetyltransferase (CAT) gene as described previously (14).
The HIV transactivator gene 'tat' derived from the HIV$_{SF-2}$
molecular clone was positioned between the SV40 early promoter and poly (A) addition site yielding the plasmid pTAT
(12,14).  All the plasmids containing deletion and point
mutations in HIV LTR were constructed by standard recombinant
DNA techniques (15), and were described in detail earlier
(14,16,17).  The plasmids were purified through two rounds of
ethidium bromide-cesium chloride gradient centrifugation for
transfection experiments.  The HCMV immediate early-1 gene,
encoding the 72,000-dalton major IE polypeptide, was
constructed with the HSV thymidine kinase promoter directing
transcription of this gene (17).


### DNA Transfection and Virus Infection

HeLa cells were split 24 hrs before transfection.
Calcium phosphate precipitates of plasmid DNA were formed as
described (18).  Cells (1x10⁶) were exposed to the pre-
cipitate for 6 hrs followed by 90 seconds of glycerol shock
(19).  HCMV infections were initiated 24 hrs after transfection by adding the appropriate volume of viral suspension to
obtain the desired m.o.i. per cell.  In the case of MCMV,
virus infections were initiated 24 hrs prior to transfection.


### CAT Assay

CAT assays were performed by the procedures described by
Gorman et al. (20).  The cell extracts were normalized for
degree of cell lysis by monitoring A$_{260/280}$ ratio before cell

extract was added to the enzyme assay mixture.  Enzyme assays were continued for 1 hr before ethyl acetate was added.  The products of the reaction were separated by ascending thin-layer chromatography, visualized by autoradiography, and quantitated by scintillation counting.

## Reverse Transcriptase Assay

Cells (1x10^6) were transfected with the indicated concentrations of HIV proviral DNA (21) as described. Viruses released into medium were quantitated by reverse transcriptase assay.  Cell-free supernatant after initial clarification, was centrifuged at 35,000 rpm for 1 hr and the pellet was dissolved in 50ul of virus solubilizing buffer. An aliquot (20ul) was taken for the assay using poly(rA)•(dT)$_{12-18}$ as the template (2).  Incorporation of radiolabeled thymidine into cDNA reaction products was measured by liquid scintillation spectroscopy of trichloroacetic acid precipitates.  The assay was carried out with culture medium collected 72 hrs after transfection.

## Oligonucleotide Primer Extension

Total cytoplasmic RNA was isolated from HeLa cells at 48 hrs post transfection (15).  30ug RNA was used as template for in vitro cDNA synthesis using AMV reverse transcriptase and 0.1ug of a CAT gene-specific oligonucleotide as primer. The 32-base oligonucleotide contained the chloramphenicol acetyltransferase gene sequence 5'-CTGGATATTACGGCCTTTTAAAGACCGTAAAG-3' from the coding strand. The cDNA products were resolved by electrophoresis on 8% polyacrylamide gels and by autoradiography.

## RESULTS

### Activation of HIV LTR-Directed Expression by HCMV and MCMV

Cells were transfected with pLTR-CAT (10ug) plasmid alone or in combination with the 'tat' gene plasmid pTAT. HIV LTR-directed CAT expression in the absence of transactivators was low in HeLa cells, human foreskin fibroblasts and TE671 cells.  The levels of CAT activity in cells cotransfected with pLTR-CAT and pTAT increased significantly (approximately 500 fold) relative to that in pLTR-CAT transfected cells. pLTR-CAT transfected cells were infected with HCMV or MCMV (m.o.i.=10 or 20 pfu/cell, respectively); LTR-directed CAT expression was stimulated by infection with either virus and exhibited cell type specificity (Table 1).

**Table 1**
Activation of HIV LTR-directed expression by HCMV and MCMV

| Cell line used for transfection and virus infection | Percent chloramphenicol acetylated | |
|---|---|---|
| | HCMV | MCMV |
| HeLa | 48.5 | 34.2 |
| Human foreskin fibroblasts | 13.4 | N/D |
| TE671 | N/D | 4.1 |

Cells transfected with pLTR-CAT plasmid showed CAT values in the range of 0.1 to 0.6%. N/D, not done.

## HCMV Immediate Early (IE) Gene Region Transactivates HIV LTR-Directed Expression

The immediate early genes of herpesviruses have been shown to be involved in activating a variety of promoters in trans (22,23). Based on this, we tested the effect of HCMV-IE gene region on HIV LTR-directed expression. HCMV-IE plasmid was cotransfected in different concentrations with pLTR-CAT (10ug). The results are shown in Figure 1. The extent of activation was linear with respect to the concentration of immediate early gene plasmid.

## Localization of Sequences in HIV LTR needed for Activation by HCMV and MCMV

Similar to eukaryotic and viral promoters, the HIV LTR contains transcriptional regulatory sequences including a TATA box, Sp1 binding sites, a core enhancer region, and negative regulatory regions (16,24). A number of HIV LTR mutants containing deletions, insertions, and point mutations were constructed in the pLTR-CAT plasmid. The details of the LTR mutants used in this study are given in Tables 2 and 3. HeLa cells were transfected with wild type or mutant pLTR-CAT

alone or in combination with either pTAT or HCMV-IE.
Transactivation of HIV LTR-directed expression by HCMV-IE was
completely abolished when sequences upstream of -48 were
deleted (Table 2). Mutations in all three Sp1 binding sites
decreased activation by HCMV-IE and MCMV. These experiments
demonstrate that sequences in the U3 region of the LTR are
critical for activation by HCMV and MCMV. Mutations
localized in the 'tar' sequences (-17 to +80) (25) did not
reduce the extent of activation by HCMV-IE and MCMV (Table
3). All of the 'tar' region LTR mutants exhibited
inordinately higher levels of CAT activity than that
exhibited by the wild type LTR in the absence of
transactivators; the mechanism responsible for these higher
CAT activities noted with the 'tar' mutants was not apparent
in these experiments. The small reduction in CMV
transactivation observed in LTR 'tar' mutants did not
indicate that these HIV sequences were necessary for
interaction with CMV regulatory polypeptides.

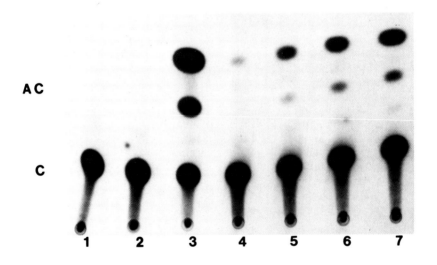

**Figure 1.** Effect of HCMV-IE gene on HIV LTR-directed
expression. 10ug LTR-CAT was used in combination with
various concentrations of HCMV-IE. Lane 1, No DNA; lane 2,
pLTR-CAT; lane 3, pLTR-CAT+pTAT (.5ug); lane 4, pLTR-
CAT+HCMV-IE (2ug); lane 5, pLTR-CAT+HCMV-IE (4ug); lane 6,
pLTR-CAT+HCMV-IE (8ug); lane 7, pLTR-CAT+HCMV-IE (10ug.). C,
chloramphenicol; AC, acetylated chloramphenicol.

**Table 2**
Transactivation of HIV-LTR harboring mutations in U3 region by HCMV-IE and MCMV

| Plasmid designation | Nature of mutation in the LTR U3 sequences | CAT activity (fold increase) | |
|---|---|---|---|
| | | + HCMV-IE | + MCMV |
| HIV-LTR CAT | none | 54.8 | 7.5 |
| HIV-LTR -278 CAT | deletion of sequences upstream of -278 | 31.8 | N/D |
| HIV-LTR -176 CAT | deletion of sequences upstream of -176 | 27.2 | N/D |
| HIV-LTR -117 CAT | deletion of sequences upstream of -117 | 24.9 | N/D |
| HIV-LTR -103 CAT | deletion of sequences upstream of -103 | 35.2 | N/D |
| HIV-LTR -65 CAT | deletion of sequences upstream of -65 | 29.3 | 7.6 |
| HIV-LTR -48 CAT | deletion of sequnces upstream of -48 | 3.0 | 1.8 |
| HIV-LTR -17 CAT | deletion of sequences upstream of -17 | 1.5 | 1.0 |
| Sp1M1-CAT | clustered site mutations in Sp1 binding site III | 23.8 | 4.8 |
| Sp1M3-CAT | clustered site mutations in Sp1 binding sites I, II, and III | 14.8 | 3.0 |

10 ug pLTR-CAT and 10 ug HCMV-IE plasmid DNA were used in cotransfection experiments. In the case of MCMV infection, 20 m.o.i. per cell was used before pLTR-CAT DNA transfection. Fold increase was calculated by using the values obtained in the presence or absence of HCMV-IE cotransfection and MCMV infection. N/D, not done.

**Table 3**
Transactivation of HIV-LTR harboring mutations in R region by HCMV-IE and MCMV

| Plasmid designation | Nature of mutation in the LTR R sequences | CAT activity (fold increase) | |
|---|---|---|---|
| | | + HCMV-IE | + MCMV |
| HIV-LTR CAT | none | 54.8 | 7.5 |
| Ins 1-CAT | insertion of a 36 base pair polylinker between the BglII and SacI sites in the tar region (28 bp addition) | 26.3 | 12.0 |
| Ins 2-CAT | Ins 1-CAT mutant with a deletion of 21 base pairs within the polylinker (7 bp addition) | N/D | 11.2 |
| LTR/338/CAT | 6 base pair change in the 1st direct repeat sequences in the tar region | 15.2 | 6.1 |
| LTR/360/CAT | 6 base pair change in the 2nd direct repeat sequences in the tar region | 12.0 | N/D |

See table 2 for methods.

## RNA Analysis

To understand the mechanism of activation by cyto-megalovirus, RNA was analyzed from the transfected cells. Total RNA was extracted from cells cotransfected with pLTR-CAT and HCMV immediate early gene. Primer extension analysis of the RNA is shown in Figure 2. An increase in CAT mRNA initiated from the HIV LTR promoter complex is evident and is in parallel to the CAT activity observed. HCMV-IE gene was also able to transactivate pTKCAT plasmid transcription.

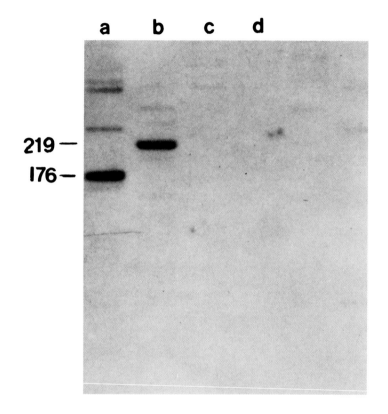

**Figure 2.** Primer extension analysis of total cytoplasmic RNA from HeLa cells using CAT-specific oligonucleotide primer.  a, RNA from cells transfected with pTKCAT
and HCMV-IE; b, RNA from cells transfectd with pLTR-CAT and
HCMV-IE; c, RNA from cells transfected with pTKCAT; d, RNA
from cells transfected with pLTR-CAT.

## Effect of HCMV Immediate Early Gene on HIV Synthesis

Activation of HIV LTR-directed expression by HCMV-IE was
further extended to the synthesis and assembly of HIV
particles.  HIV proviral DNA (pZ6Neo) was transfected alone
or in combination with HCMV-IE plasmid into HeLa cells.  HIV
particles released into the medium were monitored by reverse
transcriptase assay.  HCMV-IE increased HIV production 10-15
fold when cotransfected with HIV proviral DNA (Fig. 3).

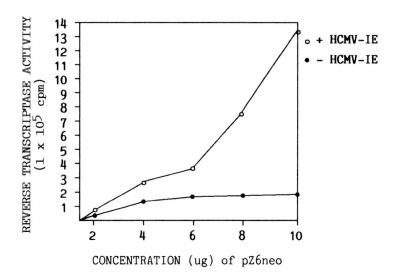

**Figure 3.** Effect of HCMV-IE on HIV production. 10ug HCMV-IE gene was transfected in combination with various concentrations of HIV proviral DNA.

## DISCUSSION

The results presented in this paper show that both human and murine cytomegalovirus infection of pLTR-CAT transfected cells enhance the HIV LTR-directed expression of the CAT gene. The transient expression assays were carried out in HeLa cells because of the low level expression of HIV LTR-CAT plasmids in these cells. The extent of activation of pLTR-CAT expression was higher in HCMV infected cells than in MCMV infected cells. In addition, subgenomic clones derived from HCMV containing the immediate early gene region transactivated the HIV LTR-directed expression. Experiments with murine cytomegalovirus also suggest that the transactivation effect may be directed by the immediate early gene products of MCMV. Although MCMV is able to replicate in murine and rabbit kidney cells, sheep brain cells, and goat fibroblasts, MCMV infection of human cells shows the expression of only immediate early gene products and not viral replication (26).

The genetic organization of HIV LTR is very similar to other retroviruses (27) and contains several features shared

by many promoters recognized by eukaryotic RNA polymerase
(Pol II) (24). Mutational analysis of HIV LTR with respect
to the HIV transactivator gene 'tat' function show that
sequences spanning from -17 to +80 with respect to the
transcriptional start site are critical for transactivation.
Our studies indicate that the target sequences of HIV LTR
needed for transactivation by cytomegaloviruses are different
from those required for transactivation by the 'tat' gene
product. Mutations upstream of the transcriptional start
site in HIV LTR show marked reduction in the activation by
cytomegaloviruses. Specifically, point mutations in all
three Sp1 binding sites decreased significantly the
activation effect.

The immediate early gene products of cytomegaloviruses
have a positive regulatory effect on HIV LTR-directed
expression (17). We and others reported that herpes simplex
viruses (HSV-1 and HSV-2), sodium butyrate, phorbol esters
and mitogens activate HIV LTR-directed expression
(12,13,28,29). The mechanism of activation of HIV LTR-
directed expression by cytomegaloviruses is not known. HCMV
immediate early gene enhancement of HIV LTR-directed CAT
activity was also paralleled by an increase in the
corresponding level of CAT mRNA. It is likely that an
increase in mRNA is brought about either by an increase in
the transcription rate of transfected pLTR-CAT or by other
mechanisms such as mRNA stabilization. Since the CMV
immediate early gene products have been shown to regulate a
number of viral and cellular promoters but have not been
shown to bind specifically to DNA sequences, (22), it is
probable that the activation effect involves interactions
with cellular transcription factors. The specific binding of
several cellular transcription factors to the HIV LTR have
been documented (29,30), and the interactions of CMV
immediate early proteins with these host factors await to be
determined.

A biological characteristic of HIV infection similar to
several DNA viruses is the protracted latency period
exhibited in many HIV-infected individuals. The overwhelming
majority of T4+ lymphocytes infected with HIV in AIDS
patients do not produce virus continuously and harbor the
proviral genome in a latent state (31). The findings of HCMV
and HIV coinfected cells (J. Nelson and R. Robinson,
unpublished results), of stimulated virus production from
cells cotransfected with HIV proviral genomes and HCMV-IE
genes, and of CMV transactivation of HIV promoter regulatory
elements presented here provide evidence for a cofactor model
for HCMV in the progression of AIDS in HIV-infected persons.

That the HCMV-IE polypeptides transactivate HIV LTR-directed gene expression indicates a transcriptional mechanism for HIV gene activation through interactions with host transcription factors.

## REFERENCES

1. Barre-Sinoussi F, Chermann JC, Rey R, Nugeryre MT, Chamaret S, Gruest J, Dauget C, Axler-Blin C, Vezinet-Brun F, Rouzioux C, Rosenbaum W, Montagnier L (1983). Isolation of a T-lymphocytic retrovirus from a patient at risk for the acquired immunodeficiency syndrome (AIDS). Science 220:868.
2. Gallo RC, Salahuddin SZ, Popovic M, Shearer GM, Kaplan M, Haynes BF, Parker TJ, Redfield R, Oleske J, Safai B, White G, Foster P, Markham PD (1984). Frequent detection and isolation of cytopathic retroviruses (HTLV-III) from patients with AIDS and at risk for AIDS. Science 224:500.
3. Levy JA, Hoffman AD, Dramer SM, Lanois JA, Shimabukino JM, Oskiro LS (1984). Isolation of lymphocytopathic retroviruses from San Francisco patients with AIDS. Science 225:840.
4. Curran JW, Morgan WM, Hardy AM, Jaffe HW, Darrow WW, Dowdle WR (1985). The epidemiology of AIDS: Current status and future prospects. Science 229:1352.
5. Rosenberg PR, Uliss AE, Friedland GH, Harris CA, Small CB, Klein RS (1983). Acquired immunodeficiency syndrome. Ophthalmic manifestations in ambulatory patients. Ophthamology 90:874.
6. Khaelem M, Kaligh SB, Goldsmith J, Fetkenhour C, O'Grady RB, Phair JP, Chrobak M (1984). Ophthalmologic findings in acquired immune deficiency syndrome (AIDS). Arch Ophthamol 102:201.
7. Kestelyn P, Van de Perre P, Rouvroy D, Lepage P, Bogaerts J, Nzaramba D, Clumeck N (1985). A prospective study of the ophthamologic findings in the acquired immune deficiency syndrome in Africa. Am J Ophthamol 100:230.
8. Henderly DE, Freeman WR, Smith RE, Causey D, Rao NA (1987). Cytomegalovirus retinitis as the initial manifestation of acquired immune deficiency syndrome. Am J Ophthamol 103:316.
9. Wong-Staal F, Gallo RC (1985). Human T-lymphotropic retroviruses. Nature (London) 317:395.

10. Pomerantz RJ, Kuritzkes DR, De la Monte SM, Rota TR, Baker AS, Albert D, Bor DH, Feldman EL, Schooley RT, Hirsh MS (1987). Infection of the retina by human immunodeficiency virus type 1. New Engl J Med 317:1643.

11. Landesman SH, Ginzburg HM, Weiss SH (1985). Special report: The AIDS epidemic. New Engl J Med 312:521.

12. Rando RF, Pellett PE, Luciw PA, Bohan CA, Srinivasan A (1987). Transactivation of human immunodeficiency virus by herpesviruses. Oncogene 1:13.

13. Mosca JD, Bednarik DP, Raj NBK, Rosen CA, Sodroski JG, Haseltine WA, Pitha PM (1987). Herpes simplex virus type-1 can reactivate transcription of latent human immunodeficiency virus. Nature (London) 325:67.

14. Peterlin BM, Luciw PA, Barr PJ, Walker MD (1986). Elevated levels of mRNA can account for the transactivation of human immunodeficiency virus. Proc Natl Acad Sci USA 83:9734.

15. Maniatis T, Fritsch EF, Sambrook J (1982). "Molecular Cloning: A Laboratory Manual". Cold Spring Harbor Laboratory: Cold Spring Harbor, NY.

16. Jones KA, Kadonaga JT, Luciw PA, Tjian R (1986). Activation of the AIDS retrovirus promoter by the cellular transcription factor, Spl. Science 232:755.

17. Bohan CA, Nelson JA, Srinivasan A, Robinson RA (1988). Human cytomegalovirus immediate early-1 gene transactivates the human immunodeficiency virus long terminal repeat. J Virol: in press.

18. Graham FL, Vander Eb AJ (1973). A new technique for the assay of infectivity of human adenovirus 5 DNA. Virology 52:456.

19. Frost E, Williams J (1978). Mapping temperature-sensitive and host-range mutations of adenovirus type 5 by marker rescue. Virology 91:39.

20. Gorman CM, Moffat LF, Howard BH (1982). Recombinant genomes which express chloramphenicol acetyltransferase in mammalian cells. Mol Cell Biol 2:1044.

21. Srinivasan A, Anand R, York D, Ranganathan P, Feorino P, Schochetman G, Curran J, Kalyanaraman VS, Luciw PA, Sanchez-Pescador R (1987). Molecular characterization of human immunodeficiency virus from Zaire: Nucleotide sequence analysis identifies conserved and variable domains in the envelope gene. Gene 52:71.

22. Roizman B, Batterson W (1985). In Fields B (ed): "Virology". Raven: NY, p497.

23. O'Hare P, Hayward GS (1985). Evidence for a direct role for both the 175,000- and 110,000- molecular weight immediate early proteins of herpes simplex virus and the transactivation of delayed early promoters. J Virol 53:751.

24. Rosen CA, Sodroski JG, Haseltine WA (1985). Location of cis-acting regulatory sequences in the human T cell lymphotropic virus type III (HTLV-III/LAV) long terminal repeat. Cell 41:813.

25. Rosen CA, Sodroski JG, Goh WC, Dayton AI, Lippke J, Haseltine WA (1986). Post-transcriptional regulation accounts for the transactivation of the human T-lymphotropic virus type III. Nature (London) 319:555

26. Walker D, Hudson J (1987). Analysis of immediate-early and early proteins of murine cytomegalovirus in permissive and nonpermissive cells. Arch Virol 92:103.

27. Sanchez-Pescador R, Power MD, Barr PJ, Steimer KS, Stempien MM, Brown-Shimer SL, Gee WW, Renard A, Randolph A, Levy JA, Dina D, Luciw PA (1985). Nucleotide sequence and expression of an AIDS - associated retrovirus (ARV-2). Science 227:484.

28. Bohan CA, York D, Srinivasan A (1987). Sodium butyrate activates human immunodeficiency virus long terminal repeat - directed expression. BBRC 148:899.

29. Nabel G, Baltimore D (1987). An inducible transcription factor activates expression of human immunodeficiency virus in T cells. Nature (London) 326:711.

30. Wu F, Garcia J, Mitsuyasu R, Gaynor R (1988). Alterations in binding characteristics of the human immunodeficiency virus enhancer factor. J Virol 62:218.

31. Hoxie JA, Haggarty BS, Rackowski JL, Pillsburg N, Levy JA (1985). Persistent noncytopathic infection of normal human T lymphocytes with AIDS associated retrovirus. Science 229:1400.

Molecular Biology of the Eye: Genes, Vision,
and Ocular Disease, pages 379–383
© 1988 Alan R. Liss, Inc.

# Discussion Summary: Molecular Biology of Ocular Viral Infections

Edmund C. Dunkel

Eye Research Institute,
Molecular Virology Laboratory
20 Staniford Street,
Boston, MA, and
Department of Ophthalmology
Harvard Medical School
Boston, MA

The workshop on ocular Herpesvirus infections (HSV) addressed many controversial issues concerning the HSV infection including: [1] retinal infection with HSV, CMV, VZV and HIV; [2] retention and potential latent infection of end organ tissues with HSV; [3] detection of RNA complementary to the ICP-0 region of the HSV genome and the functional role of this transcript in regulating HSV latent ganglionic infection; and [4] molecular characterization of active and latent VZV infection in an experimental model of ocular Varicella zoster virus infection.

Knowledge concerning the molecular interactions of HSV and VZV with the host cell both in the end organ (cornea) and in the ganglion (neuron) is expanding and new findings are focusing research efforts away from functional clinical and virus recovery parameters and towards a redefinition of the HSV and VZV latent infection. This definition will involve ultimately the molecular analysis of the latency state and will indicate the presence and/or absence of HSV and VZV gene transcripts (either sense or anti-sense messages). Continued molecular evaluation will afford the opportunity to characterize these serious ocular infectious diseases at a basic biological level. New information on gene transcripts responsible for establishment and maintenance of HSV latency as well as initiation of the HSV reactivation will be essential in directing traditional and new therapies to combat these viral infections.

The discussion summary for this workshop is divided into 4 sections.Each workshop participant has contributed a i page summary of their presentation area.

Dr. Jay Pepose
Georgetown University Medical Center
Department of Ophthalmology
Washington, DC

## The Viral Retinidies

There are at least eight well characterized forms of viral retinitis--
herpes simplex retinitis, cytomegalovirus retinopathy, varicella zoster
retinitis, measles (SSSP) retinopathy, Rift Valley fever retinitis, the acute
retinal necrosis (ARN) syndrome, rubella retinopathy and HIV retinopathy.
This presentation focuses on CMV, HIV and the ARN syndrome.

Cytomegalovirus retinopathy results from the hematogenous seeding
of CMV to the retina, occuring in immunocompromised patients such as
AIDS victims, organ transplant recipients or those undergoing
chemotherapy for treatment of malignancies. CMV retinopathy is the most
frequent infectious finding in AIDS, occurring bilaterally in 50% of cases,
and may be associated with acute inflammation and hemorrhage.
Cytomegalovirus retinopathy may be treated with the nucleoside analogue
ganciclovir. Despite its virustatic effect, ganciclovir is not virucidal. We
have been able to localize cytomegalovirus nucleic acid and antigens in the
retinas of patients with AIDS who died while undergoing ganciclovir
chemotherapy accounting for the recurrence of the lesions upon cessation of
therapy. Thus, in the presence of ganciclovir, some viral genes are
expressed and atypical particles are formed, but cytomegalovirus DNA does
not appear to be effectively packaged into infectious units.

In collaborative sutdies with Pomerantz, et al., we have isolated
HIV from the retinas of AIDS patients, as well as HIV seropositive
individuals with no clinical signs of AIDS. HIV was isolated from these
retinas within 1 week of culture, indicating a very heavy viral inoculum.
The role of HIV in producing the small retinal vessel vasculopathy and
possible transactivating effects of concurrent CMV infection of the retina is
now under investigation.

The acute retinal necrosis (ARN) is characterized by necrotizing
retinitis, obliterative vasculitis, optic neuritis and papillitis occuring in
otherwise healthy patients. In collaborative studies with Culbertson and
others, we have isolated varicella zoster virus in the retinas of two patients
with this syndrome and have demonstrated by restriction enzyme analysis
that the isolate has the characteristics of a typical varicella virus strain. In
addition, this antiviral activity against a panel of antiviral drugs are similar to
OKA strain of varicella. This virually devastating syndrome was not
reported prior to 1972. Therefore, it remains an enigma why an old virus
would cause a new syndrome. It is possible that subtle mutations in the
genome have occurred but are too small to be noticed by restriction enzyme
analysis.

AIDS, HIV retinopathy and the acute retinal necrosis syndrome are all evidence of the evolution of infectious diseases that we are witnessing in our lifetime. The application of molecular virology techniques may grant important insights into elucidating the pathogenesis of these syndromes and may lead to therapeutic interventions.

Dr. Deborah Pavan-Langston
Eye Research Institute and Department of Ophthalmology
Harvard Medical School
Boston, MA

## Can HSV establish a Latent Infection In the Cornea ?

It is a well established fact that herpes viruses invade superficial nerve endings in the periphery (cornea) and travel by axopasmic flow to ganglionic and central nervous system neuronal nuclei. Here, the virus establishes a lytic infection and in some neurons, the infection is converted into a latent state by mechanisms yet incompletely undertstood. Both a static and dynamic state have been postulated to describe HSV latency and the truth may lie somewhere in between. Molecular biology techniques, specifically in situ and dot blot nucleic acid hybridization to HSV probes have demonstrated conclusively the presence of specific herpetic nucleic acid sequences such as the ICP-0 region, and sense and anti-sense RNA in the trigeminal ganglia and in brain nucleic acid extracts. The functional importance of these fragments durning latent infection is now being further characterized.

Neural tissue however may not be the only reservoir of latent virus. Other theories of HSV latent infection suggest that the HSV genome may be continuously present in a latent state in the end organ of clinically normal individual and that the genome can reactivate in situ to result in clinical disease. Virus recovery from corneal buttons removed at keratoplasty in clinically normal individuals suggests that the HSV genome may be retained at least in part in corneal foci long after acute infection and this retention may represent herpetic latency in non-neuronal tissues. Studies from our laboratory using cloned HSV DNA probes have indicated the presence of the HSV genome in both experimentally induced HSV stromal infection in the rabbit and in total nucleic acid extracts from human corneas at transplant. Our results indicate that the HSV genome is retained in cells in all layers of the rabbit cornea through 90 days post infection (basal epithelium, stromal keratocytes, and endothelium). In the human corneal samples, HSV DNA was detected in 50% of the samples with a documented clinical history of chronic HSV keratitis. Interestingly, no correlation between clinical HSV ocular disease type and HSV DNA detection was noted. However, most of the positive hybridization signals were obtained from keratoplasty samples of patients with a >10 year history of HSV ocular infection. Additional molecular investigation and characterization of end organ HSV latency is needed to answer more completely the HSV-host cell interactions involved in establishing and maintaining these peripheral latent foci.

from these investigations, a new molecular definition of HSV latency both in the ganglia and potentially in the end organ (eye) can be established that is based on HSV gene expression and retention of HSV-induced RNA during latent infection.

Dr. Y. Jerold Gordon
Department of Ophthalomology, University of Pittsburgh
Pittsburgh, PA

## RNA Complementary to the HSV ICP-0 Gene is Retained in Human Trigeminal Ganglia.

Recent animal studies demonstrated abundant RNA transcripts which are complimentary (antisense) to the herpes alpha gene ICP-O in latently infected ganglia. We investigated the situation in unselected human trigeminal ganglia (TGs). Strand-specific 2.7 kb HSV-1 ICP-O RNA probes were prepared and their sense determined in prodctively infected cells. While in situ hybridization demonstrated ICP-O antisense RNA transcripts in the nuclei of neurons in ll of 24 ganglia (46%), ICP-O messenger RNA was not detected in any of the 24 ganglia (0%). The percentage of positive neurons per ganglion was low (0.l7%-l.22%). As all subjects with positive neuronal hybridization were also seropositive, we conclude that HSV-1 RNA complimentary (antisense) to ICP-O mRNA is present in human trigeminal ganglia during latency. The exclusive presence of ICP-O antisense RNA in TGs from seroposivtive cadavers has also been independently shown by others (Croen et al, N. Engl. J. Med., 3l7:l427-32, l987, Haarr, L., personal communication). The role of ICP-O antisense RNA during human ganglionic latency is currently unknown. A regulatory role is possible through an antisense mechanism, a trans-acting protein or a direct cis or trans acting mechanism of the RNA transcript. The current study  is significant as it provides a new molecular definition of herpetic ganglionic latency. HSV latency models in rabbits and mice are appropriate models to study human ganglionic latency as the molecular findings appear to be identical in all three species. Finally, we believe that all latency models (in vitro, end organ, etc) must satisfy the new molecular definition of latency in order to be considered authentic.

prior ocular stimulus (14).

## PATHOGENESIS OF EXPERIMENTAL AUTOIMMUNE UVEITIS

Immunization of experimental animals with S-antigen leads to both humeral and cell-mediated responses. T-cell mediated responses play a major role in the pathogenesis of EAU since the disease does not develop in athymic nude rats, the disease develops following the adoptive transfer of T-cells from rats previously immunized with S-antigen, and the disease can be inhibited by cyclosporin A.

The importance of T-cells in the pathogenesis of EAU was shown by Salinas-Carmona and associates (15) who showed that homozygous nude rats (rnu/rnu) failed to develop EAU, while heterozygous rats (rnu/+) were good responders to S-antigen. In addition, EAU could be induced in the non-responder (rnu/rnu) nude rats by the adoptive transfer of lymphocytes from responders (rnu/+).

More direct evidence for the participation of T-cells in EAU has been provided by adoptive transfer experiments. Faure and de Kozak (16) transferred EAU to naive Lewis rats from donor rats previously immunized with bovine or guinea pig S-antigen. The process has been made more efficient recently by Mochizuki and associates (17) who cultured donor lymph node cells in the presence of S-antigen prior to adoptive transfer. Furthermore, they characterized the lymphocytes that transferred disease as W3/25+ T-helper/suppressor cells rather than OX8 T-suppressor/cytotoxic lymphocytes. Uveitopathogenic T-cell lines have been generated from Lewis rats immunized with native S-antigen (18,19), S-antigen cyanogen bromide peptide fragments (20), or synthetic peptides which correspond to the amino acid sequence of S-antigen (Merryman, et al, in preparation).

Cyclosporin A, an immunosuppressive agent that selectively inhibits T-lymphocytes, is an effective inhibitor for the induction of EAU in Lewis rats (21). The effect appears to be related to the inhibition of the T-lymphocyte to release interleukin 1 or interleukin 2 (22).

T-cells appear to play a role in the pathogenesis of some forms of human uveitis such as sympathetic ophthalmia (23) and birdshot retinochoroidopathy (24). Furthermore, an EAU can be induced in subhuman primates by S-antigen (16,25) and in some patients T-cell mediated immune responses to either bovine or human S-antigen can be elicited (26).

## UVEITOPATHOGENIC SITES IN S-ANTIGEN

The nature of the uveitopathogenic sites in bovine S-antigen was initially investigated using proteolytic digests of the molecule. Stein (27) showed that bovine S-antigen could be digested into smaller fragments with Staphlococcus aureus V8 protease and that the digest was uveitopathogenic in Lewis rats. Kamada and associates (28) extended these observations to show that an EAU could be induced in Lewis rats with a 24Kd peptide fragment obtained by chymotryptic digestion of S-antigen followed by gel filtration chromatography. Although the nature of these peptide fragments were not characterized with regard to amino acid composition or sequence, these studies suggested that polypeptides were sufficient to induce an EAU in Lewis rats without a conformationally intact, native S-antigen.

A knowledge of the amino acid sequence of bovine S-antigen (4,5,6) made it possible to more precisely localize uveitopathogenic regions in S-antigen by synthesizing peptides, corresponding to the entire 404 amino acid sequence, and testing each for its ability to induce an EAU in Lewis rats as summarized in Table 1.

TABLE 1

PATHOGENECITY OF SYNTHETIC PEPTIDES CORRESPONDING TO AMINO ACID SEQUENCE OF S-ANTIGEN[a]

| Peptide Number | Amino Acid Position | Amino Acid Sequence | Pathogenecity |
|---|---|---|---|
| 1 | (1-21) | MKANKPAPNHVIFKKIRDKS | - |
| 2 | (22-41) | VTIYLDKRDYIDHVERVEPV | - |
| 3 | (42-59) | DGGVVLVDPELVKGKRVYV | - |
| 4 | (60-74) | SLTCARFYGQEDIDV | - |
| 5 | (75-93) | MGLSFRRDLYFSQVQVIPS | - |
| 6 | (94-113) | VGASGDHHRLQESLIKKLGG | - |
| 7 | (114-130) | NTYFFLLTFPDYLPCSV | - |
| 8 | (131-149) | MLQPEPQNVGKSTGVNFEI | - |
| 9 | (150-167) | KAFATNSTDVEEDKIPKK | - |
| 10 | (168-183) | SSVRLLIRKVQHAPRD | - |
| 11 | (184-197) | MGPQPRAEASWQFF | - |
| 12 | (198-220) | MSDKPLRLAVSKSKEIYYHGEPI | - |
| 13 | (221-240) | PVTVAVTNSTEKTVKKIKVL | (+) |

| 14 | (241-260) | VEQVTNVGLYSSDYYIKTVA | (+) |
| 15 | (261-280) | AEEAQEKEPPNSSLTKTLTL | - |
| 16 | (281-302) | VPLLANNRERRGIALDGKIKHE | + |
| 17 | (303-320) | DTNLASSTIIKEGIDKTV | + |
| 18 | (321-338) | MGILVSYQIKVKLTVSGL | - |
| 19 | (339-355) | LGELTSSEVATEVPFRL | - |
| 20 | (356-368) | MHPQPEDPDTAKE | - |
| 21 | (369-380) | SFQDENFVFEEF | - |
| 22 | (381-390) | ARQNLKDAGE | - |
| 23 | (391-404) | YKEEKTDQEAMDE | - |

---

[a]Lewis rats were immunized with various doses of the synthetic peptides ranging from 5 to 2,000 µg/amimal in Freund's complete adjuvant supplemented with 2 mg/ ml Mycobacterium tuberculosis. Bordetella pertussis (11 x 10$^9$ dead cells) was given intraveneously at the time of immunization. Control animals received 50 µg of purified native S-antigen or an equivalent dose of saline adjuvant and B. pertussis as above. The amino acid sequence is that given by Shinohara et al. (1987). Synthetic peptides did not contain methionines.

Initially Lewis rats were immunized with 50 µg of each of the synthetic peptides as a screening dose and tested for the induction of EAU. These studies identified the region of bovine S-antigen which corresponded to one large cyanogen bromide (CNBr) peptide (amino acid positions 198 to 320) as the uveitopathic region (29,30,31,32). That this CNBr peptide is uveitopathogenic has subsequently been documented by Gregerson and associates (20). Under our experimental conditions one peptide (designated peptide M; 18 amino acids in length) corresponding to amino acid positions 303 to 320 consistently induced an EAU in Lewis rats. In order to further define this site smaller peptides, 10 to 16 amino acids in length, corresponding to the amino and carboxy terminal portions of peptide M, were synthesized and tested. These studies further localized this site to twelve amino acids corresponding to amino acid positions 303 to 314 in bovine S-antigen. We have also shown that peptide M is uveitopathogenic in guinea pigs (33). Furthermore, peptide M is also uveitopathogenic in subhuman primates (personal observation, T. Shinohara, 1987).

Another peptide, designated peptide K, corresponding to amino acid positions 241 to 260 also induced an EAU. The disease induced by this peptide, however, was highly variable and has been the subject of additional studies, as described below.

In order to further clarify the nature of other potential uveitopathogenic sites, Lewis rats were immunized with large doses (up to 2,000 µg/animal) of the synthetic peptides corresponding to amino acid positions 198 to 320. Two additional peptides induced an EAU under these experimental conditions. One peptide corresponding to amino acid positions 281 to 302, designated peptide N, consistently induced disease. This peptide is adjacent to peptide M, thus localizing this uveitopathogenic region to amino acids 281 to 314. Since the amino terminal portion of peptide M is necessary for pathogenecity, it is possible that this region of S-antigen may contain one or possibly two uveitopathogenic sites. Experiments are in progress to further refine this uveitopathogenic site. The other peptide which induced an EAU corresponded to amino acid positions 221 to 240. This peptide also lies adjacent to peptide K, and like peptide K, the EAU induced by this peptide was also highly variable.

We believe that our studies localize a major uveitopathogenic site in bovine S-antigen to the amino acid positions 281 to 320. A possible second uveitopathogenic site is localized to amino acid positions 221 to 260. Furthermore, an analysis of the primary and secondary structure of bovine S-antigen suggests that these two sites are interrelated. Certain proteins, such as proteases or lens crystallins, may exist in nature as repeated structures, perhaps by gene fusion and duplication. A computerized analysis of the amino acid sequence of S-antigen reveals a possible two-fold repeated structure with two regions of sequence similarity. These two regions correspond to peptide N and peptide M (amino acid positions 281 to 320) and to peptide 3 and peptide K (amino acid positions 221 to 260; Figure 1).

This suggests, to us, that under appropriate experimental conditions such as the immunizing dose of peptide, the proper adjuvant, or a history of prior ocular stimulus that peptide 3 and peptide K may be uveitopathogenic. The relevance of these studies to EAU, however, needs additional clarification.

28. Kamada Y, Yama M, Das ND, Samuelson D, Leverenz VR and Schichi H (1985). Preparation of a uveitogenic peptide by chymotryptic digestion of bovine S-antigen. Invest Ophthalmol Vis Sci 26:1274.

29. Donoso LA, Merryman CF, Shinohara T, Dietzschold B, Wistow G, Craft C, Morley W, Henry RT (1986). S-antigen: Identification of the MAbA9-C6 monoclonal antibody binding site and the uveitopathogenic sites. Curr Eye Res 5:995.

30. Donoso LA, Merryman CF, Shinohara T, Dietzschold B, Sery T, Smith A, Kalsow CM (1987). S-antigen: Characterization of a pathogenic epitope which mediates experimental autoimmune uveitis and pinealitis in Lewis rats. Curr Eye Res 6:1151.

31. Donoso LA, Merryman CF, Shinohara T, Sery TW, Smith A (1987). S-antigen: Experimental autoimmune uveitis following immunication with a small synthetic peptide. Arch Ophthalmol 105:838.

32. Shinohara T, Donoso L, Wistow G, Dietzschold B, Craft C and Tao R (1987). The structure of bovine retinal S-antigen: Sequence analysis and identification of monoclonal antibody epitopes and uveitogenic site. Jpn J Ophthalmol 31:197.

33. Singh VK, Yamaki K, Donoso LA, Shinohara T (1987). S-antigen: Experimental autoimmune uveitis induced in guinea pigs with two synthetic peptides. Curr Eye Res, in press.

34. Mannie MD, Paterson PY, U'Prichard DC, Flouret G (1985). Induction of experimental allergic encephalomyelitis in Lewis rats with purified synthetic peptides: Delineation of antigenic determinant for encephalitogenicity, in vitro activation of cellular transfer, and proliferation of lymphocytes. Proc Natl Acad Sci 82:5515.

35. Merryman CF, Donoso LA, Sery TW, Sciutto E, Bauer A, Shinohara T (1987). Adoptive transfer of experimental autoimmune uveitis following immunization with a small synthetic peptide. Arch Ophthalmol 105:841.

36. Gotsch F, Rothbard J, Howland K, Towsend A, McMichael A (1987). Cytotoxic T-lymphocytes recognize a fragment of influenza virus matrix protein in association with HLA-A-2. Nature 326:881.

37. Fujinami RS and Oldstone MBA (1985). Amino acid homology between the encephalitogenic site of myelin basic protein and virus: Mechanism for autoimmunity. Science 29:1043.

38.  Oldstone MBA (1987).  Molecular mimicry and autoimmune
     disease.  Cell 50:819.
39.  Carnegie PR, Weise MJ (1987).  Visna and myelin basic
     protein.  Nature 329:294.

**Molecular Biology of the Eye: Genes, Vision, and Ocular Disease, pages 399–408**
© **1988 Alan R. Liss, Inc.**

INDUCTION OF EXPERIMENTAL AUTOIMMUNE UVEORETINITIS (EAU) BY
A SYNTHETIC PEPTIDE DERIVED FROM THE RETINAL PROTEIN IRBP

T.M. Redmond, H. Sanui, L.H. Hu, B. Wiggert
H. Margalit, T. Kuwabara, G.J. Chader and I. Gery

National Eye Institute, NIH
Bethesda, MD 20892

ABSTRACT  Interphotoreceptor retinoid-binding protein
(IRBP) is a 140 Kda ocular- and pineal-specific
glycolipoprotein.  Immunization with IRBP induces
inflammation in the eye (EAU) and pineal (EAP) in
various experimental animals.  In an earlier study, we
identified three CNBr cleavage fragments of bovine
IRBP that induced EAU.  These fragments have been
localized to portions of IRBP of known amino acid
sequence by N-terminal peptide sequencing and DNA
sequence analysis.  In order to identify the putative
immunopathogenic epitopes within these fragments, nine
synthetic peptides based on the two fully sequenced
fragments were made and tested in rats for their
capacity to induce EAU and EAP and to provoke immune
responses.  A 23-residue peptide, designated R4, was
found to reproducibly induce EAU/EAP in immunized
Lewis rats.  This disease was less severe and less
acute than that induced by intact IRBP.  R9, a 27
residue peptide differing from R4 by the addition of
four N-terminal residues, caused a weaker disease than
R4 and cross-reacted very strongly with R4 in in vitro
cellular response assays.  Other tested peptides did
not induce disease but some were found to provoke
considerable cellular immune responses as measured by
the lymphocyte proliferation assay.  Additional
peptides based on these fragments are being synthesized in order to further circumscribe the epitope
represented in R4 and R9 and to localize other
epitopes.

## INTRODUCTION

Experimental autoimmune uveitis (EAU) is an animal model for the spectrum of human ocular inflammatory diseases termed uveitis. It is induced in a number of animal species by ocular-specific antigens including retinal S-antigen (S-Ag) (1), rhodopsin (2) and interphoto-receptor retinoid-binding protein (IRBP) (3-5). IRBP, the major soluble protein component of the interphotoreceptor matrix is an ocular-specific glycolipoprotein of apparent $M_r$ of about 140 Kda on sodium dodecyl sulfate-polyacryla-mide gel electrophoresis (SDS-PAGE) thought to be involved in retinoid transport between the photoreceptor cells and the retinal pigment epithelium (6). In addition to ocular tissues it is also found in the pineal (6).

IRBP induces reproducible EAU and its corollary, experimental autoimmune pinealitis (EAP) in Lewis rats immunized with doses less than 1 μg (3). Cell-mediated mechanisms are important in the pathogenesis, and the disease may be adoptively transferred to naive animals by injection of helper T-cells from immunized animals (7).

In an effort to localize the uveitogenic epitope(s) within IRBP we have purified a number of cyanogen bromide fragments of the protein (8). CNBr digestion of reduced, S-carboxymethylated IRBP gives rise to about 25 peptide fragments. Of these, three fragments have been purified and shown to induce EAU when injected into Lewis rats. These findings appear to indicate that there are multiple uveitogenic sites within bovine IRBP. In this paper we report on the further localization of the uveitogenic epitopes of IRBP using synthetic peptides based on two of these uveitogenic CNBr fragments.

## EXPERIMENTAL

Choice of Synthetic Peptides

As derived by amino-terminal sequence and DNA sequence data (see Nickerson et al., this volume), the sequences of two uveitogenic CNBr fragments CB-58 and CB-71 (58 and 71 residues in length, respectively) are shown in Figure 1. In order to further circumscribe the uveitogenic epitope within these fragments and to study the immunology of these fragments, synthetic peptides were made based on these

**Molecular Biology of the Eye: Genes, Vision, and Ocular Disease, pages 409–417**
© **1988 Alan R. Liss, Inc.**

# DEVELOPMENTAL OCULAR DISEASE IS MEDIATED BY MACROPHAGES IN GM-CSF TRANSGENIC MICE[1]

R. Andrew Cuthbertson[2], Richard A. Lang[3], Ashley Dunn[3], Jennifer D. Penschow[2], Ian Lyons[2], Gordon K. Klintworth[4], Donald Metcalf[5] and John P. Coghlan[2]

[2]The Howard Florey Institute for Experimental Physiology and Medicine, University of Melbourne, Parkville, Victoria, 3052, Australia.

[3]Ludwig Institute for Cancer Research (Melbourne Tumour Biology Branch), P.O. Royal Melbourne Hospital, 3050, Victoria, Australia.

[4]Duke Eye Center, Duke University Medical Center, Durham NC 27710.

[5]The Walter and Eliza Hall Institute for Medical Research, P.O. Royal Melbourne Hospital 3050, Victoria, Australia.

ABSTRACT   We made transgenic mice that develop eye disease with the murine granulocute-macrophage colony stimulating factor (GM-CSF) structural gene driven by the Moloney virus promoter. Ocular disease, characterized by retinal destruction, cataractogenesis, corneal opacity and vitreous neovascularization, was present when affected animals opened their eyes 14 days after birth (A14). The disease was mediated by destructive intraocular cells which were phagocytic and stained with monoclonal antibodies F4/80 and anti-Mac1, which with their morphology suggested that they were macrophages.

[1]   Dr. R. Andrew Cuthbertson is a National Health and Medical Research Council Australian Post-doctoral Fellow. This work was supported by grants in aid from the National Health and Medical Research Council, the Ian Potter Foundation and the Howard Florey Biomedical Foundation.

Hyalocytes are resident intraocular macrophages with a
physiological role that includes the removal of the
hyaloid vasculature during development.  Hybridization
histochemistry, using $^{32}$P-labeled single strand RNA
probes to GM-CSF and to a transcribed $\phi$X 174
bacteriophage DNA marker present in the $3^1$-
untranslated region of the transgene, showed that
ocular disease might be caused by macrophage auto-
stimulation.  Expression of the transgene peaked
between 14 and 21 days after birth, corresponding to
the period of maximal tissue destruction.  In this
model, expression of the introduced gene during ocular
development may mediate auto-stimulation of
intraocular hyalocytes resulting in severe ocular
disease.


## INTRODUCTION

The colony stimulating factors (CSFs) are a group of
glycoproteins which in-vitro act specifically to control the
proliferation, differentiation and end-cell activation of
haemopoietic cell populations [12].  One such factor, murine
granulocyte-macrophage colony stimulating factor (GM-CSF)
[5] [7], stimulates the proliferation and function of
granulocytes, macrophages and eosinophils [12].
During mammalian ocular development the vitreous
cavity of the eye is vascularised by a temporary capillary
network known as the hyaloid vasculature.  This network,
essential for normal ocular development, exists during the
latter half of intrauterine life and is removed
physiologically before ocular maturation.  Hyalocytes are
resident intraocular phagocytic cells and it has been
proposed that the hyalocytes remove the temporary hyaloid
vasculature, in a programmed fashion, during normal ocular
development [2].  This removal of capillary endothelial
cells is both tissue-specific and temporally regulated but
the physiological signals, both to instigate destruction of
the temporary capillary bed and to halt the process on
completion, are unknown.
GM-CSF transgenic mice have accumulations of activated
macrophages, eye disease and a fatal syndrome of muscle
wasting [10].  The eye disease, which in the adult mouse is
characterised by gross phagocyte infiltration, retinal
degeneration, cataract and corneal and vitreous
neovascularization, has its origin early in development.

c.

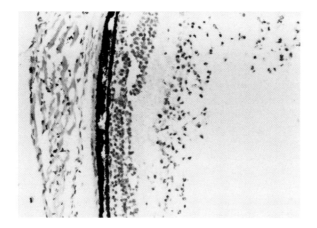

d.

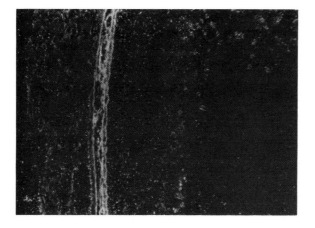

FIGURE 2c and d.  Negative control hybridizations,
using a ϕX 174 mRNA-synonymous riboprobe on a section from
the same A14 transgenic eye as in Figure 2a and b, show only
background silver grains over both vitreous macrophages and
remaining retina (x100).

Immunocytochemistry shows that these cells bear macrophage-specific antigens.

Hybridization histochemistry demonstrates that transgene expression is in the abnormal intraocular macrophages themselves, and not in the retina or other ocular tissues. Both hybridization histochemistry and Northern analysis show that measurable transgene expression begins on about A9, reaches a peak between A14 and A21 and then declines in the adult. Thus the onset of transgene expression coincides with the onset of removal of the hyaloid vasculature by hyalocytes in the normal mouse.

Normal ocular development involves both construction and destruction, dictated by signals that are poorly understood in mammals at present. Transgene expression may follow a normal developmental signal which in non-transgenic animals results in the tissue-specific and temporally regulated removal of the hyaloid vasculature. In the transgenic mice this control is lost, with an amplification, and loss of tissue-specificity and temporal regulation of the phagocytic response. Thus we propose that this ocular disease may be mediated by transgene expression, in response to a physiological developmental signal, resulting in auto-stimulation of resident intraocular hyalocytes at a crucial time in ocular development and leading to catastrophic ocular disease.

## ACKNOWLEDGEMENTS

We would like to thank Ms. Paula Darling for excellent technical advice and the secretaries of the Howard Florey Institute for typing the manuscript.

## REFERENCES

(1) Austyn JM and Gordon S (1981). A monoclonal antibody directed specifically against the mouse macrophage. Eur J Immunol 10:805.

(2) Balasz EA, Toth LZ and Ozanics V (1980). Cytological studies of the developing vitreous as related to the hyaloid vessel system. Albrecht v. Graefes Arch Klin Exp Ophthal. 213: 71.

(3) Bourne JA (1983). Handbook of immunoperoxidase staining methods. Santa Barbara, Dako Corp., USA.

(4)    Brinster RL, Chen HV, Trumbauer ME, Yagle MK and Palmiter RD (1985).  Factors affecting the efficiency of introducing foreign DNA into mice by microinjecting eggs. Proc Natl Acad Sci USA 82:4438.

(5)    Burgess AW, Wilson EMA and Metcalf D (1977). Stimulation by human placental conditioned medium of hemopoietic colony formation by human marrow cells.  Blood 49:573.

(6)    Davidson WF, Fredrickson TN, Rudikoff EK, Coffman RL, Hartley JW and Morse HC (1984).  A unique series of lymphomas related to the Ly-1$^+$ lineage of B lymphocyte differentiation.  J Immunol 133:744.

(7)    Gough NM, Gough J, Metcalf D, Kelso A, Grail D, Nicola NA, Burgess AW and Dunn AR (1984).  Molecular cloning of cDNA encoding a murine hematopoietic growth regulator, granulocyte-macrophage colony stimulating factor.  Nature 309:763.

(8)    Hsu SM, Raive L and Fanger H (1981).  Use of avidin-biotin-peroxidase complex (ABC) in immunoperoxidase techniques:  a comparison between ABC and PAP procedures.  J Histochem Cytochem, 29:577.

(9)    Lang RA, Metcalf D, Gough NM, Dunn AR and Gonda TJ (1985).  Expression of a hemopoietic growth factor cDNA in a factor-dependent cell line results in autonomous growth and tumorigenicity.  Cell 43:531.

(10)   Lang RA, Metcalf D, Cuthbertson RA, Lyons I, Stanley E, Kelson A, Kannourakis G, Williamson J, Klintworth GK, Gonda TJ and Dunn AR (1987).  Transgenic mice expressing a hemopoietic growth factor gene (GM-CSF) develop accumulations of macrophages, blindness and a fatal syndrome of tissue damage.  Cell 51:675.

(11)   Maniatis T, Fritsch EF and Sambrook J (1982). Molecular Cloning.  Cold Spring Laboratory, Cold Spring Harbor, New York.

(12)   Metcalf D (1984).  The Hemopoietic Colony Stimulating Factors.  Amsterdam, Elsevier.

(13)   Penschow JD, Haralambidis J, Aldred P, Tregear GW and Coghlan JP (1986).  Location of gene expression in the CNS using hybridization histochemistry.  Methods in Enzymology 124:534.

(14)   Southern EM (1975).  Detection of specific sequences among DNA fragments separated by gel electrophoresis.  J Mol Biol 98:503.

Molecular Biology of the Eye: Genes, Vision, and Ocular Disease, pages 419–426
© 1988 Alan R. Liss, Inc.

# MOLECULAR INTERACTIONS OF CRYSTALLINS IN RELATION TO CATARACT[1]

C Slingsby, H P C Driessen, H White, S Mylvaganam,
S Najmudin, B Bax, M A Bibby, P F Lindley, D S Moss and
T L Blundell

Birkbeck College, Department of Crystallography,
Laboratory of Molecular Biology, Malet Street,
London WC1 7HX UK

Eye lenses are packed with crystallin proteins in order to achieve the high refractive index necessary for their focussing function. Lenses must also be transparent, a word which has become synonymous with crystalline, implying order. Understanding the process of cataract, whereby a lens becomes opaque, requires knowledge of the kinds of order maintaining the transparent state. Disturbances to the regular cytoplasm-membrane lattice repeat, such as abnormal growth and broken cells, will destroy the crystalline ordering of lens fibre cells (1). Some crystallins have an internal order derived from the symmetrical folding of the polypeptide chain and aggregates of crystallins are presumed to contain centres of symmetry thereby limiting particle growth (2). Circumstances which perturb these tertiary and quaternary structures can cause unlimited aggregation resulting in light scattering centres. A theoretical analysis of the nature of the organization of proteins within lens fibre cells (3) together with low angle X-ray scattering data (4) lead to the idea that lens transparency is a function of the order achieved by close packing of protein molecules (4). In senile nuclear cataract, where membrane structure is not grossly perturbed, the loss of transparency is associated with alterations to protein packing interactions in ways which may be related to the numerous covalent modifications endured by these long-lived structural proteins (5).

[1] This work was supported by
The Medical Research Council (London) UK

Mammalian lens proteins are derived from two gene families α- and βγ-crystallins.  Although considerable information is known about primary structures of αA and αB subunits (6) and their modified forms (7,8) rather different models have been proposed for their association into large heteropolymers (9,10).   Insight into the βγ-crystallin family was gained when the three-dimensional structures of γ-II and γ-IIIb crystallins were revealed by X-ray diffraction techniques (11,12) showing that each molecule was internally quadruplicated comprising four 'Greek key' motifs arranged to form two domains and when the β-crystallins were found to be members of the same family (13).   All members have a fourfold repeat in their sequences of critical amino acids which are involved in stabilizing a folded β-hairpin between two anti-parallel β-sheet strands (14,15).   Mutations involving these conserved amino acids would be predicted to destabilize the symmetrically folded protein.  β-crystallins differ from γ-crystallins in having longer sequences (13,16) and a further subdivision occurs between basic β-crystallins having N- and C- terminal extensions and acidic β-crystallins with only an N-terminal extension (16-17).   Molecular modelling using computer graphics techniques has demonstrated that certain structural features distinguish the bilobal regions of the β-crystallins in ways which may be correlated with their sequence extensions and subunit interactions (18).  Proteolytic cleavage of N-terminal sequences of the predominant basic β-crystallin occurs in aging human lenses (19) and shortened β-crystallin polypeptides appear in selenium induced cataracts in rats (20) suggesting that modification of these extensions may lead to altered interactions.

The γ-crystallin family has several conserved cysteine thiols located in the domain cores whereas cysteines on the surface are variable (21).  Bovine γ-II crystallin has a cluster of sulphydryls in the N-terminal domain with the potential to form an intramolecular disulphide (22).  This protein reacts avidly with glutathione 'in vitro' to form stable mixed disulphides (23).   Bearing in mind the recent discoveries that some crystallin genes have evolved from other genes or share their function with another gene product (24) it is possible that γ-crystallins have evolved from redox active thiol containing enzymes.   The involvement of γ-crystallin oxidation in nuclear cataract has long been suspected (25), they being rich in reactive thiols, being located in the lens nuclear region and being the oldest proteins therein. Recent evidence continues to implicate covalent modification of Y-crystallins in human cataract formation (26).

Self-association of Y-crystallins contributes towards a reversible process called cold cataract whereby a young transparent lens becomes opaque due to minor temperature perturbation. The high protein concentration in lens cytoplasm of the nuclear region is near to a critical point where very soluble proteins undergo a low energy phase separation driven by the competing forces of protein-protein, water-water and protein-water interactions (27,28). It is now established that certain members of the Y-crystallin family have critical points ($T_c$) at temperatures well above body temperature which would result in their separation into phases of differing protein density causing light scattering if a critical concentration were reached (29,30). The Y-crystallin genes are differentially regulated (31,32). Those members of the Y-crystallin family with a propensity to phase separate are preferentially accumulated in the lens nuclear region (33, 34, 35). Cold cataract occurs when the overall cytoplasmic protein concentration is around 30% v/v at which point the light scattering centres formed from higher protein density regions are composed mainly of specific Y-crystallins at a protein concentration similar to that in their crystalline state (36,37,38). At this high protein density it would be expected that the kinds of interactions observed in the crystalline lattice would also occur in the scattering centres although the order would be short range (39).

The structure of bovine Y-IV crystallin, a protein with a high $T_c$, has been solved by molecular replacement (40) and shown to be very similar in structure to bovine Y-II and Y-IIIb crystallins. The crystals of Y-IIIb have the highest water concentration whereas the Y-IV crystals have the highest protein concentration and so are the most densely packed. Both Y-II and Y-IIIb, proteins with a low $T_c$, make heterologous contacts around symmetry axes whereby the N-terminal domain of one molecule interacts with the C-terminal domain of another molecule (14,41). For example, in Y-II crystallin residues His 14 and Cys 15 in motif 1 interact with the C-terminal domain of a different molecule related by the $4_1$ crystallographic axis. In Y-IIIb crystallin residues Met 102 and Met 103, which occur in topologically similar positions in motif 3 in the C-terminal domain to residues 14 and 15, interact around an approximate $2_1$ axis with the N-terminal domain of another molecule (41). However, in Y-IV crystallin residues Met 102 and Val 103 are involved in a crystallographic two-fold contact which radically alters the packing arrangement (42). We are currently analysing the effect on interaction sites of natural mutations specific to the high $T_c$ Y-crystallins in order to predict those residues worthy of further investigation by selective mutation.

Regulation of expression of the Y-crystallin genes results in synthesis of proteins with widely varying association behaviour. The β-crystallin gene family is more divergent with component subunits making complex specific interactions. The major subunit, βB2, can be isolated in the unfolded form, reaggregated to a stable dimer and crystallized (43). The dimer is a major component of $βL_2$-crystallin (44). However, βH-crystallin contains products of all the β-crystallin genes and their post-translational modifications leading to an extremely heterogeneous ensemble of ~200kDa aggregates. In order to understand how these β-crystallin aggregates interact with α- and Y-crystallin, the basic principles of how β-crystallin subunits interact with one another must first be elucidated. Models of β-crystallin subunits, constructed by homology with Y-crystallin, have shown that in the N-terminal domain of βB1 and βB2 there is a hydrophobic cluster on the β-sheet surface whereas βB1 and βA3 have a hydrophobic loop region in the C-terminal domain (18). We have found that the βB2 subunit can effectively solubilize other β-crystallin polypeptides leading to the suggestion that the polar C-terminal domain of βB2-crystallin may direct heteropolymer interactions. The lack of synthesis of βB2 polypeptide in the Philly mouse cataract (45) would lead to disorganization of the remaining β-crystallin subunits causing abnormal aggregation which in turn may perturb α- and Y-crystallins. In such a way it is envisaged that during the process of cataract in Philly mouse the altered β-crystallin aggregates could modulate Y-crystallin interactions, thus contributing to the elevated temperature of phase separation (46).

References

1. Duncan G, Jacob T J C (1984). The lens as a physiochemical system. In Davson H (ed): "The Eye" IB, Academic Press, p 159.
2. Slingsby, C (1985). Structural variation in lens crystallins. Trends in Biochem Sci 10:281.
3. Benedek G B (1971). Theory of transparency of the eye. Appl Optics 10:459.
4. Delaye M, Tardieu A (1983). Short-range order of crystallin proteins accounts for eye lens transparency. Nature (London) 302:415.
5. Harding J J, Crabbe M J C (1984). The lens: development, proteins, metabolism and cataract. In Davson H (ed): "The Eye" IB, Academic Press, p 207.
6. de Jong W W (1981). Evolution of lens and crystallins. In Bloemendal H (ed): "Molecular and cellular biology of the eye lens," New York: Wiley, p 221.
7. Spector A, Chiesa R, Sredy J, Garner W (1985). cAMP-dependent phosphorylation of bovine lens α-crystallin. Proc Natl Acad Sci USA 82:4712.
8. Voorter C E M, Mulders J W M, Bloemendal H, de Jong W W (1986). Some aspects of the phosphorylation of α-crystallin A. Eur J Biochem 160:203.
9. Tardieu A, Laporte D, Licinio P, Krop B, Delaye M (1986). Calf lens α-crystallin quaternary structure. J Mol Biol 192:711.
10. Augusteyn R C, Koretz J F (1987). A possible structure for α-crystallin. FEBS Lett 222:1.
11. Blundell T L, Lindley P F, Miller L, Moss D S, Slingsby C, Tickle I J, Turnell B, Wistow G (1981). The molecular structure and stability of the eye lens: X-ray analysis of γ-crystallin II. Nature (London) 289:771.
12. Chirgadze Y N, Sergeev Y V, Oreshin V D, Fomenkova N P (1981). Structure of γ-crystallin IIIb from calf lens at 5Å resolution. FEBS Lett 131:81.
13. Driessen H P C, Herbrink P, Bloemendal H, de Jong W W (1981). Primary structure of the bovine β-crystallin Bp chain. Internal duplication and homology with γ-crystallin. Eur J Biochem 121:83.

14. Wistow G, Turnell B, Summers L, Slingsby C, Moss D S, Miller L, Lindley P F, Blundell T L (1983).   X-ray analysis of the eye lens protein Y-II crystallin at 1.9Å resolution.   J Mol Biol 170:175.

15. Chirgadze Y N, Nevskaya N A, Fomenkova N P, Nikonov S V, Sergeev Y N, Brazhnikov E V, Garber M B, Lunin V Y, Urzumstsev A P, Vernoslova E A (1986).   Spatial structure of gamma-crystallin IIIb from calf eye lens at 2.5Å resolution.   Dokl Akad Nauk SSSR 209:492.

16. Berbers G A M, Hoekman W A, Bloemendal H, de Jong W W, Keinschmidt T, Braunitzer G (1984).   Homology between the primary structures of the major β-crystallin chains. Eur J Biochem 139:467.

17. Piatigorsky J (1984). Lens crystallins and their gene families.   Cell 38:620.

18. Slingsby C, Driessen H P C, Mahadevan D, Bax B, Blundell T L (1988).   Evolutionary and functional relationships between the basic and acidic β-crystallins.   Exp Eye Res 46: (in press).

19. Takemoto L, Takemoto D, Brown G, Takehana M, Smith J, Horwitz J (1987).   Cleavage from the N-terminal region of βBp crystallin during aging of the human lens.   Exp Eye Res 45:385.

20. Shearer T R, David L L, Anderson R S (1987).   Selenite cataract : a review.   Curr Eye Res 6:289.

21. Summers L J, Slingsby C, Blundell T L, den Dunnen J T, Moormann R J M, Schoenmakers J G G (1986).   Structural variation in mammalian Y-crystallins based on computer graphics analyses of human, rat and calf sequences. Exp Eye Res 43:77.

22. Summers L, Wistow G, Narebor M, Moss D S, Lindley P F, Slingsby C, Blundell T L, Bartunik H, Bartels K (1984). X-ray studies of the lens specific proteins:  the crystallins.   Pept Prot Rev 3:147.

23. Slingsby C, Miller L (1985).   The reaction of glutathione with the eye-lens protein Y-crystallin. Biochem J 230:143.

24. Wistow G, Piatigorsky J (1987).   Recruitment of enzymes as lens structural proteins.   Science 236:1554.

25. Spector A (1984).   The search for a solution to senile cataracts.   Investig Ophthalmol Vis Sci 25:130.

26. Takemoto L J, Hansen J S, Zigler J S, Horwitz J (1985). Characterization of polypeptides from human nuclear cataracts by western blot analysis.   Exp Eye Res 40:205.

27. Tanaka T, Ishimoto C, Chylack L T (1977).  Phase separation of a protein-water mixture in cold cataract in the young rat lens.  Science 197:1010.
28. Thomson J A, Schurtenberger P, Thurston G M, Benedek G B (1987).  Binary liquid phase separation and critical phenomena in a protein/water solution.  Proc Natl Acad Sci USA 84:7079.
29. Blundell T L, Lindley P F, Miller L R, Moss D S, Slingsby C, Turnell W G, Wistow G (1983).  Interactions of Y-crystallin in relation to eye-lens transparency. Lens Res 1:109.
30. Siezen R J, Fisch M R, Slingsby C, Benedek G B (1985). Opacification of Y-crystallin solutions from calf lens in relation to cold cataract formation.  Proc Natl Acad Sci USA 82:1701.
31. Moormann R J M, den Dunnen J T, Heuyerjans J, Jongbloed R J E, van Leen R W, Lubsen N H, Schoenmakers J G G (1985).  Characterization of the rat Y-crystallin gene family and its expression in the eye lens.  J Mol Biol 182:419.
32. Murer-Orlando M, Paterson R C, Lok S, Tsui L-C, Breitman M L (1987).  Differential regulation  of Y-crystallin genes during mouse lens development.  Dev Biol 119:260.
33. Slingsby C, Croft L R (1973).  Developmental changes in the low molecular weight proteins of the bovine lens. Exp Eye Res 17:369.
34. Siezen R J, Thomson J A, Kaplan E D, Benedek G B (1987). Human lens Y-crystallins: isolation, identification, and characterization of the expressed gene products. Proc Natl Acad Sci USA 84:6088.
35. Siezen R J, Wu E, Kaplan E, Thomson J A Benedek G B (1988).  Rat lens Y-crystallins.  J Mol Biol 199:475.
36. Carlisle C H, Lindley P F, Moss D S, Slingsby C (1977). Preliminary X-ray crystallographic study of the bovine lens protein, Y-crystallin fraction II.  J Mol Biol 110:417.
37. Chirgadze Y N, Nikonov S V, Garber M B, Reshetnikova L S (1977).  Crystallographic study of Y-crystallins from calf lens.  J Mol Biol 110:619.
38. Blundell T L, Lindley P F, Moss D S, Slingsby C, Tickle I J, Turnell W G (1978).  The low resolution structure analysis of the lens protein Y-crystallin.  Acta Cryst B34:3653.

426    Slingsby et al.

39. Bernal J D (1964). The structure of liquids. Proc Roy
    Soc A280:299.
40. White H E, Driessen H P C, Slingsby C, Moss D S, Turnell
    W G, Lindley P L (1988).  Structural analysis of the
    bovine lens protein γIVa-crystallin. Acta Cryst B44.
    (In press).
41. Sergeev Y V, Chirgadze Y N, Driessen H P C, Slingsby C,
    Blundell T L (1987).  The key role of residue 103 in the
    surface interactions of γ-crystallins. Mol Biol (USSR)
    21:377.
42. White H E, Driessen H P C, Slingsby C, Moss D S, Lindley
    P F (1988).  Structural analysis of the bovine lens
    protein γIVa-crystallin.  Internal symmetry and lattice
    interactions. (In preparation).
43. Slingsby C, Miller L R, Berbers G A M (1982).
    Preliminary X-ray crystallographic study of the
    principle subunit of the lens structural protein, bovine
    β-crystallin. J Mol Biol 157:191.
44. Berbers G A M, Boermann O C, Bloemendal H, de Jong W W
    (1982).  Primary gene products of bovine β-crystallin
    and reassociation behaviour of its aggregates.  Eur J
    Biochem 128:495.
45. Carper D, Shinohara T, Piatigorsky J, Kinoshita J H
    (1982).  Deficiency of functional messenger RNA for a
    developmentally regulated β-crystallin polypeptide in a
    hereditary cataract. Science 217:463.
46. Clark J I, Carper D (1987).  Phase separation in lens
    cytoplasm is genetically linked to cataract formation in
    the Philly mouse.  Proc Natl Acad Sci USA 84:122.

Molecular Biology of the Eye: Genes, Vision,
and Ocular Disease, pages 427–436
© 1988 Alan R. Liss, Inc.

# A COMMON MUTATIONAL SITE FOR RETINOBLASTOMA SUSCEPTIBILITY GENE INACTIVATION[1]

Robert Bookstein, Eva Y.-H. P. Lee, T. W. Sery[2], and W. H. Lee

Experimental Pathology Program & Center for Molecular Genetics
Department of Pathology M-012, University of California, San Diego
La Jolla, California 92093

ABSTRACT A gene in chromosome region 13q14 has been
identified as the human retinoblastoma susceptibility (RB) gene on
the basis of altered gene expression found in virtually all retinoblastomas. By restriction analysis of genomic clones, the RB gene
consisted of at least 20 exons distributed over 150 kb of cloned
DNA; however, two large introns (each larger than 40 kb) have
not yet been completely spanned. Three retinoblastoma cell lines
(Y79, RB355, and WERI-27) expressed shortened RB mRNA
transcripts but no normal-sized (4.7 kb) transcripts. A genomic
library made from Y79 DNA yielded clones demonstrating a
deletion joining introns 1 and 6 in one RB allele. A unique
sequence DNA probe in intron 1 detected similar and possibly
identical heterozygous deletions in genomic DNA from these three
retinoblastoma cell lines, thereby explaining the origin of their
shortened RB mRNA transcripts. The same probe detected
genomic rearrangements in fibroblasts from two hereditary
retinoblastoma patients, indicating that intron 1 includes a
frequent site for mutations predisposing to retinoblastoma.
Identification of commonly mutated regions will contribute
significantly to genetic diagnosis in retinoblastoma patients and
families.

## INTRODUCTION

Retinoblastoma is an intraocular cancer of early childhood that arises
from the developing retina. In a substantial minority of cases, suscep-

---

[1]Supported by grants from the National Eye Institute to W. H. L.
(EY 05758) and R. E. B. (Physician Scientist Award EY 00278).
[2]Wills Eye Hospital, Ninth & Walnut St., Philadelphia, PA 19107.

tibility to retinoblastoma can be inherited from a parent who was previously cured of the tumor (1,2). In such families, the inheritance pattern (about 50% of offspring affected) indicates transmission of a single dominant autosomal gene. This gene (the retinoblastoma susceptibility [RB] gene) was localized to chromosome band 13q14 by linkage analysis of retinoblastoma pedigrees and examination of cases having cytogenetic deletions in somatic cells (3,4). Based on a statistical analysis of clinical data, Knudson inferred that retinoblastoma could result from as few as two mutational events (5). Cavenee *et al* (6) demonstrated specific loss of heterozygous chromosome 13 markers in retinoblastomas compared to somatic cells from the same patients, and suggested that the tumor might be caused by inactivation of both alleles of a single gene on chromosome 13. At the molecular level, Dryja *et al* (7) found two retinoblastomas with small homozygous deletions limited to region 13q14. These studies indicated that a mutant RB allele is "recessive" to its normal counterpart within a cell, and that the latter essentially functions to prevent tumor formation during retinal development. A class of such "cancer suppressor" genes has been postulated to explain other forms of heritable cancer predisposition and chromosomal abnormalities analogous to those seen in retinoblastoma (8,9).

Recently, a gene in band 13q14 encoding an mRNA of 4.7 kb was identified as the RB gene based on tumor-specific alterations in expression, and apparent recessive nature at the cellular level (10). Complementary DNA (cDNA) segments representing the RB gene transcript have been cloned (10,11,12) and sequenced (10). All hereditary and nonhereditary retinoblastomas examined to date have demonstrated altered RB gene expression: RB mRNA transcripts are either markedly reduced in quantity, or abnormal in length (10-12). About 40% of retinoblastomas show DNA deletions detectable by RB cDNA probes, while the rest appear normal. Antibodies generated against the RB gene product, pp110[RB], show complete absence of this nucleophosphoprotein in five out of five retinoblastomas, while it was easily detected in all normal or neoplastic cells containing a normal RB mRNA transcript (13). This data further strengthens the hypothesis that the absence of functional RB protein is potentially oncogenic.

Given the different patterns of genetic alteration observed in retinoblastomas, it is evident that the RB gene is subject to a variety of mutational mechanisms, the details of which are as yet unknown. In order to further characterize the RB gene and some of its mutations, we constructed a restriction and exon map of the intact RB gene based on analysis of genomic DNA clones. The derived map contains all exons present in the full-length cDNA sequence (4757 nucleotides) (13). A genomic library made from retinoblastoma cell line Y79 yielded two clones containing an intragenic deletion junction that was not previously detected by cDNA probes for the RB gene. Using a single-copy probe

Molecular Biology of the Eye: Genes, Vision,
and Ocular Disease, pages 437–443
© 1988 Alan R. Liss, Inc.

# IDENTIFICATION OF MUTATIONS IN THE PUTATIVE RETINOBLASTOMA GENE [1]

Brenda L. Gallie, James M. Dunn, Audrey Goddard, Andrew Becker and Robert A. Phillips

Hospital for Sick Children Research Institute and the Departments of Ophthalmology and Medical Genetics, The University of Toronto, Toronto, Canada M5G 1X8

ABSTRACT Retinoblastoma (RB) tumors develop when both alleles of a gene (RB1) are mutated and unable to function normally. In some cases, one mutant allele in the germline results in a hereditary predisposition to development of RB tumors in infancy, and sarcoma tumors in adolescence. In other cases, with no hereditary tendency, both alleles of the same gene are mutated only in the somatic retinal cell that becomes malignant. Friend et al. have reported the cloning of a gene, 4.7R, with some properties expected of the RB1 gene (1). We observed that 78% of RB and OS tumors from RB patients show normal genomic DNA restriction patterns for 4.7R, and normal size and amounts of 4.7R mRNA on Northern blots. However, using RNase protection, point mutations or small deletions were identified in four of eight RB tumors. Comparison of the constitutional cells and tumor cells by RNase protection of 4.7R resulted in detection of the germline mutation in one bilateral, heritable case, and exclusion of a germline mutation in a unilateral case. This data confirms that the 4.7R gene is very likely to be the RB1 gene.

[1] This work was supported by grants from the National Cancer Institute of Canada and the Medical Research Council of Canada. ADG is supported by MRC studentship. BLG is a Research Associate of the Ontario Cancer Foundation.

## INTRODUCTION

Knudson hypothesized in 1971 that all RB tumors are induced by two mutations: in the hereditary cases the first mutation is present in the germline and individual tumors develop when a somatic second mutation occurs in the retinal cells (2).      Non-hereditary tumors arise by two somatic mutations in the same individual retinal cell.

When restriction fragment length polymorphic (RFLP) markers were developed for chromosome 13 (3,4), the location of RB1, it was demonstrated that both of the mutations predicted by Knudson involve the same locus (5).      Predisposed retinal cells carrying a germline mutation in the RB1 gene become malignant only when the normal homologous allele is also damaged.    Frequently, the mutant chromosome 13 in RB tumors is duplicated with most RFLP on the long arm of chromosome 13 becoming homozygous; occasionally a single mutant chromosome remains in the tumor; and in 30% of RB tumors no change in the chromosome 13 haplotype is detectable using RFLP markers on either side of the RB1 gene locus.    It has been presumed that these 30% of tumors carry point mutations or small deletions in the normal allele that are not detectable by studies of the flanking regions of chromosome 13.

A candidate gene for RB1, 4.7R, was cloned by Friend et al. (1). Homozygous deletion of this gene has been noted in several RB tumors (1,6,7).      Since the majority of these deletions extended beyond the boundaries of the 4.7R gene, the possibility remained that the true RB1 gene was located adjacent to the 4.7R gene.

Using a 4.7R cDNA (1) we have studied normal and tumor cells from RB patients by Southern and Northern blots and RNase protection, to assess the eligibility of 4.7R as RB1.

## DETECTION OF MUTATIONS IN NORMAL AND TUMOR CELLS OF RB PATIENTS

Southern Blot Analysis.

By Southern blot analysis of 32 RB tumors not previously studied, four tumors were identified with genomic abnormalities of 4.7R (8).    Two RB tumors (RB530 and RB537) were homozygously deleted for the entire 4.7R gene.    One tumor (RB414) showed a decrease in intensity of two Hind III fragments known to correspond to the 3' end of the 4.7R gene, suggesting a 3' hemizygous deletion.    The fourth RB tumor (RB369E) showed a similar hemizygous 3' deletion, but, in addition, digestion of the DNA with several restriction enzymes showed large junction fragments.    Further characterization of the abnormality in this tumor indicated that the mutation was an insertion in the 5' end of

11. Forrester K, Almoguera C, Han K, Grizzle WE, Perucho M (1987). Detection of high incidence of K-*ras* oncogenes during human colon tumorigenesis. Nature 327: 298.
12. Myers R, Lumelsky N, Lerman L, Maniatis T (1985). Detection of single base substitutions in total genomic DNA. Nature 313:495.
13. Wiggs J, Norenskjöld M, Yandell D, Rapaport J, Grondin V, Janson M, Werelius B, Petersen R, Craft A, Riedel K, Liberfarb R, Walton D, Wilson W, Dryja TP (1988). Prediction of the risk of hereditary retinoblastoma, using DNA polymorphisms within the retinoblastoma gene. New Engl J Med 318: 151.

Molecular Biology of the Eye: Genes, Vision,
and Ocular Disease, pages 445–448
© 1988 Alan R. Liss, Inc.

# SV40 T ANTIGENS CAUSE PHAKOMA, C-*MOS* A DEFECT IN LENS FIBER DIFFERENTIATION IN TRANSGENIC MICE

Heiner Westphal

Section on Mammalian Gene Regulation,
Laboratory of Molecular Genetics,
National Institute of Child Health and Human Development,
National Institutes of Health, Bethesda, Maryland 20892

ABSTRACT    The transgenic technology affords a unique possibility of directing specific gene products to predetermined tissues of the live mouse. Lens-specific expression of SV40 T antigens results in malignant lens tumors, that of c-*mos* in a characteristic defect of lens fiber differentiation.

## INTRODUCTION

Transgenes are defined gene constructs inserted in the mouse germ line, most commonly via embryo microinjection (1). The chance to observe such genes at work in the living organism is the chief reason for the enthusiasm with which the transgene technology has been received in virtually any field of biomedical research, including the molecular biology of the eye. The study to be described below contrasts the action of an oncogene and a protooncogene in the lens. There are several advantages of examining genes that perturb cell growth in this tissue. The lens has a simple architecture and consists exclusively of ectodermal epithelia differentiating into fibers. The embryonic development of the lens has been studied in great detail. If the transgene product is deleterious, the lens can be removed without affecting the general health of the animal.

Our studies allow us to observe transgene-mediated changes in cell differentiation and growth properties from their initiation in the embryonic lens to terminal stages in the adult animal. This experimental series complements work of other laboratories who study the expression of similar genes in more complex tissues and organ systems (see 1-3 for recent reviews).

# RESULTS AND DISCUSSION

## Oncogenesis of the lens

My colleagues Kathleen Mahon, Ana Chepelinsky, Jaspal Khillan, Paul Overbeek, Joram Piatigorsky and myself have studied oncogenesis in the lens. Experimental details may be found in a recently published article (4). We constructed the "αT" transgene, consisting of murine αA-crystallin enhancer/promoter sequences fused to the coding sequence of the SV40 T antigens. These powerful oncogenes had previously been shown to cause tumors in the transgenic mouse (5,6). Since tumors of the lens had never been observed in vertebrates, we asked whether our experimental approach would succeed in overriding the apparent tumor immunity of this tissue. If so, when and in which cells would cancer arise and how would it progress in space and time?

Our previous results had shown that the regulatory sequences of the murine αA-crystallin gene which we incorporated in our gene construct direct gene expression specifically to lens epithelia and fibers, beginning at the time of primary lens fiber differentiation (7). When observing embryos bearing the αT gene we detected transformed cells in the anterior hemisphere of the lens shortly after primary fiber differentiation had initiated. In several of our αT lines, tumors developed rapidly and invaded neighboring tissues. Tumor cells expressed the SV40 T antigens. Animals died shortly after reaching sexual maturity. However, one of our αT lines, generated by my colleague A. Dey, is characterized by a much more protracted tumor progression, and progeny of this line have normal life expectancy. My colleague T. Nakamura has recently been able to establish αT lens cell lines in culture which produce SV40 T antigens and retain the ability to synthesize lens crystallins (unpublished).

We conclude that lens tumor immunity can be overridden by lens specific expression of SV40 T antigens in the transgenic mouse. Cell lines can be established from these lenses which retain their ability to produce highly specialized crystallin gene products.

## A Defect in Lens Fiber Differentiation

My colleagues Jaspal Khillan, Fritz Propst, Marianne Oskarsson, Toichiro Kuwabara, George Vande Woude and myself have examined the genetic effects in the lens of a hybrid gene which contains the murine c-*mos* protooncogene under the control of the long terminal repeat (LTR) of Moloney murine sarcoma virus (Mo-MSV). Experimental details may be found elsewhere (8).

This hybrid gene scores highly positive in the 3T3 cell transformation assay (9) but, as a transgene, has failed to cause any noticeable malignancies. However, three transgenic mouse lines which we generated are characterized by a unique type of lens pathology. Shortly after birth, insufficient posterior elongation of differentiating lens fibers and lack of basement membrane secretion leads to the breakdown of the posterior lens capsule. This, in turn, results in a posterior protrusion and swelling of lens tissue which remains nucleated. In the course of the first three weeks after birth, globular cells begin to fill the entire anterior and posterior chambers of the eye. Concomitantly, there is massive expression of c-*mos* RNA in the lens of the transgenic animals whereas it is absent from wild-type lenses. Hyperplasia or neoplasia of tissues have not been detected in any progeny carrying and expressing the v-*mos* transgene. Rather, c-*mos* expression results in an inhibition of proliferation of equatorial lens epithelia which normally give rise to secondary fibers. Such inhibition could cause the described chain of events.

We conclude that the genuine murine protooncogene c-*mos*, fused to the LTR of Mo-MSV, elicits a specific defect in lens fiber differentiation, without causing hyperplasia or neoplasia.

## REFERENCES

1. Palmiter RD, Brinster RL (1986). Germ-line transformation of mice. Annu Rev Genet 20:465.

2. Hanahan D (1986). Oncogenesis in transgenic mice. In Graf T, Kahn P (eds): "Oncogenes and growth control," Heidelberg: Springer-Verlag, p. 349.

3. Westphal H (1987). Transgenic mice. BioEssays 6:73.

4. Mahon KA, Chepelinsky AB, Khillan JS, Overbeek PA, Piatigorsky J, Westphal H (1987). Oncogenesis of the lens in transgenic mice. Science 235:1622.

5. Brinster RL, Chen HY, Messing A, Van Dyke T, Levine AJ, Palmiter RD (1984). Transgenic mice harboring SV40 T antigen genes develop characteristic brain tumors. Cell 37:367.

6. Hanahan D (1985). Heritable formation of pancreatic β-cell tumors in transgenic mice expression recombinant insulin/simian virus 40 oncogenes. Nature (London) 315:115.

7.  Overbeek PA, Chepelinsky AB, Khillan JS, Piatigorsky J, Westphal H (1985). Lens-specific expression and developmental regulation of the bacterial chloramphenicol acetyltransferase gene driven by the murine αA-crystallin promoter in transgenic mice. Proc Natl Acad Sci USA 82:7815.

8.  Khillan JS, Oskarsson MK, Propst F, Kuwabara T, Vande Woude GF, Westphal H (1987). Defects in lens fiber differentiation are linked to c-*mos* overexpression in transgenic mice. Genes & Development 1:1327.

9.  Blair DG, Oskarsson M, Wood TG, McClements, WL, Fischinger PJ, Vande Woude GF (1981). Activation of the transforming potential of a normal cell sequence: A molecular model for oncogenesis. Science 212:941.

**Molecular Biology of the Eye: Genes, Vision, and Ocular Disease, pages 449–456**
© **1988 Alan R. Liss, Inc.**

ABNORMAL REGULATION OF N-RAS EXPRESSION:
A POTENTIAL ROLE IN PROLIFERATIVE
VITREORETINOPATHY

David K. Wilcox

Department of Ophthalmology,
The Eye and Ear Institute
University of Pittsburgh
Pittsburgh, Pennsylvania  15213

Retinal pigmented epithelial cells incubated in
vitreous undergo a metaplasia from an epithelial to
fibroblast-like phenotype.  We studied the levels of
n-ras in normal and metaplastic RPE.  In control
cells n-ras RNA levels peaked at 6 hours returning to
prestimulation levels at 12 hours.  In metaplastic
RPE n-ras levels peaked at 6 hours at levels 2 fold
over controls; and remained 2-4 fold higher than
control levels at 18 hours. Elevated levels of n-ras
may play a role in the RPE metaplasia associated with
proliferative vitreoretinopathy.

Introduction

Proliferative vitreoretinopathy(PVR) is a disorder
characterized by the formation of membranes on the sub and
epiretinal surfaces.  The contraction of these membranes
leads to recurring retinal detachment.  The ability of
retinal pigmented epithelium(RPE) to participate in
membrane formation in proliferative vitreoretinopathy is
well established( 1-4 ).

Supported by       Grant NEI  R01  EY06479 To D.K. Wilcox
                   and by an unrestricted grant from
                   Research to Prevent Blindness to the
                   Department of Ophthalmology

Numerous studies both in animal models and in culture have demonstrated the ability of RPE cells to undergo a metaplasia to a fibroblast-like cell type(5,6,7). These fibroblast-like RPE cells are also found in epiretinal membranes which are analyzed following surgical removal in individuals with PVR.

Studies in which RPE cells were injected into the vitreous cavity revealed that the cells proliferate and form epiretinal membranes which result in retinal detachment(4). The exposure of RPE cells to vitreous in culture results in the proliferation and metaplasia to a fibroblast-like cell type(6,7). The factors which initiate the metaplasia are not known but serum components, the vitreous itself, retinal derived factors and interaction with extracellular matrix materials such as collagen are known to stimulate some of the metaplastic changes(6,8).

Recent advances in the studies of the transforming genes involved in neoplasia have led to a better understanding of the processes of normal growth and differentiation. The identification of the class of genes termed "protooncogenes"( the normal cellular equivalent of the retroviral transforming genes) has greatly aided these studies. The products of protooncogenes have been implicated in the normal mechanisms which regulate cellular growth and differentiation(9).

Our laboratories efforts have focused on identifying protooncogenes which may be involved in the metaplasia of the RPE cell during the initiation and progression of PVR. The regulation of n-ras RNA production is abnormal in metaplastic RPE cells. Both the timing and levels of production are altered during metaplasia.

## Results

In order to better understand the metaplasia of RPE during proliferative vitreoretinopathy we have employed an in vitro tissue culture technique which mimics the in vivo situation. Earlier work has shown that exposure of RPE cells in culture to vitreous results in a metaplasia from an epithelial to a fibroblast-like phenotype(6,7).

**A** **B**

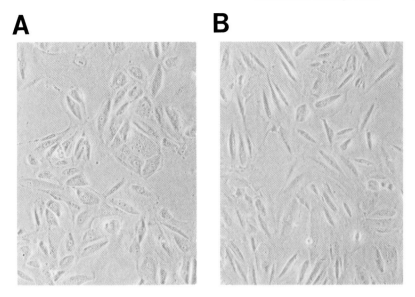

FIGURE 1. RPE Morphology A. Control cells at 24 hours B. Vitreous treated cells at 24 hours.

We too find that in the presence of vitreous the RPE cell undergoes a morphological alteration to an elongated spindle shaped cell similar to a fibroblast(figure #1.). The morphological alteration is observed only as long as vitreous is present since its removal results in a return to a normal morphology within 24 hours (data not shown).

Both DNA synthesis and cell division are stimulated in the presence of vitreous.(Table 1 )

As we have previously demonstrated(10), the levels of cytoplasmic RNA complementary to n-ras are altered in both proliferating normal RPE cells and vitreous-induced metaplastic RPE cells. RPE cells were incubated with 500 ul/ml of cell free vitreous. The cytoplasmic RNA was collected, electrophoresed and hybridzed with a $^{32}$p-labeled fragment from the 3' non-coding region of the n-ras gene (11,12,13). In normal proliferating RPE cells there is a loss of n-ras RNA within one hour post stimulation. This is followed at 2 hours by an increased accumulation which peaks at approximately 6 hours. This proliferation induced n-ras RNA accumulation gradually decreases, and by 18 hours poststimulation RNA levels have returned to normal (Figure 2).

TABLE 1

Addition[1]          cpm X 10-5/10-5 cells

---

Control (N/A)[3]                   63 + 7
Vitreous (500 ul/ml)              193 + 12.8
Serum (10% FCS)                   176 + 13.2

---

[1]Supplement to basal
media(DMEM:Hams F-12, 1:1 with 0.5% FCS)
[2] [3]H Thymidine TCA precipitable counts
incorporated in a 24 hour period.
[3] N/A = no addition, cells remained in
DMEM:Hams F-12, 1:1, plus 0.5% FCS.

In contrast, in metaplastic RPE the levels of
cytoplasmic n-ras RNA remain nearly constant during the
first hour poststimulation, and by 2 hours are
approximately 2-4 fold over the levels observed in the
normal cells.  At 6 hours poststimulation the levels of
n-ras RNA are 2 to 4 fold over control levels.  There is a
total increase of 20 fold compared to the one hour control
levels.  N-ras levels decrease; however, the levels remain
2-4 fold higher than in the control cells at 18 hours
poststimulation (Figure 2).

Rehybridization of these blots with the protooncogene
"neu" showed a constant low level of expression in both
normal and metaplastic RPE at all the time points tested.
In addition, staining of parallel gels with ethidium
bromide showed equal staining(data not shown).  These two
results indicate that the changes observed in figure 2 are
due only to alteration in n-ras RNA levels.

# Index